WD500

EXERCISE PHYSIOLOGY FOR
HEALTH PROFESSIONALS

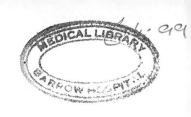

FORTHCOMING TITLES

THERAPY IN PRACTICE SERIES

Edited by Jo Campling

This series of books is aimed at 'therapists' concerned with rehabilitation in a very broad sense. The intended audience particularly includes occupational therapists, physiotherapists and speech therapists, but many titles will also be of interest to nurses, psychologists, medical staff, social workers, teachers or volunteer workers. Some volumes are interdisciplinary, others are aimed at one particular profession. All titles will be comprehensive but concise, and practical but with due reference to relevant theory and evidence. They are not research monographs but focus on professional practice, and will be of value to both students and qualified personnel.

Exercise Physiology for Health Professionals

STEPHEN R. BIRD

Senior Lecturer, Departments of Occupational Therapy and Sport Science, Christ Church College, Canterbury, UK.

CHAPMAN & HALL
London · New York · Tokyo · Melbourne · Madras

Published by Chapman & Hall, 2-6 Boundary Row, London SE1 8HN

Chapman & Hall, 2-6 Boundary Row, London SE1 8HN, UK

Chapman & Hall, 29 West 35th Street, New York NY10001, USA

Chapman & Hall Japan, Thomson Publishing Japan, Hirakawacho Nemoto Building, 7F, 1-7-11 Hirakawa-cho, Chiyoda-ku, Tokyo 102, Japan

Chapman & Hall Australia, Thomas Nelson Australia, 102 Dodds Street, South Melbourne, Victoria 3205, Australia

Chapman & Hall India, R. Seshadri, 32 Second Main Road, CIT East, Madras 600 035, India

First edition 1992

© 1992 Stephen R. Bird

Typeset in 9/11 Times by Mews Photosetting, Beckenham, Kent
Printed in Great Britain by St Edmundsbury Press, Bury St Edmunds, Suffolk

ISBN 0 412 35430 6

A catalogue record for this book is available from the British Library

Library of Congress Cataloging-in-Publication data
Bird, Stephen R., 1959–
    Exercise physiology for health professionals / Stephen R. Bird.
        p.   cm. – (Therapy in practice : 26)
    Includes bibliographical references and index.
    ISBN 0-412-35430-6 (pb.)
    1. Exercise therapy. 2. Exercise–Physiological aspects.
3. Physical fitness. I. Title. II. Series: Therapy in practice
series : 26.
    [DNLM: 1. Exercise–physiology. 2. Physical Fitness–physiology.
WE 103 B61783e]
RM725.B57   1992
615.8'2–dc20
DNLM/DLC
For Library of Congress   91-13784
                                                               CIP

Contents

Acknowledgements

I would like to thank my wife Jackie for all her support and assistance throughout the production of this book. I should also like to thank my family, colleagues and friends, to all of whom I owe so much. Finally, a special 'thank you' to Dave Cartwright for being a very 'understanding' illustrator.

1

Introductory aspects of exercise physiology

EXERCISE PHYSIOLOGY AND THE HEALTH PROFESSIONAL

For the health professional a knowledge of exercise physiology and its practical application is becoming increasingly important. Exercise is commonly used as a form of treatment by those working in the fields of occupational therapy, physiotherapy and health promotion. In many cases the desired effects of a prescribed exercise programme will be physiological, whilst in others the benefits may extend beyond this, with the therapist utilizing exercise to provide the participant with various social and psychological benefits. For some an exercise programme may be clinically based, whilst for others it may occur in a wider social context. Indeed, for many it will involve a combination of the two and perhaps a progression from the clinical to the social.

In the clinical setting, exercise may be used as a form of therapy in the treatment, prevention and rehabilitation processes of a wide range of disorders and problems, both physical and mental. When incorporated into a treatment programme, exercise has to be shown to reduce the amount of medication required to control disorders such as hypertension and diabetes. Exercise also has an important role to play in minimizing the effects of degenerative diseases and in some cases may be utilized as a form of 'preventive medicine'. So for many individuals exercise will be incorporated into a basic rehabilitation programme after injury or illness, or in the case of degenerative diseases it may be used to minimize the decline in their physical capabilities. The improvement or maintenance of people's physical capacity may result in their being able to lead a more independent lifestyle in which they are able to perform standard household tasks and do daily activities more easily. In other situations exercise may provide the stimulus for them to develop their physical, social and mental capabilities. In this context an improvement in an individual's physical capacity may be viewed in the context of a more recreational or sporting environment. Such leisure-orientated activities may convey important benefits to many individuals, not just the élite competitive performer. For example, basic recreational activities such as walking and swimming are used as a form of therapy for many individuals, including both the physically and mentally handicapped, and as such may convey numerous social as well as physical benefits to the participants. It should also be remembered that exercise can provide a valuable form of rehabilitation and recreation for those who may be considered to be disabled. The value of such activity is most apparent with the increasing numbers of participants in 'disabled sports'. Wheelchair sports, blind runners, amputee and mentally disabled sportspeople, to name but a few of the groups involved, are now beginning to receive a higher media profile with major international competitions taking place between participants from all over the world.

One of the roles of the therapist will be to optimize an individual's physical capacity; an appropriate level of physical fitness is important for everyone if they are to fulfil their potential and get the most out of life. Physical fitness may be considered as a measure of a person's capacity to cope with the physical demands of his or her lifestyle. Depending upon the individual, this could be viewed as an ability to move around the home and do basic household chores, to cope adequately with the physical demands of an active lifestyle or, with more active individuals, it may refer to their capacity to participate in recognized forms of physical activity, including sports. It can therefore be seen that precisely what is meant by physical fitness depends on the individual. Factors such as age, inherent physical capabilities, acquired dysfunctions, injury, general aspirations and lifestyle all affect an individual's current and potential physical capabilities and, hence, physical fitness.

If the physical capacity of individuals is impaired, then so may their lifestyle; or, on a more positive note, if their physical capabilities can be improved (perhaps through participating in an appropriate exercise programme) then their lifestyle may be enhanced. This concept can be applied to virtually everyone whether they are suffering from a major physical disability, are recovering from a disease or traumatic accident, or alternatively are generally 'well' but have fallen below their physical potential due to inactivity. In all cases an increase in their physical capabilities will almost certainly improve their self-esteem, satisfaction in what they achieve and the overall quality of their life. This can be seen most clearly in the physically disabled where an increase in their physical capabilities may be realized as an improvement in their ability to move around the house and perform basic household chores. In virtually everyone (disabled or not), any physical improvement is likely to result in their finding basic activities such as shopping or gardening less demanding and tiring. An improved physical capacity is also likely to increase their overall feeling of 'well-being' and thus make them more able to cope with the physical demands of their lifestyle. One of the functions of people involved in a health promotion, treatment or rehabilitation programme will be to maximize the physical capacity of the individuals involved as appropriate to their needs. Although physical fitness is important for all, quite clearly the physical activity programme needed to achieve 'fitness' will be quite different in the cases of a coronary rehabilitation patient, a muscular dystrophy sufferer, an obese individual, an amputee and a professional footballer who may have simply strained a muscle. Physical fitness can be viewed as a spectrum: for some, the idea of physical fitness simply means being free from disease, whilst for others it may mean taking positive steps to avoid or reduce the debilitating effects of a disease; for some it may mean attaining a physical capacity within the restrictions of a disease or disability, whilst for others it may mean reaching the peak of physical excellence.

Improvements in the physical capabilities of individuals may be attributable to changes in a variety of factors, including an increase in their range of movement, an improvement in their muscular strength or an improvement in their coordination. In some cases, it may even be the result of an improvement in the condition of their heart or circulation. The science of exercise physiology is, of course, also applied to those seeking sporting excellence, and whilst this text is not aimed primarily at this group of individuals it is applicable for those professionals who may come into contact with them at certain times. Despite a long historical association between exercise, therapy and health much confusion still exists over the reported benefits of exercise both within the health professions and amongst their patients. When prescribing exercise as a form of therapy, therapists or practitioners need to be fairly precise with their exercise recommendations and specific individualized programmes need to be devised for each individual in accordance with his or her needs. This is because different forms of exercise convey very specific benefits. For the patient some forms of exercise may be more beneficial than others, and not only is the type of exercise important but also its intensity, frequency and duration as well as other considerations such as a prior warm-up and a knowledge of the level at which to start. A knowledge of basic exercise principles and the effects of exercise upon the body are therefore important for health professionals if they are to ensure that the 'patient' is to gain the most benefit from the exercise programme they prescribe. Conversely, it may be argued that the therapist who does not have an adequate understanding of exercise physiology and its application may be restricted and be unable to provide patients or clients with an optimal therapy or rehabilitation programme.

The use of terms such as 'exercise programmes' and 'training effects' often conjures up visions of the competitive sporting individuals who are seeking physical excellence. However, it must be remembered that exercise programmes and exercise physiology have a wider application than the sporting context. Indeed, the élite competitive sportsmen and sportswomen form only a relatively small percentage of the population. For a much larger group of individuals, exercise physiology and its implications will be linked with recreation, physical therapy and various forms of treatment programmes and thus will often be associated with the promotion of good health or the minimizing of ill health. The sporting individuals do, however, form a specific group which often come into contact with the health professional, especially when they have an exercise-related injury. For these individuals the inclusion of exercise into a rehabilitation programme has specific significance. To some extent these individuals form a special case and when treating them appropriate types of exercise may be prescribed which enable the injured part to recover whilst going someway towards satisfying the individual's desire to continue exercising and remain 'fit'. Some of the injuries occurring in this group may be as a result of overuse caused by doing too much or inappropriate forms of training, whilst other examples of exercise-related injuries the therapist or doctor may encounter include those of a more traumatic nature such as pulled muscles, damaged ligaments and strained tendons. Such individuals will frequently be treated by physiotherapists and sports doctors who have to cope with the additional complication that the patient will wish to return to sport as rapidly as possible. In such cases a gradual progressive exercise programme forms an essential component of the treatment process and needs to be incorporated and designed in such a manner that the chances of the injury recurring are minimized.

The role of this text is to provide health professionals with a basic understanding of exercise physiology and of how it may be applied in the context of their professional work. This is not to say that there is any magic formula that will ensure success but that there are certain guidelines that can be used when applying a knowledge of exercise physiology to an individual and his or her circumstances. Having this information should enable health professionals to utilize their professional judgement about individuals and make appropriate, informed decisions about the incorporation of exercise into their treatment programme and/or lifestyle.

Exercise physiology, as the name implies, is the area of study that primarily looks at the physiological aspects of the body before, during and after exercise. This can be seen to include:

(a) the body's immediate responses to exercise;
(b) the more long-term physiological adaptations the body makes following a bout of exercise, which may be described as the 'training effect' and has implications for the individual's physical capacity and health; and
(c) the physical factors that determine the physical capacity of the individual and how exercise may alter these factors.

Observing the responses of the human body to exercise has led to an understanding of how exercise may be used to convey various benefits upon the body. That is to say: firstly, whether an individual would benefit from participating in some form of exercise; secondly, the form of exercise that would convey most benefit; and, thirdly, the practical aspects such as how often the individual should undertake the exercise, how 'hard' it should be and how long it should last. A knowledge of these factors can then be applied practically in the designing of exercise programmes that will bring about the desired benefits to the individual. If designed appropriately and adhered to, such exercise programmes will enable individuals to optimize their physical capacity according to their individual needs and realistic goals as determined by their own individual circumstances. It must also be remembered that an increasing number of 'disabled' individuals are participating in physical activity and sport, not simply as a means of physical treatment but for recreation and the sheer enjoyment of participating in competitive sport. In such cases a knowledge of exercise physiology becomes important as it can be applied to not only minimize their disability but also to maximize their sporting prowess.

As can be seen, therefore, from these general examples, fitness is specific to the individual and therefore any form of physical therapy or physical training programme prescribed for an individual must be specific if that individual is to gain the most benefit from it. In order to do this the professionals working in the fields of occupational therapy, physical therapy, physiotherapy, health promotion and sports medicine must have a good understanding of the workings of the body. Indeed, in attempting to apply an exercise programme they must have a good understanding of the body from an exercise perspective. Hence, in addition to a knowledge of the more traditional aspects of anatomy and physiology a good practical knowledge of exercise physiology and aspects relating to physical fitness now have far-reaching implications for those working in the fields of health and health promotion.

THE COMPONENTS OF PHYSICAL FITNESS

In order to fully understand the concept of an individual's 'physical capacity' and hence the aims and objectives of an exercise programme it is first necessary to describe the constituents of physical fitness in some detail. A good comprehension of the components of physical fitness should thereby enable the reader to appreciate the specific objectives and implications of particular forms of exercise. An individual's physical potential and/or physical capacity to move their limbs and perform motor activities is determined by a large number of factors, including:

- their muscular strength
- their muscular endurance
- the condition of their cardiovascular system (including the heart, lungs, blood and blood vessels)
- the mobility of their joints and flexibility
- their coordination.

All these factors are important in determining someone's capacity to perform basic movements and/or exercise. Whilst these contributing factors may be considered under separate headings it needs to be emphasized that in reality they are all interrelated and all are required to a greater or lesser extent in any form of physical movement. A lifting activity (such as lifting a bag) may require a greater strength contribution than a stretching activity (such as reaching up into a cupboard), which will require more mobility. However, a degree of strength and mobility are needed in both. The relative importance of each aspect will depend upon the type of movement being performed. For the therapist it is important to realize which factor(s) may be limiting a person's ability to perform a physical movement or activity and hence the type of therapy/exercise most likely to improve the limiting factor(s). Undertaking the appropriate form of exercise should then increase the participant's ability to perform the desired movement or activity.

Muscular strength

Muscular strength refers to a muscle's, or group of muscles', capacity to exert force. Everyday examples include the lifting of an object or moving one's body or limb against a force (often gravity). A lower than desirable level of muscular strength can occur if a muscle or group of muscles are not exercised or used regularly. This can result in a reduction in the size of the muscle (muscular atrophy) and may be extreme in situations where a limb has been immobilized for some time. An example would be a broken bone, where the limb has been put in a cast. Alternatively, a lack of use of the muscle due to a failure of the nervous system to stimulate it adequately can also result in atrophy and reduced muscular strength. The cause of this may vary from that of a serious medical condition to a simple lack of use brought on by a more sedentary lifestyle. Regardless of the cause, the effect of reduced muscle strength may inhibit an individual's capacity to climb stairs or lift objects and, in general, can make many common activities difficult or even impossible. Exercise programmes designed to improve muscular strength should have the reverse effect, improving the condition of muscles, increasing their strength and generally increasing the individual's capacity to perform activities that require muscular strength. In many cases muscular strength exercises will also reverse the process of atrophy and cause an increase in the size of the muscles (hypertrophy) along with the accompanying increase in strength. However, certain medical conditions may limit the amount of 'improvement' that is possible and in certain circumstances the exercises may be primarily aimed at minimizing a degenerative process rather than seeking to produce specific increases in strength.

Muscular strengthening exercises that are prescribed on a therapeutic basis are not likely to result in the participant developing excessively large muscles even if weights, pulleys and multigyms are used. The large muscles possessed by powerful 'athletes' are only obtained through large amounts of training with very heavy weights. Any patient who may be concerned about developing such a physique through a basic therapeutically orientated exercise programme need not be concerned. Indeed, it takes much effort to increase muscle mass, therefore women (who are often more concerned about developing large muscles than their male counterparts) need not worry especially since they tend to have significantly lower levels of anabolic hormones than do men.

Cardiovascular fitness and muscular endurance

Cardiovascular, or as it is sometimes known, 'aerobic' fitness refers to an individual's capacity to perform prolonged forms of physical activity. It is therefore an integral part of an individual's endurance capabilities. Cardiovascular fitness is a complex phenomenon: it depends upon the condition of the heart, lungs, blood, blood vessels and muscles. It refers to the capacity of the cardiovascular system to deliver oxygen to the working muscles, and to the capacity of these muscles to utilize that oxygen during muscular activity. The muscles of an individual with a poor cardiovascular system and little endurance will have an impaired supply of oxygen and, as a result, that individual will tire quite rapidly even when undertaking tasks that would be considered by others as relatively undemanding. Examples of such activities include walking, cycling, climbing stairs and almost any activity that requires repetitive muscular contractions over a prolonged period of time.

Flexibility or mobility

Flexibility, mobility or suppleness refers to the amount of movement attainable at a joint or over a number of joints (as in the case of the spine). An individual's flexibility may be considered under two subheadings:

1. Active flexibility
2. Passive flexibility.

Active flexibility refers to the amount of movement individuals are capable of when using their own muscular contractions. An example of this would be how far they could bend to the side (unaided) or how high they could raise their arms (unaided).

Passive flexibility refers to the range of movement possible at a joint or over a series of joints when the joint or limb movement is aided by an external force, such as help from a therapist or assistant.

Owing to the assisted nature of passive flexibility more movement is usually possible under passive conditions than through active contractions alone. However, both are important for the individual in terms of their physical capacity (fitness) and as a means of therapy or physical training. Quite clearly a reduced amount of active flexibility will impede most individuals in various basic movements and improving the flexibility of individuals may produce a number of benefits in the type and range of movement that they can achieve as well as the ease with which they are able to produce those movements.

Coordination

Coordination refers to the integrated working and movement of body systems and body parts. A lack of coordination at whatever level will result in impaired movement and, hence, a reduced ability to perform physical tasks. The development of 'coordination' is physiologically complex but through practice (training) improvements can occur thereby improving the physical functioning of the individual.

Appropriate forms of exercise may be used to enhance and/or maintain all of these components of physical fitness. With some individuals it may be a relatively simple task of using exercise to compensate for a somewhat sedentary lifestyle. Alternatively it may be used to facilitate a comprehensive recovery from an enforced period of inactivity and help restore a person's physical capacity. In other situations the process may be more complex, as would be the case with a rehabilitation programme after a serious accident or illness. Another example would be an exercise programme that was designed to minimize the debilitating effects of a persistent disease or disability. Very often the effects of such diseases and traumas greatly reduce the physical capacity of patients, and whilst it may not be possible to cure those individuals or return them to their previous level of motor activity, appropriate exercises can often help them to reach their physical potential, albeit somewhat reduced. Therefore, in some cases the aim of an exercise programme may be to return the individual to 'normal'; in others it may be to slow down the process of degeneration and loss of function, and, in yet others, it may be to try to improve the motor functioning of the individuals to something in excess of what they had previously attained.

MOVEMENT TERMINOLOGY

Planes and axes

When describing the movements of the body a specific terminology is required to prevent confusion. For instance, if the therapist was to record that Mr X experienced pain when he 'bent his elbow' the precise movement that caused the pain could be interpreted and visualized by another practitioner in a number of different ways. For instance, it could refer to the patient bending his elbow so that his forearm came across his body; alternatively, it could refer to bending it to the side away from his body, out in front of his body or even behind his back. Clearly such confusions need to be avoided when describing a patient's condition to another therapist or when making notes that may be read at a later date or by another practitioner. So in order to prevent such confusion a specific vocabulary is used, one aspect of which is to describe movements with reference to specific planes and axes. For this purpose there are

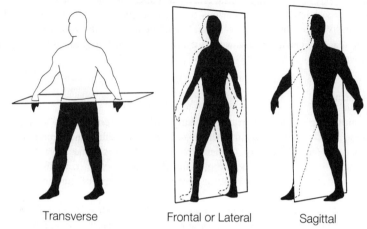

| Transverse | Frontal or Lateral | Sagittal |

Figure 1.1 Illustrating the three major planes.

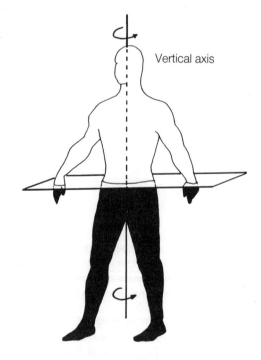

Vertical axis

Transverse plane

Figure 1.2 Illustrating the transverse plane.

three major planes, also referred to as primary or cardinal planes. The three primary planes are: the transverse plane, the sagittal plane and the frontal or lateral plane (Figure 1.1). These planes may be visualized as three panes of glass. A particular movement is said to be in that plane if it runs parallel to that pane of glass. Each pane has a corresponding axis which passes perpendicularly through it. Movements may therefore be described as occurring in a plane and about an axis.

One plane can be visualized as passing horizontally through the body dividing it into a top and bottom half; this is referred to as the transverse plane. Passing through this plane from the top of a person's head down to between the feet runs the longitudinal or vertical axis. To assist with the visualization of these planes and axes along with the movements that occur in them it often helps to use models made of stiff cardboard or plasticine. A wire or pencil passing through the model can be used to represent the axis. If the pencil is spun in the transverse plane and longitudinal axis (Figure 1.2), the model would be seen to rotate about the axis rather like an ice skater performing a spin. Movements in the transverse plane about the longitudinal axis include rotating the head, twisting the body or moving the forearm across the body (Figure 1.3).

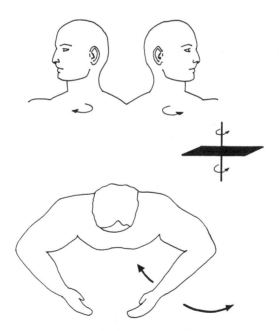

Figure 1.3 Illustrating movements in the transverse plane.

A second plane, extending down the centre of the body and dividing it into left and right halves, is referred to as the sagittal plane. The sagittal plane has its corresponding axis, the bilateral axis passing through the body from one hip to another

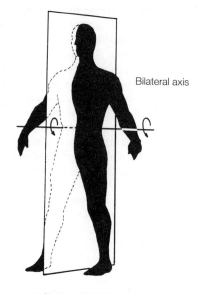

Sagittal plane

Figure 1.4 Illustrating the sagittal plane.

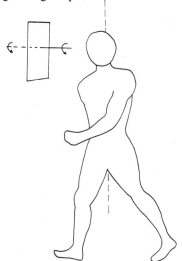

Figure 1.5 Illustrating movements in the sagittal plane.

(Figure 1.4). If the body were to rotate about this axis it would rotate forwards or backwards, as occurs in a somersault. The use of models may again help to aid the visualization of this movement. Basic movements in the sagittal plane include those of the legs when walking (Figure 1.5).

The third major plane passes through the body dividing it into front and back halves. This is referred to as the frontal or lateral plane and its corresponding anteroposterior axis passes through the body from front to back (Figure 1.6). Movements in this plane and about this axis are illustrated in Figure 1.7.

However, whereas these planes and axes are useful as terms of reference, most of the movements made by the body do not correspond exactly with these planes but

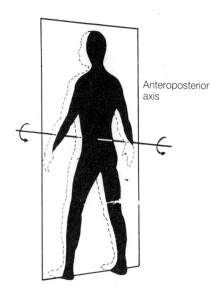

Anteroposterior axis

Figure 1.6 Illustrating the frontal or lateral plane.

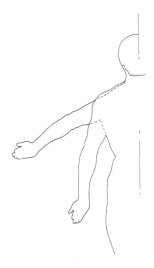

Figure 1.7 Illustrating movements in the frontal or lateral plane.

fall between and across them. For instance, when walking the arm action is not quite in the sagittal plane since the arms tend to swing slightly across the body rather than going directly forwards and back. Therefore, the movement is really in a plane between sagittal and frontal. Any movement that does not occur in one of the major planes may be described as occurring in a diagonal or 'oblique' plane about an 'oblique' axis and the position of this oblique plane of movement may be described relative to the major planes. Thus, the arm action used during walking may be described as occurring in an oblique plane which is approximately at 10 degrees to the sagittal plane. However, to further clarify the exact movement it is then necessary to specify that at the end of the forward swing the hands are closer to the midline of the body than they were at the start, and not vice versa.

It should also be noted that if the subject moves, then so do the planes. For example, if the subject is lying in a horizontal position then the sagittal plane still extends forwards, dividing the body into left and right halves, whilst the transverse plane still divides the body into top and bottom halves, and the frontal plane divides it into front and back halves. In practice most bodily movements are complex, involving many body parts which may be moving in slightly different planes. However, by systematically breaking down the movement into its component parts and utilizing the basic terminology unnecessary confusions may be avoided. Thus a basic knowledge of the vocabulary of kinesiology (the study of movement) is an important asset for anyone dealing with movement analysis and exercise therapy.

Describing movements as rotations

Reference to planes and axes provides one method of describing movements; however, there are others and when describing movements the most convenient method of description is always used. For instance, an alternative method of description may

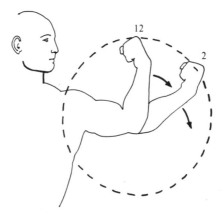

Figure 1.8 Illustrating how rotatory movements may be described with reference to a clock face.

involve the use of the term rotation. This is because the movement of a limb may be compared to the movement of the hands of a clock; that is to say, one end can be visualized as being fixed at a joint whilst the other end of the limb (or bone) moves (Figure 1.8).

To minimize the risk of confusion when describing rotatory movements the end of the limb or bone nearest the centre of the body is referred to as being proximal, whilst the end furthest from the centre of the body is described as being distal. So when describing movements of the forearm, the ends of the radius and ulna that are nearest the elbow are referred to as being proximal whilst the ends furthest from the elbow nearest the hand are referred to as being distal. Similarly in the example of the leg, the top of the femur would be referred to as proximal whilst the foot would be considered as distal. So when relating the movement to a clock face it is usually the proximal end of the limb that is imagined to be at the centre of the clock face whilst the distal end of the limb is imagined to be at the periphery. In most movements it is the proximal end which remains fixed whilst the distal end is seen to move. However, there are a few examples where the positions are reversed and the distal end remains fixed (at the centre of the clock) whilst the proximal end moves.

In order to give a description of the movements in terms of rotation, it is first necessary to standardize the position of the imaginary clock. This is essential since the action of raising a glass to one's lips may be seen as a clockwise rotation of the forearm in the sagittal plane when viewed from one side of the subject but as an anti-clockwise action in the sagittal plane when viewed from the opposite side. Therefore, for all rotations in the sagittal plane the subject is viewed as looking to the right with the clock facing the observer (Figure 1.9).

Hence, even if in reality the subject is not being viewed from this angle when the movement is being described, the assessor must in effect imagine moving themselves

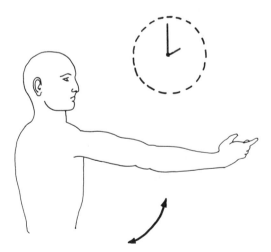

Figure 1.9 Illustrating how clockwise and anticlockwise movements may be described in the sagittal plane.

in order to describe the movement in the standard manner with the subject facing to the assessor's right, i.e. the assessor always 'sees' the right-hand side of the subject's body. Similarly, when describing movements in the transverse plane about the longitudinal axis, the assessor must visualize the movement from above with a clock

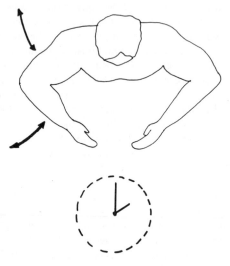

Figure 1.10 Illustrating how clockwise and anticlockwise movements may be described in the transverse plane.

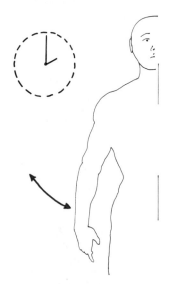

Figure 1.11 Illustrating how clockwise and anticlockwise movements may be described in the frontal or lateral plane.

placed at the foot of the subject, facing upwards (Figure 1.10) and, finally, for rotations in the frontal plane about the anteroposterior axis the assessor must visualize the subject to be directly facing them with a clock above the subject's head, also facing front (Figure 1.11).

Describing body parts and movements

When describing movements the use of planes and axes will enable an accurate description of the direction of a movement. This description can be enhanced by the use of a more extensive and specific vocabulary that refers to the types of movement that are possible within those planes. For example, common everyday expressions such as 'to bend' or 'to move' may be interpreted in a number of ways. To prevent this, those working in the fields of exercise therapy and exercise promotion should have a basic kinesiological vocabulary which will enable them to describe certain movements accurately. Common terms used to describe forms of movement include; flexion, extension, abduction, adduction, elevation, depression, eversion, inversion, rotation, supination and pronation. In addition, other standardized terms may also be required to describe precisely the body part that is being moved and, in this context, the terms anterior, posterior, lateral, medial, distal, proximal, superior, inferior, deep and superficial may be utilized. When these terms are used in conjunction with the planes and axes described earlier, a precise description of any movement can be made. Finally, in order to describe a movement it is necessary to have a starting point as

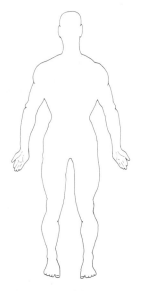

Figure 1.12 Illustrating the anatomical position.

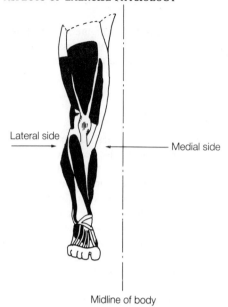

Midline of body

Figure 1.13 Illustrating the use of the terms lateral and medial.

a frame of reference. In kinesiology the starting point is referred to as the anatomical position (Figure 1.12). When describing movements, many need to be visualized as beginning from the anatomical position even if in reality they have not. This helps to clarify the description of certain movements and its value will be illustrated in the following sections.

Lateral and medial

The term lateral refers to the body part furthest from the midline of the body, whereas medial refers to the body part nearest the midline of the body (Figure 1.13). Hence particular ligaments in the knee are referred to as being lateral ligaments (running down the outside of the knee) and medial ligaments (running down the inside of the knee). Similarly, the foot may be described as having a lateral border and a medial border.

Distal and proximal

When referring to parts of the limbs of the body the term distal refers to the part furthest away from the centre of the body whilst proximal refers to the part nearest the centre. This can be illustrated using the example of the radius and ulna of the forearm. The distal ends of these bones form part of the wrist joint whereas their proximal ends form part of the elbow joint.

Anterior and posterior

Anterior refers to the body part nearest the front of the body whilst posterior refers to the body part nearest the back or dorsal side of the body.

16

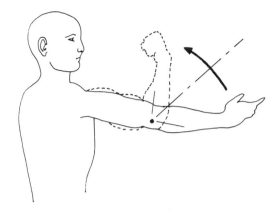

Figure 1.14 Illustrating flexion of the elbow joint.

Superior and inferior

Superior refers to the part nearest the head whilst inferior refers to the part furthest away from the head.

Deep and superficial

Deep refers to the part furthest from the surface of the body whilst superficial refers to a part near the surface. Thus a muscle may be described as having superficial muscle fibres and deep muscle fibres. Alternatively, muscle damage may be described as deep or superficial.

Flexion and extension

Flexion refers to a movement which reduces the angle of a joint. A simple flexion movement in the sagittal plane would be elbow flexion (Figure 1.14). Other examples include hip flexion (lifting the thigh whilst walking), flexing the knee, flexion of the back (leaning forward) and flexing the ankle.

Movement of the arm about the shoulder joint is a little more difficult to define since it is not very clear when the angle of the joint is decreasing. However, as with all other movements in the sagittal plane (bar the knee) a forward movement from the anatomical position is deemed to be flexion. Therefore, raising the arm from the anatomical position is considered to be shoulder flexion (Figure 1.15).

With such a movement it is important to remember the rule that the movement is deemed to have begun from the anatomical position, whether in reality it did or did not. For example, if in reality the movement being described began with the arm already extended forwards in the sagittal plane and parallel to the ground, the initial movement of the arm from this position would be up and back. This would then contradict the rule that a flexion of the shoulder joint requires the arm to move forwards. However, because the movement is imagined to have started from the anatomical

17

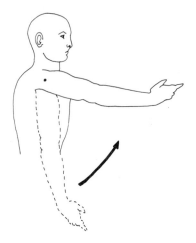

Figure 1.15 Illustrating shoulder flexion.

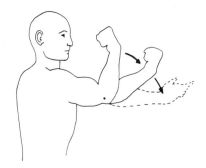

Figure 1.16 Illustrating extension of the elbow.

position and a movement is described according to the initial action, it would still be referred to as shoulder flexion and thus would not contravene the rule.

The opposite to flexion is extension and any movement that increases the angle at a joint is therefore referred to as an extension movement. Extending the ankle, knee and hip are all movements that occur in the sagittal plane whilst walking as the foot pushes against the ground and the 'leg' straightens. Similarly, lowering the arm and straightening the elbow are also extension movements (Figure 1.16).

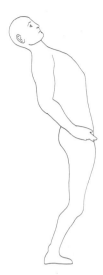

Figure 1.17 Illustrating hyperextension of the back.

In the sagittal plane the movement of the fingers may be considered in a similar manner to the movement of the limbs and trunk. This consistency is ensured since, in the anatomical position, the palms of the hands face forwards. As with all the other movements described in the sagittal plane (bar the knee joint) the 'bending' of the fingers is referred to as flexion and their straightening as extension. Movements of the foot at the ankle joint in the sagittal plane may also be described using the terms flexion or extension. Alternatively, the specific terms of dorsiflexion and plantarflexion may be applied to describe ankle flexion and ankle extension respectively. Dorsiflexion refers to the ankle movement that brings the toes nearer to the knees whilst plantarflexion refers to the ankle movement that occurs when a dancer 'points her toes' or stands on the balls of her feet.

The term hyperextension is often used to refer to an extension movement that is beyond the normal anatomical position. Hyperextending the back would result in a participant 'leaning' backwards (Figure 1.17). In addition, some individuals will also exhibit an ability to hyperextend other joints beyond the 'normal' expected range of movement, in which case the term hyperextension may again be applied. An example of this would be hyperextending a joint such as the elbow.

It can be seen from the diagrams that flexion and extension movements may also be described as rotations in the various planes. This alternative mode of description is covered in a later section.

Lateral flexion

Flexion movements may also occur in the frontal plane. For example, bending to the side may be described as a lateral flexion of the trunk (Figure 1.18). If the

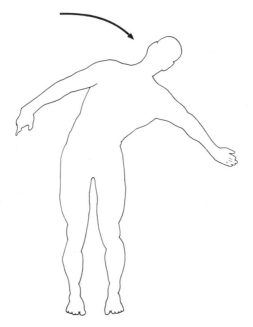

Figure 1.18 Illustrating lateral flexion of the back.

subject bends to the right, thereby decreasing the angle of the trunk on that side, it is called 'right lateral flexion of the trunk'. Conversely, bending to the left would be 'left lateral flexion of the trunk'. In addition to their use in describing movements of the trunk, left and right lateral flexion may also be used to describe movements of the neck in the frontal plane.

Abduction and adduction

These are terms used to describe movements in the frontal plane about the anteroposterior axis. In order to describe these movements it is first necessary to visualize the body in the anatomical position with a 'midline' running down the centre of the body from the top of the head to the floor. Beginning in the anatomical position, any movement of a body part away from the midline of the body is referred to as abduction whereas any movement towards the midline of the body is referred to as adduction. Examples of adduction and abduction are presented in Figure 1.19.

As with the flexion movements in the sagittal plane described earlier, movements in the frontal plane must be envisaged as starting from the anatomical position. Thus when crossing the feet (left leg over right leg) the left foot will initially move to the subject's right, towards the midline of the body, cross the midline of the body and then continue moving to their right away from the midline of the body. However, since the movement is envisaged to have started from the anatomical position and the initial movement is clearly towards the midline of the body and hence an

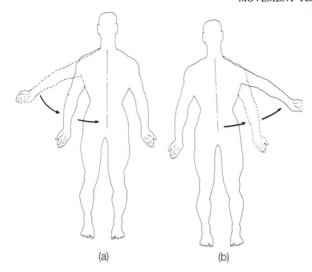

Figure 1.19 Illustrating adduction and abduction of the arm.

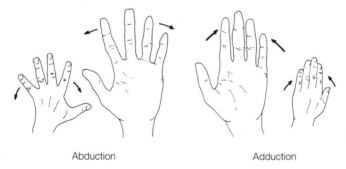

Abduction   Adduction

Figure 1.20 Illustrating abduction and adduction of the fingers.

adduction, the entire movement, regardless of where it was initiated in reality, is referred to as an adduction. The movement of the arms in the frontal plane may be described in a similar manner to those of the legs.

The movements of the fingers in the frontal plane are considered separately to those of the limbs or trunk. When describing movement of the fingers in the frontal plane a midline is imagined running through the middle finger of the hand. Any movement of the other fingers or thumbs away from the middle finger is referred to as abduction of the fingers whilst the movement of fingers or thumbs towards the middle finger is referred to as adduction (Figure 1.20).

*Horizontal extension (horizontal abduction) and horizontal flexion
(horizontal adduction)*

These movements are performed in the transverse plane and, unlike most other actions,

21

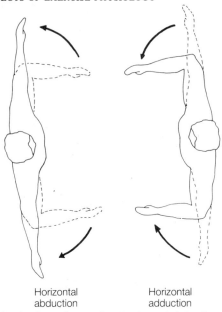

Horizontal
abduction

Horizontal
adduction

Figure 1.21 Illustrating horizontal extension (horizontal abduction) of the elbows in the transverse plane and horizontal flexion (horizontal adduction).

cannot be performed directly from the anatomical position. To perform these movements the limb must first be abducted or flexed until in a horizontal position. Horizontal extension and horizontal flexion may be performed by both the upper and lower limbs. However, strength and flexibility are required to perform such movements with the lower limbs. Without assistance, many individuals will only be able to perform them with the upper limbs. Horizontal extension (horizontal abduction) refers to a movement of the limb in the transverse plane away from the midline of the body. Horizontal flexion (horizontal adduction) refers to a movement of the limb in the transverse plane towards the midline of the body (Figure 1.21).

Elevation and depression

The terms elevation and depression are commonly used to describe movements of the shoulder, the simplest example being the case of 'shrugging' the shoulders. In such an action, the upward movement of the shoulders is referred to as elevation whilst the downward movement is known as depression. Elevation and depression may also be used to describe movements of the foot – for example, the 'elevation of the lateral border of the foot' (Figure 1.22). However, in such cases it is often more usual to describe such movements of the foot with the specific terms 'eversion' and 'inversion'.

Eversion and inversion

These are terms commonly used to describe movements of the foot. Eversion refers to the raising of the lateral border such that, if standing, the weight is placed on the medial border of the foot. The opposite to eversion is inversion, where the medial border is raised and weight is placed on the lateral border of the foot.

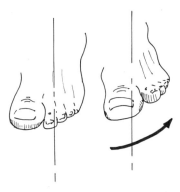

Figure 1.22 Illustrating elevation of the lateral border of the foot.

Supination and pronation

These are somewhat more complex movements and their exact meaning will depend upon the body part being moved and the plane in which it is being moved. Pronation of the arm is best illustrated by considering the subject to be in the anatomical position and having his or her hands turned such that the palms now face backwards not forwards. This is achieved by rotating or twisting the right hand anticlockwise and the left hand clockwise (for movements in the transverse plane imagine the clock at the feet of the subject). The opposite to pronation is supination. Supination would describe the action used to tighten a screw (if using the right hand), whereas a pronating action with the right hand would loosen the screw. The terms pronation and supination are also often used to describe movements of the foot. In this case the movement occurs in an oblique plane. Pronation of the foot is used to describe the combination of moving the toes away from the midline of the body and raising the lateral border so that the weight tends to be placed on the medial side of the foot. Supination refers to the opposite action – that of moving the toes closer to the midline of the body and raising the medial border such that the weight is placed on the lateral border of the foot.

Clockwise and anticlockwise rotations

Such terms may be effectively used to describe twisting movements such as rotating the spine in the transverse plane (Figure 1.23). However, when describing such movements it must be remembered that the movement has to be imagined to be 'viewed' from above the subject. The use of the terms clockwise and anticlockwise rotations may also be used to describe flexion and extension movements in the sagittal, frontal and oblique planes, thereby providing an alternative mode of description. Similarly, certain movements of the arms and legs may also be described as inward and outward rotations. Thus, if starting in the anatomical position, a clockwise rotation of the right limbs would be described as an outward rotation. Conversely, an outward rotation of the left limbs would require an anticlockwise rotation. Inward rotations

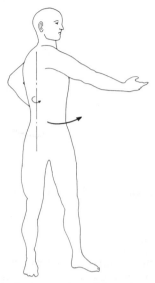

Figure 1.23 Illustrating an anticlockwise rotation of the spine.

would therefore be achieved by a clockwise rotation of the left limbs and an anticlockwise rotation of the right.

Circumduction

Circumduction refers to a rotatory movement of a body part such that its movement traces a cone. An example would be the circumduction of the shoulder joint (Figure 1.24) where the arm rotates from the shoulder joint (which forms the point of the cone) whilst the hand traces a circle (forming the base of the cone).

Summary

It can therefore be seen that, in practice, any one particular movement may be described in a number of different ways and it is up to the individual to decide which is the most appropriate in terms of clarity. The correct application of such terms will provide the user with a means of precisely and unambiguously describing movements. The use of this form of movement terminology also enables the classification of muscles and muscle groups by function. For practical purposes muscles may be described in simple terms as being hip flexors, elbow flexors, ankle flexors and so on. This provides a simple, practical means of description which may be used instead of, or to complement, their Latin names, depending upon the circumstances in which reference is being made.

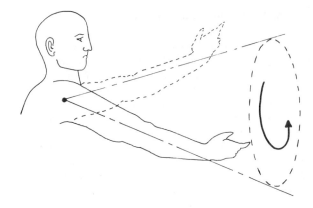

Figure 1.24 Illustrating circumduction of the shoulder joint.

TYPES OF MUSCLE CONTRACTION

For those wishing to use exercise within their professional work a clear understanding of the workings of the body is essential. When studying exercise physiology a sound knowledge of muscle function forms a central part of that understanding. Muscles fulfil many roles – some obvious, others not so obvious. They contract to initiate movement of the whole body or a body part, regulate movement that is being caused by another force or even prevent movement that is being caused by another muscle or an external force such as gravity. Basic coordinated movements require many muscles to contribute in a variety of ways to produce the desired action. To gain an understanding of the complex and varied roles that muscles fulfil in movement sequences it is first necessary to review their functions in isolation, always remembering that in reality muscles work in coordinated groups rather than separately.

When an appropriate nerve impulse is sent to a muscle, tension builds up in that muscle. This process is more commonly described as a muscular contraction. The physiological details associated with the process of muscle contraction are dealt with in a later chapter. Muscles may contract in a number of different ways in different circumstances. If there is a change in the length of the muscle, and hence the build up of tension is associated with movement, the contraction is described as being dynamic or isotonic. Alternatively, if tension builds up in the muscle but its length remains unaltered and there is therefore no movement, the contraction is described as static or isometric. The different types of muscle contraction may be classified as follows:

1. Dynamic (isotonic) concentric
2. Dynamic (isokinetic) concentric
3. Dynamic (isotonic) eccentric
4. Static (isometric).

Dynamic (isotonic) concentric contractions

A muscle contraction is said to be dynamic (isotonic) and concentric when the resulting tension in the muscle causes it to shorten and cause movement. The term isotonic means 'same tension'. In such a contraction the speed of the resulting movement may vary owing to the physiology and biomechanics of the body. For example, the movement may be relatively slow in the early stages of its initiation, be quite rapid during the middle phase, and then be slow towards the end. Many body and limb movements will fall into this category. Such movements occur when the tension in the muscle, and thus the force of contraction, exceeds that of an opposing force or resistance applied to it. The resistance (or opposing force) may be in the form of the weight of a limb or the weight of an object that the individual is attempting to lift. In summary, if the force of the contraction exceeds that of the resistance, then the muscle will shorten in length and cause movement. An example would be the contraction of the hip flexors which raise the leg in the process of walking, or the contraction of the biceps when raising a glass to one's mouth. The change in speed during the movement is attributable to a number of factors including differences in the strength of the muscle at different lengths, changes in the effective angle of pull of the muscle on the bones during the movement, and the general inertia of the part providing the resistance.

Dynamic (isokinetic) concentric contractions

An isokinetic contraction is in many respects similar to an isotonic contraction. However, during an isokinetic contraction the speed of the movement remains constant, hence the name isokinetic. This is achieved by altering the tension in the muscle during the movement or providing an accommodating resistance which enables a constant speed to be produced throughout the range of movement. Such movements may occur when the participant is working against an applied resistance such as the therapist's arm which may be used to resist the movement and, hence, dictate the limb speed throughout the entire range of movement. To achieve this the therapist may need to alter the resistance applied at various stages of the movement. Alternatively, resistance may be applied using specially designed isokinetic machines which can be programmed to allow the limb to move at a predetermined speed throughout the full range of move-ment. In this method the machine provides a variable/accommodating resistance which is consistently just less than that produced by the muscle. As with isotonic concentric contractions, the movement observed under isokinetic conditions is achieved by the muscle generating a force which exceeds that of the resistance thereby causing the muscle to shorten and hence cause movement.

Dynamic (isotonic) eccentric contractions

An eccentric contraction is said to take place when tension is present in the muscle but it lengthens rather than shortens. This occurs when the muscle is already in a shortened or semi-shortened state and the force generated by the muscle is less than that of an opposing external force. In such movements the opposing force causes the muscle to lengthen, despite the muscle generating a force which would otherwise have caused it to shorten. Eccentric contractions are commonly used by the body to regulate movements caused by external forces such as gravity. This form of contraction is common in controlling such actions as the lowering of an object onto a table. Here the movement is caused by the force of gravity but the eccentric contractions of the biceps control the lowering action. By generating a tension in the bicep which is slightly less than that of the external force (gravity acting upon the arm and object being held) the muscle slowly lengthens, thereby gradually lowering the object. If the biceps did not contract eccentrically during the movement the object would effectively be lowered very rapidly in an uncontrolled manner. Another example of an eccentric contraction occurs when lowering oneself into a chair. In this example the eccentric contractions of the hip and leg extensors permit a controlled lowering action. If the eccentric contractions did not take place we would simply fall into the chair rather than lowering ourselves in a controlled manner.

A similar form of eccentric contraction occurs when someone walks or runs. When the foot strikes the ground and begins to take the weight of the body, the hip and knee joints tend to flex. If this flexion were not checked then we would simply collapse onto the floor. To prevent this the hip and knee extensors contract to oppose the flexion movement. In the early stages of this 'checking process' the amount of force generated by the contraction of hip and knee extensors is less than that caused by gravity. Hence the hip and knee extensors lengthen despite the tension being generated in them, and thus the hip and knee joints continue to flex (albeit at a slower rate). The hip and knee extensor muscles can therefore be said to be working eccentrically. A fraction of a second later in the movement, as the muscular contractions of the knee extensors continue, they begin to exceed that of the force of gravity and the downward (flexion) movement is slowed down. The flexion movement is then stopped for a brief instant and as the force of the muscular contractions continue to exceed that of gravity the extensor muscles start to shorten and cause the leg to straighten. Hence, when walking, the hip and knee extensors will work eccentrically to check the downward movement caused by gravity as the weight is placed on the leg, the movement (flexion) will be stopped for an instant and then the extensors will start to work concentrically as their force of contraction exceeds that of gravity, and they shorten, causing the hip and knee to be extended.

Static (isometric) contractions

If the resistance or opposing force applied to a muscle is equal to the force of contraction that the muscle is generating, then, although tension is present in the muscle, no movement will take place. This form of muscle contraction is referred to as a static or isometric contraction. Many muscles and muscle groups function in this manner during various bodily activities. For example, although the muscles of the trunk may be used to move the body they also spend much of their time maintaining the trunk in a relatively fixed position, combating the force of gravity and retaining the individual's posture. Other muscles within the body may work in a similar manner to prevent unwanted movement caused either by external forces such as gravity or by the action of other muscles that may be contracting dynamically. Consequently, although an activity such as walking occurs through the dynamic contraction of various muscles, the activity also requires numerous other muscles to contract isometrically in order to maintain body posture during the activity.

DESCRIBING THE RANGE OF MOVEMENT

The movement of a limb or body part may be described according to its motion within the full range of movement that the joint can produce. The full range of movement of a joint is from the position where it is fully flexed to the position where it is fully extended. Alternatively, it may be from the position of maximal abduction to maximal adduction and so on, depending on the specific movement being considered. The outer range of movement of a joint refers to the movement in the region where the muscle causing the movement is close to being at its longest possible length. Conversely, the inner range of movement of a joint corresponds to movement in the range where the muscle causing the movement is close to being fully contracted. The middle range of movement lies between the two. Figure 1.25 illustrates how the movement at the elbow joint may be described in terms of its inner, middle, outer and full range. In a further example – that of elbow flexion and extension – movement from a fully extended to a partially flexed position is described as its outer range of movement as during the motion the biceps is close to being at its maximum length. As the flexion movement continues the biceps moves the elbow through its middle range into its inner range of movement, at which point it is close to being fully shortened. Conversely, the extension movement caused by the triceps muscle would be described in the following manner: the initial movement from the fully flexed position (when the triceps is close to its maximum length) is described as its outer range; and the region during which the elbow is almost fully extended and the triceps is fully contracted as its inner range. In this way the description of a range of movement at a joint depends upon the muscles that are acting to cause the movement.

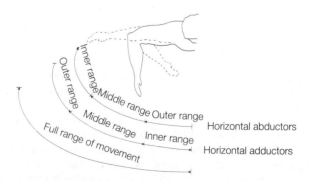

Figure 1.25 Illustrating the range of movement at a joint.

THE VARIED ROLES THAT MUSCLES FULFIL

Having briefly covered the different forms of muscle contraction it is now possible to discuss the various roles of muscles and the functions they fulfil in initiating, controlling and preventing movement. For discussion purposes the roles that muscles fulfil may be considered under the following headings:

1. Agonists or movers
2. Antagonists
3. Fixators including
   (i)   stabilizers
   (ii) supporters
4. Regulators
5. Neutralizers
6. Synergists

However, in such a discussion it must be remembered that in different circumstances a muscle or muscle group may fulfil many roles, even during what may at first appear to be the same movement. For instance, the biceps of the arm may be considered as an agonist when lifting an object, a regulator when lowering it, a supporter when holding an object steady and an antagonist when the elbow is being extended by the triceps. Similarly, if the movement in Figure 1.26 is considered, the initial flexion movement will be caused by the biceps acting as an agonist whilst the triceps remains relaxed and lengthens, thereby being by definition an antagonist. However, once the forearm has passed the vertical then the movement would automatically continue under the force of gravity but may need to be controlled by the eccentric contraction of the triceps, which would then be acting as a regulator.

Conversely, the reverse movement during which the elbow was extended would initially involve the triceps working as the agonist whilst the biceps remained relaxed and lengthened, thereby being the antagonist. However, in the second phase of the

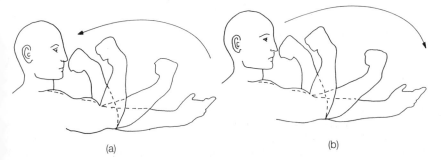

(a)   (b)

Figure 1.26 Illustrating how the roles which muscles fulfil may alter during a single movement. (a) Biceps acts as agonist and the triceps as antagonist until the movement reaches the vertical, whereupon gravity continues the movement whilst the triceps works eccentrically as a regulator. (b) The triceps acts an an agonist and the biceps as an antagonist during the early phase of the movement; once beyond the vertical gravity will continue the movement whilst the biceps works eccentrically as a regulator.

movement the biceps may be required to act as regulator in order to control the lowering movement. This example also serves to illustrate the fact that when muscles are used they usually work in pairs or groups, not singularly. This requires complex coordination and cooperation between muscle groups. Failure to achieve this co-ordination for whatever reason will result in uncoordinated and/or impeded movement.

When describing a movement and relating it to the muscle groups involved it is important to ask a number of questions: 'Is the movement being caused by muscular contraction or gravity?' 'If the movement is being caused by gravity, is it being regulated by eccentric muscular contractions?'; and 'Which joints are involved, and hence, which muscle groups are active during the movement?'. Another factor to be considered is whether any other muscle groups are involved in stabilizing either the joint or other parts of the body during the movement.

Agonists

Agonists are muscles which cause a movement; they are therefore sometimes described as movers. When flexing the elbow from the anatomical position in the sagittal plane the elbow flexors would be referred to as the agonists, with the major muscle involved being the biceps brachii: hence in such an action it may be referred to as the prime mover. Other examples of agonists include the hip flexors when raising the leg upwards and forwards during walking, or the knee and ankle extensors during walking when pushing against the ground.

Antagonists

An antagonist is a muscle which would oppose a movement if it contracted. Therefore, in order to permit a free movement the antagonist must relax and lengthen. If it does not, as can happen in certain neuromuscular disorders such as spasticity, the movement will be impeded. Examples of antagonists include the elbow extensors (triceps brachii) when the elbow is flexing and the ankle extensors such as the gastrocnemius when the ankle is being flexed.

Fixators

A fixator is a muscle which contracts to prevent unwanted movement. There are two classes of fixator; stabilizers and supporters. Stabilizers contract to prevent movement that would occur due to the contraction of another muscle, whereas supporters contract to prevent movement that would occur due to an external force such as gravity.

Stabilizers

A stabilizer is a muscle which prevents an unwanted movement that may be caused by the active contraction of another muscle. Movement may be brought about by the shortening of muscle groups which are attached to bones. Often the desired action will be the movement of a joint at the distal end of the bone, whilst the joint at the proximal end of the bone remains steady or fixed. Any unwanted movement at the proximal end of the bone may reduce the effectiveness of the action. Therefore a stabilizing muscle may contract to hold the proximal end of a bone in position. During many actions a limited amount of movement at the proximal end of the bone is necessary and hence stabilizers will often work both isometrically and isotonically to achieve the desired effect. The stabilizing actions of muscles operate at the unconscious level and illustrate the complexity of coordinated movement.

Supporters

In contrast to a stabilizer, which fixes a bone in position and opposes a movement that would occur due to the action of another muscle, a supporter fixes a body part in position against an external force such as gravity. This requires the muscles to contract statically, opposing the force of gravity with an equal force. Many muscles work in this manner to maintain posture and body position, especially those of the back.

Regulators

A regulator is a muscle which controls a movement caused by the force of gravity. In doing so it must contract eccentrically. Examples of regulating actions would include the lowering of a heavy pan or weight onto a table or the lowering of oneself into a chair. If the muscles did not contract eccentrically to control/regulate the movement, a person would fall into a chair in an uncontrolled manner or lower a pan too rapidly onto a table.

Neutralizers

A neutralizer contracts to prevent the unwanted action of another muscle whilst permitting the desired action of that muscle. An example of this can be seen with the triceps brachii which can have a neutralizing action on the biceps brachii. The biceps brachii not only flex the elbow but can also supinate the forearm. When turning a door handle or tightening a screw (with the right hand) the desired action would be that of supination. However, if the action of forearm flexion were to occur at the same time it would prove to be most inconvenient with the hand being pulled away as it turned. Therefore in order to prevent forearm flexion the elbow extensors (triceps brachii) also contract. This therefore neutralizes the unwanted flexion movement whilst permitting the desired supination. Another example would be that of moving from a lying to a sitting position in bed. In the movement of sitting up a number of abdominal muscles are involved, including the right and left external obliques. Depending upon which other muscles contract at the same time, the contraction of the external obliques can result in flexion, lateral flexion or rotation. If the external obliques were to contract separately then the right external obliques would cause the body to rotate to the left whilst the left external obliques would cause the body to rotate to the right.

This rotatory action is really a combination of forward flexion and rotation. However, if both the left and right external obliques contract together they neutralize each other's opposing rotatory actions whilst permitting the desired forward flexion of the trunk.

Synergists

Synergists are muscles which operate in a complex manner to assist with a movement. They work on an unconscious level and make the actions of the agonists stronger. Synergists often act to prevent unwanted movement, steady the action caused by the agonists and help to maintain a muscle at its optimum length.

THE MAJOR MUSCLE GROUPS AND THEIR ACTIONS

The human body contains over 600 muscles which act on the 206 bones of the skeleton to stabilize it and produce effective movement. Thus, the muscles of the body affect the actions which occur at more than 200 joints or articulations. To describe such actions in detail would require a separate text, therefore the aim of this section is to present a brief overview of these aspects rather than an in-depth study. This overview should provide therapists and other health professionals with a suitable basic background and insight into the topic from which they may then wish to pursue the subject in greater detail. In summary, the section presents a basic coverage of the muscles that are used in the major movements of the limbs. These movements are those which are most likely to be incorporated into an exercise programme when the

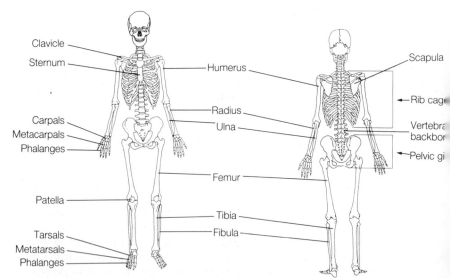

Figure 1.27 A labelled skeleton illustrating the major bones of the body.

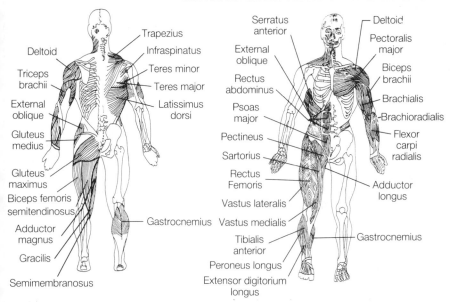

Figure 1.28 Illustrating the position of the major muscle groups of the body.

practitioner prescribes exercise as a form of therapy or gives advice on aspects related to exercise and movement.

When reading this section it should be remembered that body movements are complex, involving many muscles which fulfil many roles. Indeed, the exact role which a muscle fulfils at any one time may depend upon many factors, including:

1. The fibres that are contracting within the muscle. This has an effect since, in certain muscles, the contraction of different parts of the same muscle can produce different results and, in addition, the number of fibres contracting within the muscle will influence the amount of force it. generates.
2. Other muscles that are contracting at the same time. These may be assisting with the movement, opposing it or stabilizing a joint or body part during the movement.
3. The external forces that are acting upon the body.
4. The position of the body part when the muscle contracts.

Such differences can have a profound effect upon the resulting action, making the study of such aspects far from simple. It should also be realized that some muscles extend over two joints and thus their actions will affect the movements at more than one joint, thereby complicating the topic still further.

In order to assist with the coverage of the major muscle groups and their actions a labelled skeleton is presented in Figure 1.27 and the positions of a selection of the major muscles of the body are illustrated in Figure 1.28. For the sake of clarity, Figure 1.28 illustrates the major superficial muscle groups and not the deeper muscles which are positioned behind those illustrated. For more detailed information on the specific actions of particular muscles the reader should refer to the recommended further reading.

Muscles involved in movements of the hip

Two of the major muscle/muscle groups involved with movements of the hip are the quadriceps femoris and hamstrings. The quadriceps femoris consists of four distinct parts: the rectus femoris, vastus lateralis, vastus medialis and vastus intermedius. The functions of these constituent parts differ, and they are therefore described separately in this section. Likewise the actions of the three constituent muscles of the hamstring muscle group (the biceps femoris, semitendinosus and semimembranosus) are also described separately.

1. Hip flexion: psoas, iliacus (also stabilizes hip), sartorius, rectus femoris, pectineus, tensor fasciae latae, gluteus medius (anterior fibres), gluteus minimus (anterior fibres), adductor longus (assists), adductor brevis (assists when in standing position), adductor magnus (flexion and inward rotation when upper fibres contract alone) and gracilis (when knee is extended).
2. Hip extension: biceps femoris, semitendinosus, semimembranosus, gluteus maximus, gluteus medius (posterior fibres), gluteus minimus (posterior fibres), adductor brevis (if hip is already in flexed position it extends and adducts the hip) and adductor magnus (extension and outward rotation when lower fibres contract alone).
3. Hip adduction: pectineus, adductor longus, adductor magnus (when whole muscle contracts), gracilis, adductor brevis (when in standing position, but if hip is in flexed position it extends and adducts the hip) and gluteus maximus (lower portion assists).
4. Hip abduction: sartorius, rectus femoris, tensor fasciae latae, gluteus maximus (upper third), gluteus medius and gluteus minimus.
5. Hip inward rotation: tensor fasciae latae, semitendinosus, gluteus medius (anterior fibres), gluteus minimus (anterior fibres), gracilis and adductor magnus (inward rotation and flexion when upper fibres contract alone).
6. Hip outward rotation: sartorius, gluteus maximus, obturator externus, obturator internus, gemellus superior, gemellus inferior, quadratus femorus, piriformis, gluteus medius (posterior fibres), gluteus minimus (posterior fibres), adductor magnus (outward rotation and extension when lower fibres contract alone), adductor longus (assists), biceps femoris (assists) and pectineus (weak assistor).

Muscles involved in movements of the knee

1. Knee flexion: biceps femoris, sartorius, semitendinosus, semimembranosus, gracilis, popliteus, plantaris (weak assistor) and gastrocnemius (assists when plantarflexion occurs at the same time).
2. Knee extension: rectus femoris, vastus lateralis, vastus intermedius and vastus medialis.

3. Knee inward rotation (only possible when knee is flexed): sartorius and semitendinosus.
4. Knee outward rotation (only possible when knee is flexed): biceps femoris.

Muscles involved in movements of the foot and ankle

1. Foot flexion (dorsiflexion): tibialis anterior, extensor digitorum longus, extensor hallucis longus and peroneus tertius.
2. Foot extension (plantarflexion): gastrocnemius, soleus, peroneus longus, peroneus brevis, flexor digitorum longus (assists), flexor hallucis longus (assists) and tibialis posterior (assists).
3. Eversion (usually accompanied by abduction to produce pronation): peroneus longus, peroneus brevis, peroneus tertius and extensor digitorum longus.
4. Inversion (usually accompanied by adduction to produce supination): tibialis anterior, tibialis posterior and flexor digitorum longus.
5. Foot supination: tibialis anterior, extensor hallucis longus, tibialis posterior, flexor digitorum longus (assists) and flexor hallucis longus (assists).
6. Foot pronation: extensor digitorum longus, peroneus tertius, peroneus longus and peroneus brevis.

Muscles involved in movements of the shoulder joint (including the humerus)

1. Shoulder flexion: biceps brachii, deltoid (anterior portion and anterior fibres of middle portion), pectoralis major (clavicular portion), subscapularis (assists) and coracobrachialis (assists).
2. Shoulder extension: deltoid (posterior fibres of middle portion assist), deltoid (posterior portion), pectoralis major (sternal portion), latissimus dorsi, teres major, teres minor and triceps brachii (assists).
3. Shoulder abduction: deltoid (middle portion), deltoid (anterior portion assists), pectoralis major (clavicular portion abducts humerus when above horizontal), pectoralis minor, supraspinatus, subscapularis (assists) and biceps brachii (assists).
4. Shoulder adduction: pectoralis major (sternal portion), latissimus dorsi, teres major, deltoid (posterior portion assists) and triceps brachii (assists).
5. Horizontal flexion: deltoid (anterior portion), pectoralis major, coracobrachialis, deltoid (anterior fibres of middle portion assist) and biceps brachii (assists).
6. Horizontal extension: deltoid (posterior portion), teres minor and infraspinatus.
7. Inward rotation: subscapularis, pectoralis major (clavicular portion), teres major and deltoid (anterior portion assists).
8. Outward rotation: teres minor, deltoid (posterior portion assists) and biceps brachii (assists).

Muscles involved in movements of the scapula

Various muscles involved including: trapezius, rhomboid major, rhomboid minor, levator scapula, pectoralis minor and serratus anterior.

Movements of the elbow

1. Elbow flexion: biceps brachii, brachialis, brachioradialis, coracobrachialis, flexor carpi radialis (assists) and flexor digitorum sublimis (assists).
2. Elbow extension: triceps brachii and anconeus.
3. Supination: supinator (forearm supination) and biceps brachii (when triceps brachii contract at the same time to prevent elbow flexion).
4. Pronation: pronator teres and pronator quadratus (forearm pronation).

Movements of the wrist and hand

1. Wrist flexion: flexor carpi radialis, flexor digitorum sublimis, flexor carpi ulnaris and palmaris longus (assists).
2. Wrist extension: extensor carpi radialis longus, extensor carpi radialis brevis, extensor carpi ulnaris and extensor digitorum.
3. Supination: biceps brachii (when triceps contract at the same time to prevent elbow flexion).
4. Abduction: flexor carpi radialis, extensor carpi radialis longus and extensor carpi radialis brevis.
5. Adduction: extensor carpi ulnaris and flexor carpi ulnaris.

Movements of the trunk

1. Flexion: rectus abdominus, external obliques (when both sides contract) and internal oblique (when both sides contract).
2. Extension: intertransversarii (when both sides contract together), interspinales, multifidus (when both sides contract together), semispinalis thoracis (when both sides contract together), semispinalis cervicis (when both sides contract together) and psoas (hyperextension of the lumbar region).
3. Lateral flexion: quadratus lumborum (when only one side contracts), rectus abdominus (when only one side contracts), external obliques (towards the opposite side if one side contracts alone), intertransversarii (when only one side contracts), multifidus (towards the opposite side when only one side contracts), semispinalis thoracis (towards the opposite side when only one side contracts) and semispinalis cervicis (towards the opposite side when only one side contracts).
4. Rotation: external obliques (towards the opposite side if one side contracts alone), internal oblique (towards the same side if one side contracts alone), multifidus (towards the opposite side when only one side contracts), semispinalis thoracis (towards the opposite side when only one side contracts) and semispinalis cervicis (towards the opposite side when only one side contracts).

2

Physiological aspects of nerves and muscles

INTRODUCTION TO THE NERVOUS SYSTEM

The nervous system provides the body with a vastly complex information system and a means of coordinating its activities. In the context of movement and exercise the functions of the nervous system include:

(a) stimulating the muscles to contract;
(b) coordinating the contraction and relaxation of muscles to produce effective movement;
(c) monitoring and adjusting posture or movement in response to stimuli;
(d) increasing the supply of oxygen and nutrients to the muscles and the removal of metabolic wastes, which is achieved by increasing the activity of the heart and adjusting the blood flow to the muscles;
(e) functioning with the endocrine system to produce the various responses that are needed to maintain body homeostasis during exercise – which includes maintaining an acceptable body temperature and ensuring an appropriate level of body chemicals such as glucose, ions and water.

The components of the nervous system include:

(a) sensors which are sensitive to a whole range of stimuli including electro-magnetic radiation such as heat, light, sound as well as stretch, movement, touch, various chemicals and pH;
(b) neurons which conduct information around the body;
(c) neuroglia which support and protect the neurons.

The information detected by the sensors is conveyed via neurons to the central nervous system where the information is passed between neurons and processed. This may then result in information/instructions being sent out of the central nervous system via neurons to an effector such as a muscle or gland. This information, in the form of a nerve impulse, will then cause the muscle or gland to make an appropriate response to the initial stimuli. Such responses occur constantly, with many of them operating at a subconscious level so that we are unaware of them.

This initial summary is obviously a great simplification of the overall situation where any stimulus has the potential to produce a large number of complex responses.

For example, a particular stimulus may illicit a movement in response to it. For this movement to occur a number of different muscles will need to contract in different ways to produce the desired response. This coordinated response requires each of the muscles involved to receive the appropriate signals in the correct temporal sequence. The nervous system, therefore, has to ensure that the contractions (a) are appropriate, (b) take place in the correct muscles, (c) are of an appropriate strength and (d) occur in the correct sequence. Any such response is also likely to require certain muscles to relax whilst others are contracting: failure to achieve this will result in a less effective movement.

A further example of the role of the nervous system can be illustrated by describing the function of proprioceptors. Proprioceptors are sensors which detect the position and movement of the limbs, joints and muscles. They are sensitive to movement and stretch. When a person attempts to pick up an object he or she will have some expectation of the weight of the object and, hence, how strong the muscle contractions need to be in order to lift it. However, if the object is slightly heavier than 'expected', then these initial contractions may not be strong enough to move the object. This will result in the proprioceptors detecting a discrepancy between the 'expected' position of the limbs (which were expected to have lifted the object) and the actual position of the limbs (which had not moved because the object was too heavy). This discrepancy will cause an automatic response and may cause the central nervous system to send stronger impulses to the muscle thereby increasing the strength of contraction and hence the object may then be moved accordingly. These modifications to the strength of contraction occur within a fraction of a second bringing about an instantaneous adjustment to the strength of contraction. Proprioceptors constantly monitor body position and muscle contractions at a subconscious level to produce effective movement and the maintenance of posture.

The examples presented above serve to illustrate the ways in which the nervous system brings about complex responses to certain stimuli. For most people these responses are automatic and we are unaware of them. For the therapist the importance of such automatic responses is often highlighted in cases of disfunction when the neuromuscular system is not functioning appropriately. In such situations the therapist may try to help patients to learn these responses and to make the required adjustments to their movement processes. The following section presents an outline of the structure and function of the nervous system related to its involvement in movement. This should provide a basis for understanding the nature of certain disfunctions, the role of the nervous system in exercise and the way in which exercise may be applied by the therapist in the treatment of injury or disease.

STRUCTURE OF THE NERVOUS SYSTEM

The nervous system contains two broad categories of cells: (i) neurons which carry information in the form of nerve impulses and (ii) neuroglia or glial cells which are approximately 5 to 10 times more numerous than the neurons. The neuroglia fulfil a variety of functions including providing physical protection and support for the neurons; others have phagocytic properties and protect the neurons by engulfing microbes. Some neuroglia also form a myelin sheath that surrounds the axons and dendrites of the neurons. This not only provides protection and insulation for the neuron but also increases the speed of impulse transmission along these processes. Neurons may be considered under three broad categories:

(a) afferent neurons (also called sensory neurons) which carry information from sensors towards the central nervous system;
(b) interneurons which are found in the central nervous system and are involved with the processing of the information by passing impulses from one neuron to another; and
(c) efferent neurons which conduct information from the central nervous system to the effectors (muscles or glands).

The basic structure of each of these neurons is illustrated in Figure 2.1.

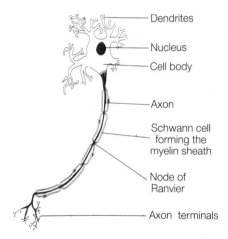

Figure 2.1 Illustrating the basic structure of neurons.

Each neuron consists of a cell body and various processes which conduct the nerve impulses. The cell body contains the nucleus of the neuron and is responsible for the general organization and maintenance of the cell. Those cellular processes which conduct impulses towards the cell body are called dendrites. In the case of afferent neurons the dendrites will conduct impulses that originated in the associated sense organs. The dendrites of interneurons and efferent neurons conduct impulses that they have received from other neurons. Those cellular processes which conduct impulses away from the cell body are called axons. The axons of afferent neurons and inter-neurons pass impulses on to other neurons whilst the axons of efferent neurons conduct their impulses towards the effector organs, which can be either a muscle or a gland. In this way muscle fibres and glands are stimulated by the impulses that they receive from the axons of their associated efferent neurons.

The major nerves of the body consist of many neurons. A nerve may be considered to have a structure that is similar to that of an electric cable, being made up of many individual strands of wire. Schwann cells (also called neurolemmocytes) are a type of neuroglia which is found wrapped around the axons of neurons. The Schwann cells produce a substance called myelin which acts as an insulator. In some neurons (mainly the smaller neurons) the Schwann cell will surround the axon in a single layer forming a thin covering that contains little myelin. These neurons are said to be unmyelinated. In unmyelinated neurons the impulses travel along the length of the axon in a continuous manner. The transmission of impulses along these axons is described as being 'continuous conduction'. In other neurons (mainly the larger neurons) the Schwann cells wrap themselves around the axons many times, producing a thick protective layer called the myelin sheath because of the presence of large amounts of myelin. Neurons possessing this covering are said to be myelinated. The Schwann cells covering myelinated axons do not form a complete covering and small gaps exist between the cells. These gaps are referred to as the nodes of Ranvier (Figure 2.1) and in myelinated neurons the nerve impulses jump between these nodes speeding up the transmission of the impulse. This form of nerve impulse transmission is referred to as 'saltatory conduction'. Myelinated neurons are capable of transmitting nerve impulses at a very rapid rate, which can be up to 120 m/s (approximately 250 miles per hour) in the larger neurons. So, in summary, the myelination of a neuron conveys to it certain properties which affect the speed and way in which it transmits nerve impulses. In diseases such as multiple sclerosis this myelin covering is damaged; this interferes with the transmission of nerve impulses and ultimately affects the signals that are sent to the muscles.

In some neurons, such as those involved with stimulating the muscles of the foot, the axons may be in excess of three feet long. Conversely, the neurons found in the central nervous system may possess axons that are only a fraction of a millimetre in length, whilst in other cases they may be absent altogether.

ORGANIZATION OF THE NERVOUS SYSTEM

The nervous system of the body is a highly organized integrated system which, for discussion purposes, may be subdivided into separate sections. However, it must be remembered that these subdivisions are closely associated with one another and have many links between them, thereby producing a coordinated functional system. Different authorities may vary slightly in the way in which they choose to divide up the nervous system. However, such slight variations only serve to illustrate the integral nature of its component parts. In this text the organization of the nervous system will be considered under the headings illustrated in Figure 2.2.

Initially the nervous system may be divided up into the central nervous system (brain and spinal cord) and the peripheral nervous system. The peripheral nervous system may then be considered under the headings of the afferent system which brings information from sensors to the central nervous system and the efferent system which carries information away from the central nervous system towards the effectors (muscles and glands). The efferent system may then be divided into the somatic or voluntary system and the autonomic or involuntary system. The somatic system is involved with voluntary or conscious actions such as walking or moving an object.

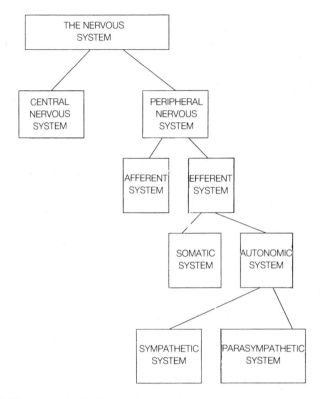

Figure 2.2 Illustrating the basic organization of the nervous system.

It is involved with bringing about actions over which there is some voluntary control. The autonomic system is involved with unconscious, involuntary activities such as controlling the movement of food through the gut and regulating the heart rate. Finally, the autonomic system may itself be divided into two branches: sympathetic and parasympathetic. These two systems tend to oppose one another, thereby bringing about the precise control of body functions; for example, the sympathetic system increases the heart rate whilst the parasympathetic system decreases the heart rate. The two systems are also involved in the vasodilation and vasoconstriction of blood vessels in the body, where again they will tend to oppose one another with one causing dilation whilst the other causes constriction (their exact action depending upon the site of the blood vessel in the body). In this manner these two systems also work in close coordination with the hormones of the body effecting their secretion. However, as previously emphasized all divisions of the nervous system work in a complex integrated manner to produce appropriate coordinated responses to stimuli.

ACTION POTENTIALS AND NERVE IMPULSES

In order to discuss how the nervous system is involved in the process of coordinated movement it is first necessary to understand the basic nature of nerve impulses. Nerve impulses may be regarded as a form of electrical activity which is caused by the movement of charged ions across the membrane of the neuron. This electrical activity travels along the length of the neuron in the form of a wave. This wave may proceed in a continuous manner in unmyelinated neurons or jump between the nodes of Ranvier in myelinated neurons (saltatory conduction). In reality, a nerve impulse comprises repeated short bursts of electrical activity called action potentials, with each action potential lasting a few milliseconds. A series of action potentials may proceed down a neuron in quick succession, forming a 'chain' of action potentials or an impulse. The length of this chain of action potentials determines the strength of the impulse. A relatively weak nerve impulse may be considered as being composed of a relatively short chain or short burst of action potentials, whilst a relatively strong impulse would be composed of a much longer chain or burst of action potentials.

In a resting neuron, sodium and potassium ions are unequally distributed across the membrane of the neuron (Figure 2.3). Throughout the length of a resting neuron there are more sodium ions outside than inside (approximately 14:1). Conversely, there are more potassium ions inside the neuron than out (approximately 28:1). Therefore, two diffusion gradients exist, one for sodium ions which would cause them to diffuse into the neuron and one for potassium ions which would cause them to diffuse out of the neuron. In the resting neuron the two diffusion gradients are maintained by the structure of the membrane which is relatively impermeable. However, the membrane is not entirely impermeable and the ions may gradually leak across it. The gradients are therefore maintained by sodium–potassium pumps which are situated in the membrane. These pump sodium ions out of the neuron whilst pumping in potassium ions.

In addition to these concentration gradients there also exists an electrical gradient across the membrane. This is partially due to the relative difference in the membrane's

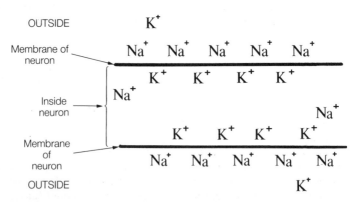

Figure 2.3 Illustrating the distribution of ions across the membrane of a neuron.

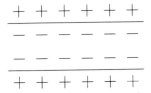

Figure 2.4 Illustrating the overall distribution of charge across the membrane of a neuron.

permeability to sodium and potassium ions and to the presence of many negative ions inside the neuron. The overall effect makes the outside of the membrane more positively charged than the inside (Figure 2.4). This electrical difference is referred to as the (electrical) potential and the membrane is said to be polarized. The electrical difference has been measured to be about 70 millivolts and, since the inside of the cell is less than the outside, is said to be -70 mV. This is the resting potential of the neuron. An action potential represents a disturbance of this resting potential caused by the rapid movement of ions across the membrane. An action potential is comprised of three phases:

1. Depolarization
2. Repolarization
3. Refractory period.

An action potential may be initiated by a variety of stimuli, including stretch in a proprioceptor, light, touch or an action potential from another neuron. If the stimulus is strong enough it is said to exceed a threshold level and the sequence of events illustrated in Figure 2.5 will result. (These events are initially very localized but changes in the electrical activity in one small area of the neuron's membrane induce similar changes in a neighbouring area, resulting in the action potential being transmitted along the length of the neuron).

Initially certain gaps or 'sodium channels' open up in a small localized area of the membrane. This causes sodium ions to rush into the neuron, through these channels, down their concentration gradient. This influx of positively charged sodium ions (along with the already present positively charged potassium ions) causes the inside of the membrane (in this localized area) to become more positively charged than the outside. During this temporary change (reversal of polarity) the inside of the neuron becomes 30 mV more positive than the outside. At this point the membrane potential is therefore registered as being about $+30$ mV. This change in the polarization of the membrane (when the inside becomes more positive) is referred to as depolarization. Depolarization in one area of the membrane will initiate the opening up of sodium channels in the neighbouring area and, hence, the movement of sodium ions into the neuron in the neighbouring area causing it also to become depolarized. This activity is repeated along the neuron forming a wave of depolarization which travels along the membrane of the neuron. The propagation of the action potential is unidirectional since an area that has just undergone depolarization needs a short time in which to recover (a refractory period) before it can be depolarized again, by which time the action

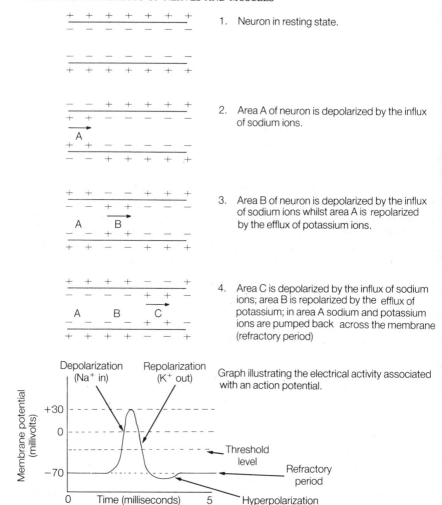

Figure 2.5 Illustrating the sequence of events associated with an action potential.

potential has proceeded along the membrane and is no longer in its immediate vicinity.

Immediately a section of membrane has been depolarized (by the influx of sodium ions) potassium channels open up in the membrane permitting the movement of potassium ions out of the neuron. These ions move out of the neuron down their concentration gradient and the loss of these positive ions from the inside of the neuron makes the inside once again less positively charged than the outside. This process is referred to as repolarization. The processes of depolarization and repolarization occur so rapidly that one region of the membrane will be depolarizing whilst the preceeding region is repolarizing. During repolarization there may be a slight overshoot whereby the membrane potential can temporarily fall below its resting potential, and this is referred to as hyperpolarization. Following the transmission of an action potential the processes of depolarization and repolarization will have resulted in certain sodium ions being inside the neuron and certain potassium ions being outside the neuron. If the neuron is to continue to function these ions must be returned to their starting positions or their diffusion gradients will gradually diminish. In order to maintain the required diffusion gradients the sodium–potassium pumps situated within the membrane pump the sodium ions out of the neuron and pump in the potassium ions, thereby returning the neuron to its resting state.

In summary, an action potential consists of the phases of depolarization, repolarization, hyperpolarization and a refractory period, all of which last approximately 5 milliseconds. When looked at in detail the phases of depolarization and repolarization can last for less than 1 ms each, with the refractory period lasting between 0.4 and 4 ms depending upon the neuron concerned. The speed at which these processes take place means that large axons are capable of transmitting up to 2500 action potentials per second whilst smaller axons may transmit up to 250 action potentials per second.

The size and strength of action potentials are not affected by the strength of the stimulus. A stimulus which is not strong enough to initiate an action potential is referred to as a subthreshold stimulus, whilst any stimulus which is strong enough to initiate an action potential is said to exceed the threshold of the neuron. Different neurons will have different threshold values, and this is important in the process of recruiting muscle fibres to contract and, hence, in determining the strength of muscle contraction. However, whereas the size of an individual action potential may be the same for any stimulus regardless of how far in excess of the threshold level it is, the difference in the strength of the stimulus is reflected by the number of action potentials it generates and, hence, the size of the impulse. Strong stimuli will produce long chains of action potentials whilst weaker stimuli will produce shorter chains.

SYNAPSES AND NEUROMUSCULAR JUNCTIONS

In order for the nervous system to be an effective communications system it must pass information from one neuron to another. In addition, appropriate information must also be passed from neurons to muscles and glands if effective responses are to be made. The point at which information is passed between two neurons is referred to as a synapse. The point at which information passes from a motor (efferent) neuron to a muscle fibre is called a neuromuscular junction.

Structure of a synapse

A synapse (Figure 2.6) may be considered to consist of:

   (i) a neuron which conducts nerve impulses towards the synapse (the presynaptic neuron);
   (ii) a gap between the neurons (the synaptic cleft); and
   (iii) a neuron which conducts nerve impulses away from the synapse (the post-synaptic neuron).

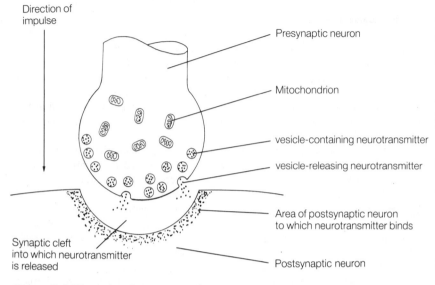

Direction of impulse

Presynaptic neuron

Mitochondrion

vesicle-containing neurotransmitter

vesicle-releasing neurotransmitter

Area of postsynaptic neuron to which neurotransmitter binds

Synaptic cleft into which neurotransmitter is released

Postsynaptic neuron

Figure 2.6 Illustrating the structure of a synapse.

Neurons may synapse with a large number of other neurons: it is calculated that in parts of the brain certain neurons may synapse with, and hence pass on information to or receive information from, up to 100 000 other neurons. The synapses of the body are known as 'chemical synapses'. This is because the information crosses the gap between the two neurons (the synaptic cleft) in the form of chemical transmitters called neurotransmitters. There are several types of neurotransmitters including acetyl choline, dopamine, noradrenalin (norepinephrine), adrenalin (epinephrine), gamma-aminobutyric acid (GABA), serotonin, glutamic acid, aspartic acid, glycine, enkephalins, endorphins, somatostatin, histamine substance P and dynorphin. Neurotransmitters are stored in small sacs (synaptic vesicles) at the end of the presynaptic neuron. The arrival of a nerve impulse at the end of the presynaptic neuron (the synaptic terminal) causes the synaptic vesicles in the synaptic terminal to become agitated and release the neurotransmitter into the synaptic cleft. The neurotransmitters then diffuse across the synaptic cleft, which is approximately 20 nm wide, and attach themselves to the membrane of the postsynaptic neuron. The binding of the neurotransmitter then affects the membrane potential of the postsynaptic neuron. This change in membrane potential will influence whether or not the postsynaptic neuron transmits the impulse further.

Transmission by the postsynaptic neuron depends upon a number of factors: firstly, the strength of the impulses it is receiving (usually from a large number of presynaptic neurons) and, secondly, whether the impulses it receives have an excitatory or inhibitory effect upon it. If the impulses being transmitted across a synapse have an excitatory effect they will promote and enhance the chances of the postsynaptic neuron transmitting the impulse. However, if the impulses have an inhibitory effect they will reduce the chances of the postsynaptic neuron conducting an impulse. In an excitatory synapse the binding of the neurotransmitter causes a slight depolarization of the membrane of the postsynaptic neuron. Conversely, in an inhibitory synapse the binding of the neurotransmitter causes a slight repolarization/hyperpolarization of the post-synaptic neuron. In reality the arrival of a single action potential at the presynaptic neuron will not be sufficient to cause the transmission of an impulse in the postsynaptic neuron. However, the arrival of a chain of action potentials may have a cumulative effect (temporal summation) which can provide a strong enough input to cause the postsynaptic neuron to conduct an impulse. Alternatively, efferent and interneurons receive inputs from many other neurons, and for any particular postsynaptic neuron it will be the integrated combination of all the excitatory and inhibitory synaptic inputs coming from many different neurons that ultimately determine whether or not the post-synaptic neuron will conduct an impulse. In this respect it should also be noted that certain synapses will have a stronger effect than others; this means that certain neurons will have a greater influence in determining the activity of the postsynaptic neuron.

Excitatory and inhibitory synapses work in the following way: an action potential is initiated by a stimulus that causes the neuron to depolarize in excess of its threshold level. If, however, the stimulus is weak then only a small amount of initial depolarization will occur (relatively few sodium ions will diffuse into the neuron). A small amount of depolarization will not exceed the neuron's threshold level and will not be sufficient to cause the complete opening of the sodium channels. Hence a full action potential will not occur and no impulse will be transmitted along the postsynaptic neuron. A weak stimulus such as this is said to produce a subthreshold amount of depolarization. If, however, the stimulus was strong, then a considerable amount of depolarization would occur in the post-synaptic neuron and if it exceeded the neuron's threshold level then a positive feedback cycle would occur, opening the sodium channels. In this situation the entry of a certain number of sodium ions facilitates the entry of further ions until eventually a full action potential results. When the threshold level is exceeded the membrane depolarizes very rapidly and the resulting action potential proceeds down the length of the neuron.

At an excitatory synapse the binding of the neurotransmitter will promote the influx of sodium ions into the postsynaptic neuron and hence a small amount of depolarization of the membrane, thereby moving it closer towards its threshold level and thus promoting the likelihood of its transmitting the impulse. Conversely, the binding of the neuro-transmitter at an inhibitory synapse will promote the efflux of potassium ions out of the postsynaptic neuron causing repolarization/hyperpolarization and thus moving the membrane potential further from the threshold level, making it less likely to reach the required level (threshold) of depolarization. This is illustrated in Figure 2.7.

Since all action potentials transmitted by a given neuron are the same size, the strength of a nerve impulse is determined by the number of action potentials which make up the nerve impulse. This brings in the concepts of temporal and spatial sum-mation, which refers to the fact that the arrival of a single action potential at the synaptic terminal will cause the release and binding of only a relatively small amount of neurotransmitter. In the case of an excitatory synapse this will cause a small amount of depolarization (excitatory postsynaptic potential, EPSP) but is unlikely to be suffi-cient for the postsynaptic neuron to reach its threshold level. However, if a series of action potentials from the same neuron arrive in quick succession they will cause the rapid release of many molecules of neurotransmitter. A considerable amount of neurotransmitter will then bind to the postsynaptic neuron, which will be depolarized to the extent that it may exceed its threshold level and transmit a nerve impulse. This is referred to as temporal summation as the action potentials arrive in quick succession

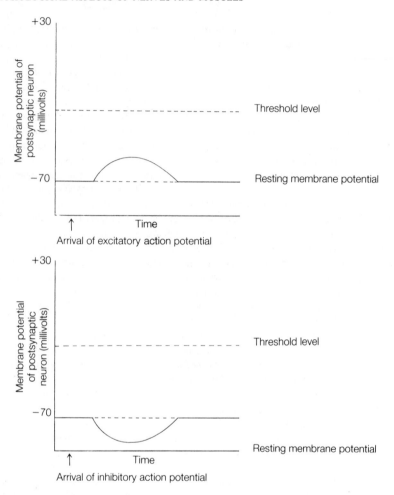

Figure 2.7 Illustrating the effects of excitatory and inhibitory action potentials upon the membrane potential of a postsynaptic neuron.

from the same presynaptic neuron. The process of spatial summation may also result in the postsynaptic neuron being depolarized sufficiently to conduct an impulse. This is where impulses arrive at the postsynaptic neuron from more than one presynaptic neuron. Here again the combined effects of their released neurotransmitter may be sufficient to depolarize the postsynaptic neuron beyond its threshold level.

The processes of temporal and spatial summation can also be applied to inhibitory synapses where the arrival of an action potential may cause a slight amount of repolarization/hyperpolarization (inhibitory postsynaptic potential, IPSP). In such instances the inhibitory inputs may counteract the excitatory inputs, preventing the threshold level from being reached and hence preventing the postsynaptic neuron from transmitting an impulse (Figure 2.8).

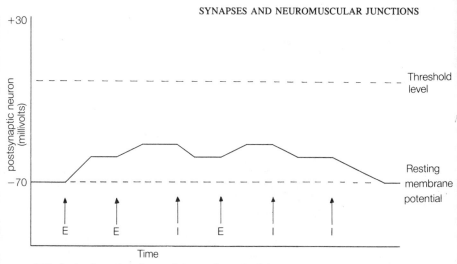

'E' indicates the arrival of an excitatory action potential.
'I' indicates the arrival of an inhibitory action potential.

Figure 2.8 Illustrating how inhibitory inputs may prevent the postsynaptic neuron from reaching its threshold level.

In summary therefore;

1. It is the summed effect of the excitatory and inhibitory inputs which determines whether or not the postsynaptic neuron conducts an impulse.
2. If the postsynaptic neuron's threshold level is exceeded then the relative strengths of the impulses from the presynaptic neurons determine the strength of the impulse conducted by the postsynaptic neuron.
3. All the action potentials conducted by an individual neuron are of the same size, and it is therefore the number of action potentials within a nerve impulse that determines its strength.

The neuromuscular junction

A neuromuscular junction represents the point of association between a motor neuron and the muscle fibre it innervates. The structure of a neuromuscular junction (Figure 2.9) is similar in many respects to that of a synapse. However, at a neuromuscular junction there is only one input – that of the motor neuron – and it is always excitatory. This means that if a motor neuron transmits an impulse it will be transmitted to the muscle fibre across the neuromuscular junction and will ultimately lead to the contraction of the muscle fibre. Therefore, if a muscle fibre or muscle needs to be inhibited from contracting, the process of inhibition must occur earlier in the neural pathway. Inhibition via IPSP must occur prior to or at the final synapse with the motor neuron. This will often be within the central nervous system where the efferent motor neuron is the postsynaptic neuron.

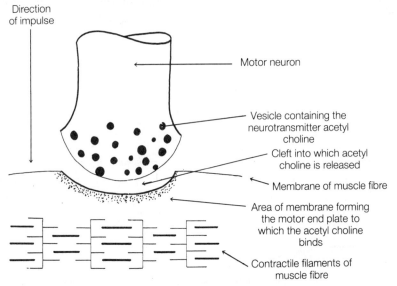

Figure 2.9 Illustrating the structure of a neuromuscular junction.

Upon entering a muscle the axon of a motor neuron may branch, forming smaller processes called telodendria. The ends of these telodendria expand slightly to form the 'synaptic end bulbs' which contain the synaptic vesicles in which are stored the neurotransmitter, acetyl choline. At a neuromuscular junction the arrival of an action potential causes the release of the acetyl choline into the gap between the synaptic end bulb and the membrane of the muscle fibre. The acetyl choline diffuses across the gap between the nerve and muscle. It then binds to a specialized section of the muscle fibre membrane called the 'motor end plate'. The binding of the acetyl choline causes the membrane of the muscle fibre to depolarize, altering its end-plate potential. This electrical activity is then transmitted along the membrane of the fibre in much the same way as an action potential is transmitted in a neuron. The wave of depolarization travels down the transverse tubules of the muscle fibre and causes the release of calcium ions from the sarcoplasmic reticulum. The release of these calcium ions will then initiate a series of reactions that will ultimately result in the process of cross-bridge cycling and the muscle fibre will contract (see The process of muscle contraction, page 56). If the acetyl choline were to remain bound to the motor end plate the fibre would remain in a state of prolonged contraction. Since this is clearly not desirable the acetyl choline is broken down and removed from the motor end plate by an enzyme called acetyl choline esterase. The component parts of the acetyl choline are then recycled into the motor neuron. This process is repeated each time the fibre is required to contract.

Since the nerve impulse in the motor neuron occurs as a result of numerous excitatory and inhibitory inputs from many other neurons, it is often referred to as the final common pathway, and it should be emphasized that once action potentials occur in the motor neuron they cannot be modified and muscular contraction will take place. Myasthenia gravis is an example of a disease which specifically affects the neuromuscular junction.

In the diseased neuromuscular junction the acetyl choline binding sites on the motor end plate are attacked by antibodies. These prevent the acetyl choline from binding and hence from depolarizing the motor end plate. This means that the muscle fibre does not contract even though nerve impulses are sent to it along its motor neuron.

INTRODUCTION TO MUSCLE TYPES

The human body contains three basic types of muscles: skeletal, cardiac and smooth. These muscle types fulfil a variety of different functions within the body and have correspondingly different structures. The diverse functions of skeletal muscle (also called striated or voluntary muscle) were discussed in some depth in Chapter 1. However, in summary skeletal muscles are used to initiate movement, prevent movement and control movement. In this context they are involved with the movement of body parts, are needed for the maintenance of posture and give the body shape. Skeletal muscles contract in a number of different ways and achieve their overall effect through their attachment to the bones of the skeleton. The muscles work in groups or pairs, with their coordinated contraction and relaxation being initiated by the nervous system. Coordinated movements and the maintenance of posture – both of which require an extremely complex interaction between numerous muscles – are normally achieved automatically by the nervous system with little or no conscious thought. For the therapist the sheer complexity of controlled and coordinated movement becomes most apparent when dealing with patients suffering from forms of neuromuscular disability or injury.

Cardiac muscle forms the major part of the walls of the heart. Its functions are therefore specific to that particular organ. The coordinated contraction of the cardiac muscle of the heart results in blood being pumped around the body. To fulfil its specialized function cardiac muscle has a specific structure which is similar to that of skeletal muscle but contains within it additional connections between its constituent muscle fibres. At rest the heart contracts approximately 72 times per minute although values for different individuals may range from below 40 to above 90 contractions or 'beats' per minute. During exercise the demands placed upon the body may cause the heart rate to increase quite considerably and during very strenuous exercise it can rise to above 180 beats per minute. The extreme demands made upon cardiac muscle require it to contract repeatedly for many years and necessitate it being fatigue resistant. This is made possible by its specialized structure, including its extensive blood supply and various other physiological properties which are specific to cardiac muscle. The extensive (coronary) blood supply provides the cardiac muscle fibres with the oxygen they need if they are not to become fatigued and hence unable to continue contracting. The muscle's specialized structure and biochemical properties ensure that it has the capacity to use this oxygen in the process of contraction.

The structure and functions of smooth (involuntary muscle) are somewhat different. Smooth muscle is found in the walls of many of the body's vessels and passageways, such as blood vessels, the gut and the airways of the lungs. Its contraction and relaxation can alter the diameter of these passageways thereby influencing the movement of their contents. The peristaltic (wave like) contractions of smooth muscle in the gut can push food through the gastrointestinal tract. Smooth muscle is also found in the sphincters which are located at various points in the gastrointestinal tract. The contraction of these sphincters can prevent the movement of material through the gut until certain digestive processes are complete. Smooth muscle also serves an important function in the cardiovascular system where it is found in the wall of many blood vessels. The relaxation of the smooth muscle causes the dilation of these blood vessels, whilst its contraction causes them to constrict. In this way, by altering the diameter of certain blood vessels the blood supply to certain areas of the body may be increased or decreased. These reflex dilations and constrictions are important in determining the distribution of blood around the body and in the control of other cardiovascular factors such as blood pressure.

During exercise there is an increase in the amount of oxygen needed by the actively contracting skeletal muscles. Much of this increased supply is achieved by the combination of a rise in heart rate and the dilation of blood vessels leading to the skeletal muscles. These responses will also facilitate the removal of waste products produced by these muscles during exercise. If the cardiovascular system did not respond in this manner then the skeletal muscles would very rapidly fatigue, preventing further muscular activity. So, in summary, it can be seen that smooth and cardiac muscle serve a number of vital functions within the body and that many of their functions are directly associated with those of skeletal muscle and exercise.

Having briefly outlined the roles of the different types of muscle the remainder of this section will concentrate upon the physiological aspects of skeletal muscle. In order to study these physiological aspects it is first necessary to outline its basic structure. This will also provide a basis for understanding particular aspects of certain dysfunctions and, hence, the objectives of certain forms of therapy.

THE STRUCTURE OF SKELETAL MUSCLE

The major components of a skeletal muscle include structural proteins, connective tissue, blood vessels and organelles such as mitochondria, which have specialized functions within the muscle cells. Nerves that conduct impulses to and from the muscle are also found within its structure. The basic structure of a skeletal muscle is illustrated in Figure 2.10.

Muscle is a highly organized and structured tissue with the individual muscle cells (muscle fibres) being highly specialized for the process of contraction. Each muscle is surrounded by a sheath of connective tissue called the epimysium. Muscle fibres within the muscle are grouped into bundles called fasciculi and are surrounded by another sheath of connective tissue called the perimysium. Within the fasciculi the individual muscle fibres are surrounded by a plasma membrane called the sarcolemma and a further sheath of connective tissue called the endomysium.

Each muscle fibre is made up of smaller units called myofibrils which are in turn made up of a highly organized arrangement of protein filaments, primarily actin filaments and myosin filaments. Structurally the actin protein forms long thin filaments within the muscle whilst the myosin protein forms thick filaments, each being composed of approximately 200 myosin protein molecules. The protein filaments are arranged to form distinct functional units along the length of the muscle and are referred to as sarcomeres (Figure 2.11). The correct alignment of these filaments within the

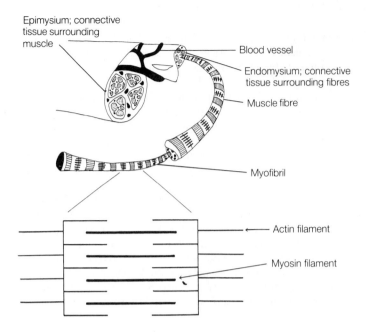

Figure 2.10 Illustrating the basic structure of skeletal muscle.

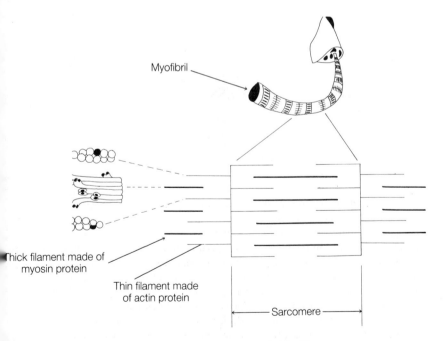

Figure 2.11 Illustrating the alignment of the thick and thin filaments.

sarcomere is vital for the process of muscle contraction. The sarcomeres are approximately 2.5 μm in length and are repeated continuously along the length of the myofibril so that within a muscle fibre the sarcomere unit may be repeated thousands of times along its entire length.

The similar alignment of groups of myofibrils and their protein filaments within the sarcomeres gives the fibres a striped or striated appearance, hence the name 'striated muscle'. As previously stated, groups of these myofibrils are bounded together by a plasma membrane (sarcolemma) and sheet of connective tissue (endomysium) to form muscle fibres (muscle cells). Within a muscle a number of muscle fibres are stimulated by the same motor neuron and form the functional unit of the muscle called the motor unit. Depending upon the function of the muscle, a motor unit may contain between 10 and 1700 muscle fibres. In muscles whose function requires a fine degree of delicate control (such as those influencing the movements of the eye) the motor units will contain relatively few fibres (between 10 and 20). Conversely, in the larger skeletal muscles where such a fine degree of control is unnecessary, as in the gastrocnemius, some motor units may contain over 1500 fibres. Passing through the muscle are the blood vessels which supply it with the nutrients and oxygen it needs as well as removing the metabolic waste products it produces. Small blood capillaries pass through the endomysium whilst the larger blood vessels are located in the perimysium.

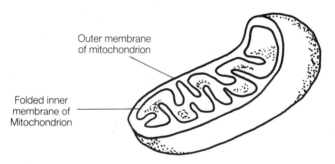

Figure 2.12 Illustrating the structure of a mitochondrion.

Also passing in and out of the muscle are various nerves. These include motor nerves, which stimulate the muscle fibres to contract, and sensory nerves, which inform the central nervous system of the position and state of the muscle. The ends of the muscle are attached to the bones of the skeleton by connective tissue in the form of tendons (shaped like ribbons or cables) or aponeuroses (sheets of connective tissue). This connective tissue runs throughout the muscle but becomes more predominant at the ends of the muscle. In this way the muscle–tendon junction is formed by a gradual change in the relative abundance of muscle fibres and connective tissue. Also found within the muscle fibres are cellular organelles and structures. These include the mitochondria (Figure 2.12), 't' tubules and sarcoplasmic reticulum (Figure 2.13). The mitochondria are specialized organelles that produce large amounts of the chemical

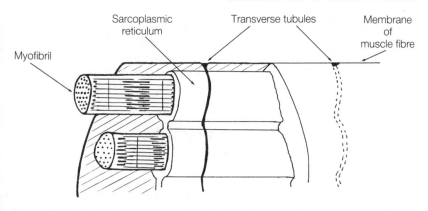

Figure 2.13 Illustrating the position of the transverse tubules and sarcoplasmic rectulum.

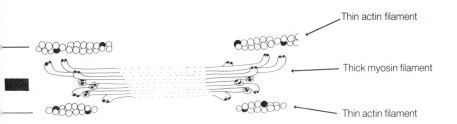

Figure 2.14 Illustrating the detailed structure of the thick and thin filaments.

ATP which is essential for muscle contraction. The transverse or 't' tubules conduct action potentials into the muscle following its stimulation by a nerve, and the sarcoplasmic reticulum are storage sacs in which calcium is stored prior to its use in the process of muscle contraction.

The process of muscle contraction is brought about by the interaction of two types of muscle protein: actin and myosin. In order to understand the process of muscle contraction it is first necessary to have a basic knowledge of the structure of the contractile filaments involved. The actin filaments are made up of two long chains of globular actin protein molecules, rather like two chains of beads twisted around each other. At certain points on the actin molecules there are specific 'binding' sites. The myosin proteins attach themselvs to these 'binding' sites during the process of muscle contraction. Myosin filaments have a very different structure with each thick filament consisting of about 200 myosin protein molecules. Each myosin molecule consists of a tail section and a globular head which can attach itself to the actin binding sites. Within a thick filament the myosin molecules are orientated so that the heads are situated at the ends of the filament (Figure 2.14). Another important feature of the myosin molecule is that it is capable of changing its shape and in effect moving its globular head. If this movement occurs while it is attached to the thin actin filament, it will pull the actin filament so that it slides past it. It is from this action that the current theory of muscle contraction derives its name 'The sliding filament model'.

THE PROCESS OF MUSCLE CONTRACTION

Skeletal muscles contract when stimulated by nerve impulses. The constituent fibres of a muscle are each associated with a particular motor neuron which conveys the nerve impulses that stimulate the muscle fibre to contract. The connection between the motor neuron and muscle fibre is referred to as the neuromuscular junction (Figure 2.9). Details of the processes which occur at a neuromuscular junction were discuussed on page 49. In summary the arrival of a nerve impulse at the neuromuscular junction initiates electrical activity in the membrane of the muscle fibre.

The electrical activity initiated in the membrane of the muscle fibre travels along the membrane and down a series of channels into the muscle fibre. These channels are called the transverse or 't' tubules (Figure 2.13). The action potentials passing through the muscle fibre cause the release of calcium ions from specific storage sacs (sarcoplasmic reticulum) within the muscle fibre and it is this release of calcium ions which ultimately results in the contraction of the muscle fibre.

In a relaxed muscle fibre there is no attachment between the actin and myosin filaments since the potential sites of connection (the 'binding' sites) on the thin actin filaments are blocked by another filamentous protein called tropomyosin. The tropomyosin protein is held in position over the binding sites by a group of proteins called the troponin complex (Figure 2.15).

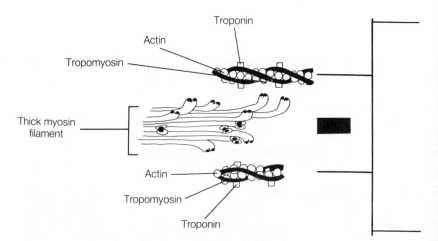

Figure 2.15 Illustrating the position of the structural proteins in a relaxed muscle fibre.

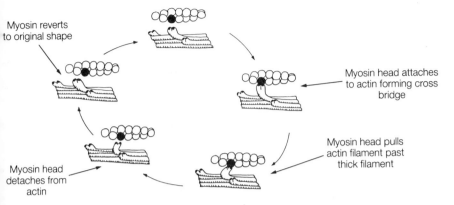

Myosin reverts to original shape

Myosin head attaches to actin forming cross bridge

Myosin head pulls actin filament past thick filament

Myosin head detaches from actin

Figure 2.16 Illustrating the process of cross-bridge cycling.

When the calcium ions are released from the sarcoplasmic reticulum they bind to the troponin protein complex causing the tropomyosin protein to move away from the binding sites on the thin actin filaments. Thus the release of calcium ions results in the binding sites on the actin filaments becoming unblocked. This enables the heads of the myosin molecules to attach themselves to the binding sites forming what are known as cross bridges. The heads of the myosin molecules will then change shape and in doing so will pull the actin filament past them (Figure 2.16). The myosin molecules may then become unattached from the actin, the heads revert to their original shape and reattach themselves to other binding sites further along the thin filament. The process of forming the attachments (cross bridges) between the actin and myosin molecules, breaking them and then reforming them, is therefore a cyclic process which is called 'cross-bridge cycling'. When a muscle fibre contracts, each myosin molecule may repeat this process of cross-bridge cycling many times with the overall result being the movement of the actin filaments as they are pulled past the myosin. Within a single muscle fibre the constituent actin and myosin filaments will undergo the process of cross-bridge cycling many times during a single muscle contraction. The process of cross-bridge cycling may therefore be likened to that of a team pulling hand over hand on a rope. However, in reality, at any instant in time the myosin molecules will be at various stages of cross-bridge formation rather than all working together in synchrony. Since the myosin molecules are orientated with their heads at opposite ends of the thick filament, their pulling action results in the actin filaments being pulled closer together. This effect can be easily visualized if it is imagined that the myosin heads at the left-hand end of the filament pull their actin filament to the right whilst the myosin heads at the right-hand end of the filament pull their actin filament to the left. The effect of this will be an overall shortening of the sarcomere during a contraction (Figure 2.17). As this shortening is repeated along the length of the muscle fibre it will result in an overall shortening of the fibre, and if sufficient muscle fibres are shortened then the length of the muscle itself will be reduced.

Upon the cessation of nervous stimulation, action potentials are no longer transmitted down the 't' tubules, which causes the calcium ions to be reabsorbed back

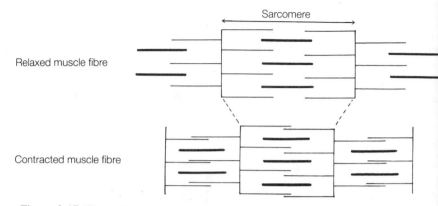

Figure 2.17 Illustrating the shortening of the sarcomere in muscle contraction.

into the sarcoplasmic reticulum. The removal of the calcium ions results in the troponin complex allowing the tropomyosin to move back over the binding sites on the actin filaments. This prevents the myosin filaments from forming any further cross bridges and, as a result, the actin filaments slide back to their original positions, the sarcomere returns to its original length and the muscle fibre relaxes. Muscle contraction requires energy because each cross-bridge cycle requires the expenditure of a molecule of adenosine triphosphate (ATP) which is the high-energy molecule used by the body during energy requiring reactions (see Chapter 3 for details of ATP synthesis).

The physiological processes occurring in isotonic concentric, isotonic eccentric and isometric contractions are essentially the same. In an isotonic concentric contraction the process of cross-bridge cycling and the shortening of the fibre may easily be related to the observed shortening of the whole muscle. However, it may initially be more difficult to relate the cross-bridge cycling process and the shortening of muscle fibres to the observed lengthening of the muscle in isotonic eccentric contractions and the maintenance of its length in isometric contractions. To explain this it needs to be emphasized that the strength of contraction and the amount of movement that is associated with the contraction largely depend upon the number of fibres that contract within the muscle rather than the amount of contraction that occurs within each fibre. In an isometric contraction cross-bridge cycling does occur, but the tension developed within the muscle does not significantly alter the length of the entire muscle because, during the contraction, the number of fibres that are contracted at any instant result in the length of the muscle being maintained. If the force against which the muscle is working increases then it must be matched by an increase in the amount of tension within the muscle. This is achieved by increasing the number of fibres that are contracting against the force. In isotonic eccentric contractions cross-bridge cycling also occurs, but owing to the greater opposing external force the entire muscle is forced to lengthen, despite the generation of tension within the muscle fibres. In this example individual muscle fibres are contracting and shortening to generate tension but within the whole muscle there is an overall lengthening. For further information on the strength of muscle contraction see the section on motor units.

In reality, muscle fibres do not contract singularly but work in groups known as motor units. A motor unit consists of a group of related muscle fibres and the motor neuron which innervates them. A knowledge of the way in which these motor units operate is central to the understanding of how the strength of muscle contractions can be altered. It is clear that for effective muscular movement and control the strength of a muscle's contraction needs to vary at different times. For example, when lifting a heavy object a much stronger contraction is needed than when lifting a light one. This difference is achieved by altering the number of motor units, and hence muscle fibres, that are used in a contraction at any instant in time and the way in which they are recruited.

MOTOR UNITS, FIBRE TYPES AND THE STRENGTH OF CONTRACTION

Motor units

When a muscle fibre contracts, it contracts fully; individual muscle fibres do not 'partially contract'. This is known as the 'all or none' principle. During the contraction of a muscle a number of motor units are activated. Within these motor units individual muscle fibres will rapidly contract and then relax, performing what is referred to as a 'twitch'. At any given time during the contraction of a muscle there will be a certain number of muscle fibres that are contracted whilst others are relaxed. As the contraction continues, the asynchronous contraction (or twitching) of these fibres ensures that the number of contracted fibres at any instant remains constant although individual fibres will go through phases of contraction and relaxation. This produces a smooth contraction of the muscle whilst providing each fibre with a period of recovery, without which the fibres would more rapidly fatigue. The factors which influence the strength of a muscle contraction may be considered under two headings:

1. The recruitment of motor units into the contraction
2. The amount of tension developed by each muscle fibre.

When motor units are recruited into a muscle contraction the strength of that contraction will be influenced by certain factors.

1. The strength will depend on which motor units are recruited. Even within the same muscle its constituent motor units will vary in the type and number of fibres they contain. In some muscles the number may vary from 25 to 400 fibres per unit, and in such cases the recruitment of the larger motor unit will result in the generation of far more tension than the recruitment of the smaller.
2. The strength of contraction will depend on the strength of neural inputs that are used to recruit the motor units into the contraction. Stronger nerve impulses will result in more fibres being contracted at any instant in time and hence a stronger contraction.

The amount of tension developed by each muscle fibre within a motor unit will also depend upon a number of factors.

1. The type of fibre. There are a number of different types of muscle fibre, each with certain characteristics. These are discussed later in this section.
2. The duration of a contraction. During prolonged or repeated muscular contractions fatigue will influence the amount of tension generated by each fibre.
3. The length–tension relationship. This is discussed in a later section but in summary it relates to the length of the muscle and degree of overlap between the contractile filaments.
4. The strength of neural inputs that stimulate the fibre. The repeated stimulation of a muscle fibre by the rapid arrival of many nerve inputs (at a rate of 20–120 action potentials per second) will cause the strength of muscle fibre contraction to increase via a process called 'summation'. Very rapid, repeated stimulation will result in a state of prolonged contraction known as tetanus. A tetanus contraction is three or four times stronger than the single twitch contraction which occurs when the fibre is stimulated by a single action potential.

In practical terms the strength of a muscle's contraction largely depends upon how many muscle fibres are stimulated to contract at any instant in time. The variation in the strength of contraction is achieved via the controlled recruitment of motor units and, hence, muscle fibres into a contraction. If a relatively weak contraction is required only relatively weak nerve signals will be sent from the central nervous system. This will result in only some of the motor neurons carrying the impulses and hence only their associated muscle fibres will be recruited into the contraction. Motor units that are recruited by relatively weak nerve impulses are said to have a low threshold. If a stronger contraction is required then stronger impulses are transmitted from the central nervous system. These will be carried by more motor neurons, hence more motor units will be recruited into the contraction. These motor units are said to have an intermediate threshold and during strong contractions will contract in addition to those with a low threshold. If a very strong contraction is required, then strong signals will be sent by the central nervous system. These will be transmitted by virtually all of the motor neurons and hence virtually all the motor units will contribute in the contraction including those with low, intermediate and high thresholds. In practical terms the motor units within a muscle have a whole spectrum of threshold values ranging from very low to very high. By altering the strength of signal sent by the central nervous system the number of motor units recruited into the contraction can be altered, as can the number of fibres that are contracted at any given time.

During a prolonged or repeated contraction there is a depletion of nutrients such as glucose and oxygen along with a build up of metabolic waste products such as carbon dioxide and lactic acid. These changes will inhibit the contractile capabilities of the muscle fibre by inhibiting certain metabolic reactions and the overall contractile process. The effect of such changes weakens the strength of contraction of the individual fibres; therefore, if the strength of muscular contraction is to be maintained, various neuromuscular adjustments need to occur. These will include an increase in the strength of nerve impulses so as to recruit more fibres into the contraction at any instant. In summary, the appropriate recruitment and activation of motor units permits the strength of a muscle's contraction to be altered, controlled and maintained even when it is fatigued.

Fibre types

Although all muscle fibres have a very similar basic structure they may be classified into two broad groups: type 1 and type 2. Motor units contain either type 1 or type 2 fibres, but not both; hence motor units may also be classified as type 1 or type 2. A muscle will contain a mixture of type 1 and type 2 fibres with the relative proportions of each type tending to reflect the role of that muscle. In this respect there is some debate as to whether the relative proportions of each fibre type are determined genetically prior to birth and are unalterable or whether exercise and general muscular activity can influence the relative abundance of each type. In general, type 1 fibres tend to be found in low threshold motor units whilst the higher threshold motor units tend to contain type 2 fibres. The work done by the low-threshold motor units tends to differ slightly in its emphasis from that of the high-threshold motor units. This difference is reflected in the physiological make-up of the fibres and is exemplified by the way in which they are biased towards certain energy pathways that are used to generate the ATP needed for their contractions. Low-threshold motor units (containing type 1 fibres) are easily recruited and perform most of the work required in low intensity, prolonged muscular activity such as maintaining posture. In accordance with this role their metabolic and structural bias makes them fatigue resistant. Conversely, the type 2 fibres which are found in high-threshold motor units are larger and more powerful than the type 1 fibres. High-threshold motor units are recruited for more powerful contractions with their type 2 fibres exhibiting a bias towards rapid powerful contractions that use anaerobic energy pathways. The general differences in fibre types are summarized below.

Type 1 fibres

Type 1 fibres, which are also called red fibres or slow twitch (ST):

(a) are located in type 1, low-threshold motor units;
(b) have a small fibre diameter;
(c) are orientated towards the aerobic production of ATP;
(d) contain a relatively large number of mitochondria;
(e) contain high levels of the chemical myoglobin which acts as an oxygen store;
(f) possess an extensive blood supply with a dense blood capillary network;
(g) have a high fatigue resistance and are suited to prolonged forms of low-intensity work;
(h) are innervated by small motor neurons with a relatively slow speed of conductance;
(i) have a slow speed of contraction (110ms).

Type 2 fibres

Type 2 fibres, which are also called white fibres or fast twitch (FT):

(a) are located in type 2, high-threshold motor units;
(b) have a large fibre diameter;
(c) are orientated towards the anaerobic production of ATP and hence contain greater concentrations of glycolytic enzymes;
(d) contain fewer and smaller mitochondria;
(e) contain less myoglobin;
(f) possess a less extensive blood supply with fewer blood capillaries;
(g) are larger than type 1 fibres containing more contractile filaments, making them stronger and suitable for short, powerful contractions;
(h) are innervated by large motor neurons with a relatively fast speed of conductance;
(i) have a fast speed of contraction (50 ms).

Following the initial classification of muscle fibres into two broad categories, research indicates that the type 2 fibres can be further subdivided into type 2a, type 2b and type 2c. Within the type 2 category the type 2a fibres are the most aerobic, having the capability of working both anaerobically and aerobically. At the other end of the type 2 spectrum the type 2b fibres are the most anaerobic, having the greatest potential for anaerobic metabolism and relatively little aerobic capability. In the opinion of many authorities the type 2c fibres are intermediate, being between the other two. It is also suggested that these fibres may shift their metabolic emphasis in accordance with the metabolic demands that are placed upon the muscle (a training effect).

Research into the relative proportions of the fibre types possessed by an individual would suggest that a high proportion of the type 1 fibres gives a muscle enduring qualities whilst a preponderance of type 2 fibres makes it more capable of short powerful bursts of activity. To support this in the sporting context, élite endurance performers appear to have a higher than average proportion of the type 1 fibres whilst individuals who excel in power events possess higher proportions of type 2 fibres. The extent to which these observed differences are due to genetic endowment and/or training remains open to debate.

TYPES OF SKELETAL MUSCLE AND MUSCULAR ATTACHMENTS

In order to fulfil their differing roles the muscles of the body need to differ in their gross and fine structure. Some need to shorten considerably in order to produce the desired range of movement whilst others need to shorten only slightly. Certain muscles are attached at a specific point on a particular bone whilst others require a much larger area of attachment in order to be effective. The diversity of functions that muscles fulfil results in a considerable variation in the size and shape of skeletal muscles. In addition, the specific arrangement of fibres within a muscle can differ. This specific alignment of fibres can substantially affect the strength of the muscle and the way it contracts. Hence the fine structure as well as the gross structure of a muscle will be linked to its basic functions.

Types of skeletal muscle

All skeletal muscles are similar in their general make up and undergo the same physiological processes during contraction. Skeletal muscles basically consist of groups of muscle fibres which function as motor units, with each fibre being largely composed of actin and myosin filaments. However, for a variety of reasons – which may be related to structure, function and the developmental constraints of the body – the actual alignment and arrangement of the muscle fibres within the muscle can vary considerably. Indeed, skeletal muscles may be described according to the arrangement of fibres within them and their overall shape.

The fibres of some muscles are aligned to run parallel to the long axis of the muscle, whilst the fibres of other muscles are aligned to run diagonally across the long axis of the muscle. Muscles in which the fibres are arranged to run parallel to the long axis are capable of a considerable amount of shortening; indeed, they may shorten by one half of their resting length. However, the amount of force that can be generated by a muscle depends upon its size and the number of muscle fibres it contains. Since muscle size is necessarily restricted within the body, this means that in order to significantly increase the strength of a muscle (without altering its size beyond its biological limitations) a different arrangement of muscle fibres is required. In muscles in which the fibres run diagonally across the long axis, more individual fibres can be fitted into the same volume. Hence, when comparing two muscles of the same size, the one with a diagonal arrangement of fibres across the long axis will be stronger than one with its fibres aligned parallel to the long axis (all other factors being equal). However, the muscle with the parallel arrangement of fibres will be capable of a greater degree of shortening than the one with its fibres arranged diagonally across the long axis. This means that where a strong contraction is required, a diagonal arrangement of fibres is preferable, but due to the multiple functions of muscles and their varied actions a compromise is often necessary. Thus, the arrangement of muscle fibres within a muscle may be a compromise in accordance with its various functions and the developmental limitations of the body. Structurally, muscles may be considered under the following headings: longitudinal, fusiform, quadrate, triangular, unipennate, bipennate and multipennate (Figure 2.18).

Muscles such as the sartorius are long strap-like muscles which have their fibres arranged parallel to the long axis of the muscle. These kinds of muscle are called 'longitudinal'. Fusiform muscles, (for example, the brachialis) are spindle shaped. Quadrate muscles have their fibres arranged in a parallel manner similar to that of the longitudinal and fusiform muscles but, as the name would suggest, they are flat muscles with four sides making them almost square or diamond shaped. An example of a quadrate muscle would be the rhomboideus major which, as the name suggests, is approximately diamond shaped. Triangular muscles have a parallel arrangement of fibres which fan out from a narrow point of attachment to a much broader area of attachment. The pectoralis major provides an excellent example of a triangular or fan-shaped muscle, and when these muscles contract they are capable of exerting a large amount of force at a small point of attachment. Muscles whose fibres are arranged across the long axis of the muscle are generally described as being penniform or pennate. The penniform muscles may then be categorized as being unipennate, bipennate or multipennate according to the number of directions in which the fibres are arranged. If the muscle fibres in a penniform muscle run in a single direction, the arrangement is referred to as being unipennate. An example of a unipennate muscle would be the extensor digitorum longus of the leg. If, however, the muscle fibres are

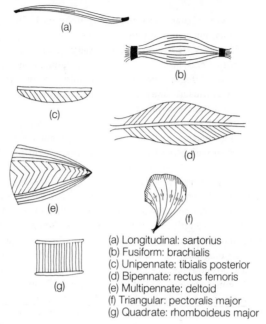

(a) Longitudinal: sartorius
(b) Fusiform: brachialis
(c) Unipennate: tibialis posterior
(d) Bipennate: rectus femoris
(e) Multipennate: deltoid
(f) Triangular: pectoralis major
(g) Quadrate: rhomboideus major

Figure 2.18 Illustrating the different types of skeletal muscle.

arranged in two directions, the muscle is referred to as being bipennate. A classic example of a bipennate muscle is the rectus femoris of the thigh. If the muscle fibres are arranged in several directions, the muscle is referred to as being multipennate with the middle portion of the deltoid muscle providing a suitable example.

Muscular attachments

In order for muscles to function effectively they need to be attached to the bones of the skeleton or, in a few cases, to other muscles. This attachment occurs via connective tissue which runs throughout the muscle but becomes more prominent at its ends. The connections between muscle and bone may be considered under two headings:

1. Tendons
2. Aponeurosis.

Tendons are cable or ribbon-like structures; the easiest example of which to visualize is the achilles tendon (also called the calcaneal tendon) which connects the calf muscles (gastrocnemious and soleus) to the calcaneus bone of the ankle. In other parts of the body a broader form of attachment is required, and this is achieved via a broad flattened sheet of connective tissue called an aponeurosis. Since tendons and aponeuroses are variations on a theme and fulfil similar functions it is not always clear when an attachment should be called a tendon and when it is an aponeurosis.

Examples of attachments which may be considered as aponeuroses include those of the external obliques and the attachment of the latissimus dorsi to the vertebrae of the back. The connective tissue found in tendons and aponeuroses is primarily made of collagen. Though it lacks the capability of contracting, it is strong since the force of the contracting muscle is conveyed through this tissue and any weakness could result in tissue damage or, in extreme cases, a rupture.

The different attachments of a muscle may be distinguished from each other and their relative positions described using appropriate terminology. When describing the attachments of muscles situated in the limbs the term proximal may be used to describe the attachment nearest the centre of the body whilst the term distal may be used to describe the attachment furthest from the centre of the body. Hence, a muscle may have a proximal attachment at the knee and a distal attachment at the ankle. Likewise a muscle could have its proximal attachment at the hip and its distal attachment at the knee. Similarly with the upper limbs a muscle could have its proximal attachment at the shoulder and its distal attachment at the elbow whilst another muscle could have its proximal attachment at the elbow and its distal attachment at the wrist. For muscles situated in the head, neck and trunk the terms upper and lower attachments may be used if their line of pull is almost vertical, while the terms 'medial' and 'lateral' may be used if the line of pull is across the body.

The terms origin and insertion may also be used to describe muscular attachments. The origin of a muscle refers to its attachment at the joint which remains relatively still when the muscle contracts, whilst the term insertion may be applied to the attachment at the end that tends to move when the muscle contracts. In the case of the limbs the origin is usually at the proximal end of the muscle whilst the insertion is usually at the distal end. However, owing to the complexity of movements in some exceptional situations the proximal end can move whilst the distal end remains relatively still.

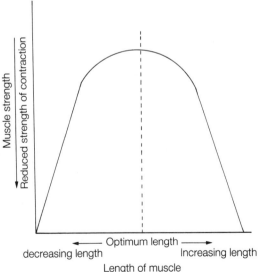

Figure 2.19 Illustrating the overlap of filaments and the length–tension relationship.

MUSCULAR LENGTH–TENSION RELATIONSHIPS AND ANGLES OF PULL

For a number of reasons the maximum amount of force a muscle can generate varies through its range of motion. These differences may be the result of the length–tension relationship of the muscle and/or the angle of pull of the muscle. The physiological basis of the length–tension relationship may be understood when the process of muscle contraction is considered. When a muscle is positioned at a certain length there will be an optimum amount of overlap between the thick and thin filaments of the muscle (Figure 2.19). In this position an optimum number of cross bridges may be formed and the muscle will be able to generate an optimal amount of tension or force. If the muscle is stretched beyond this optimal length then the amount of overlap between the thick and thin filaments will be reduced and, as a result, fewer cross bridges will be formed. Since the amount of force exerted by the muscle is dependent upon the number of cross bridges generated, the muscle will be relatively weak at this length. Conversely, when a muscle is close to its maximum amount of shortening the thick and thin filaments may interfere with one another, inhibiting cross-bridge formation and again reducing the amount of force exerted by the muscle. It can also be envisaged that in this position the thick filaments will be impeded by the Z lines at the end of each sarcomere which will further inhibit cross-bridge formation. Between these two extremes there will be an optimum length at which maximum cross-bridge formation is possible and, hence, the muscle will have the capacity to exert the greatest amount of force.

In addition to the length–tension relationship, a further cause of the observed differences in a muscle's strength at different phases of its range of motion is the 'angle of pull' of the muscle. A muscle's direction of pull is along its axis, with the resulting movement being expressed via the tendon. If the direction of pull is not directly in line with the resulting direction of movement of the bone then the pull will not be very efficient. This is best illustrated using the biceps brachii as an example (Figure 2.20).

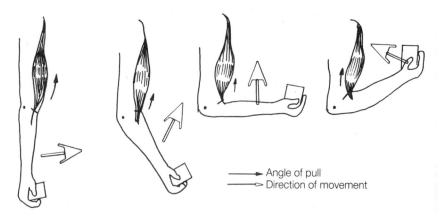

Angle of pull
Direction of movement

Figure 2.20 Illustrating the angle of pull during the phases of contraction of the biceps brachii.

When the arm is fully extended and begins to flex, the direction of pull of the muscle is upwards yet the initial direction of movement of the forearm is forwards. This results in an inefficient angle of pull. However, as the flexion movement continues the directions of pull and movement become more similar with the biceps pulling up and the arm moving in an upwards direction. This results in the force being more efficiently applied to the bone. The biceps is therefore strongest during the mid range of movement of the elbow joint. As the flexion continues beyond the mid range the direction of pull and direction of movement again become disimilar with the biceps continuing to pull up whilst the forearm moves towards the body. This makes the angle of pull less efficient and the arm not as strong during this phase of the movement.

Differences in the strength of a muscle group during different ranges of movement can also be seen in the hip and knee extensors. This is illustrated by getting someone to stand on one leg and then crouch down very slightly. This causes a slight flexion of the hips, knees and ankles. If the person then attempts to stand upright again (using only one leg) the task can usually be completed unaided and with minimum effort. However, if the person was asked to stand on one leg, crouch down in a fairly deep squatting position, and then attempt to stand upright (using only one leg), the task is likely to prove somewhat more difficult and may be impossible for many individuals. Attempting such a task from an immediate semi-squatting position is likely to require an intermediate amount of effort with a relative success rate. From these examples it can therefore be seen that the strength of a muscle is determined by anatomical, physiological and biomechanical factors.

PROPRIOCEPTORS AND THE STRUCTURE OF THE SPINAL CORD

To produce coordinated movements and maintain body posture the body/nervous system needs to be aware of the state and position of the limbs, joints and muscles of the body. This awareness of body position and body movements (kinesthetic awareness) is achieved via sense organs called proprioceptors which are found in the muscles, tendons and joints of the body. Additional information concerning body state and body position will come from other sense organs such as the eyes and the balance organs situated within the inner ear. Information about the position, state and movement of body parts is conveyed from these sense organs to the central nervous system via afferent (sensory) neurons. This information is then processed in the central nervous system which may respond by sending nerve impulses via efferent neurons (motor neurons) to the appropriate muscles which will bring about the desired adjustment in body position or body movement. This process of information sensing and body adjustment occurs continuously and enables the body to maintain its posture and/or alter the force of muscular contractions where needed when lifting objects, moving objects or moving the body itself.

Three main types of proprioceptors are found in the body:

1. Muscle spindles
2. Golgi tendon organs
3. Joint kinesthetic receptors.

67

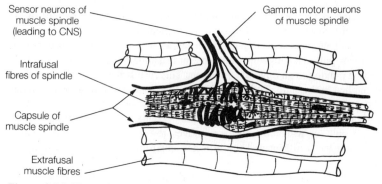

Sensor neurons of
muscle spindle
(leading to CNS)

Gamma motor neurons
of muscle spindle

Intrafusal
fibres of spindle

Capsule of
muscle spindle

Extrafusal
muscle fibres

Figure 2.21 Illustrating the structure of muscle spindles.

Muscle spindles

Muscle spindles (Figure 2.21) are found within the skeletal muscle. They are made up of modified muscle fibres called intrafusal fibres and are usually 2 to 4 mm in length but can be up to 13 mm in some cases. The intrafusal fibres of the muscle spindle are orientated so as to be parallel to the main contractile fibres of the muscle (the extrafusal fibres). Sensory neurons associated with the muscle spindles lead from the muscle spindles to the central nervous system. These sensory neurons convey information in the form of nerve impulses to the central nervous system. Also associated with the muscle spindles are gamma motor neurons which lead from the central nervous system to the intrafusal fibres of the muscle spindles. These neurons stimulate the intrafusal fibres to contract at certain times and play an important role in the adjustment of the strength of muscular contractions (see section on reflexes). In summary, when a muscle spindle is stretched nerve impulses are sent via the sensory neurons to the central nervous system conveying information on the degree and rate of stretch that the muscle spindles are experiencing. This information enables the neuromuscular system to make appropriate adjustments to muscle tone or the strength of contraction. In this context muscle spindles play a key role in the maintenance of posture and the initiation of reflexes that are used to modify movements.

Golgi tendon organs

Golgi tendon organs are found in the region of the muscle–tendon junction and are made up of a group of collagenous fibres which are surrounded by a capsule of connective tissue. Like the muscle spindles the Golgi tendon organs have sensory neurons leading from them and send information to the central nervous system when they are stretched. Golgi tendon organs provide a means of preventing muscle fibres and tendons from being damaged through being overstretched. Such overstretching could occur when the muscle attempts to contract against a resistance or, alternatively, when the muscle and tendon are both placed under stretch by another force. The Golgi tendon organs thus form part of a safety mechanism.

Joint kinesthetic receptors

Joint kinesthetic receptors, of which there are several types, are associated with the joints of the body. They are the key sense organs in informing the body of the position of the limbs and providing the sense of kinesthetic awareness. They are situated in and around the articular capsules of synovial joints and are also found in the ligaments of joints. One of their major roles is in the initiation of powerful muscular reflex contractions if the joint becomes overstretched. If a joint does exeperience excessive stretching then the joint receptors send impulses to the central nervous system which then responds by stimulating muscles associated with the joint to contract forcefully in an attempt to provide the joint with stability and inhibit further unwanted stretching of the joint.

Organization of the spinal cord

The spinal cord is a cylindrical structure extending from the inferior portion of the brain stem, the medulla oblongata, down to the level of the second lumbar vertebrae. In adults it is therefore approximately 45 cm in length. It is surrounded and protected by three layers of connective tissue, called the spinal meninges, and the bones which form the vertebral column. The spinal cord is made up of neurons and their associated neuroglia. The organization of the cells making up the spinal cord produces specific regions within the spinal cord called white and grey matter (Figure 2.22). The white matter largely consists of neuroglia and myelinated axons which extend up and down the spinal cord. The myelinated sheaths of these axons give this region its characteristic white colour. Within the white matter the neurons are grouped into bundles called columns and tracts. The columns within the spinal cord may be described according to their position within the cord, therefore the white matter may be said to consist of anterior columns, lateral columns and posterior columns. The tracts within the white matter consist of groups of neurons which have a similar function. For example, neurons which convey sensory information up the spinal cord towards the brain are grouped together into ascending tracts whilst neurons whose function it is to convey information down the spinal cord away from the brain are grouped into descending

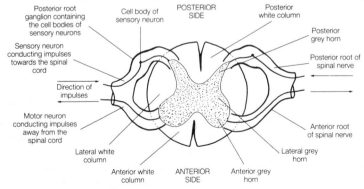

Figure 2.22 Illustrating the structure of the spinal cord.

tracts. This means that the ascending tracts convey sensory information towards the brain whilst the descending tracts convey motor information that will be passed on to efferent neurons that synapse within the spinal cord. Within white matter the constituent neurons will vary considerably in length; some will convey information from the brain down the length of the spinal cord, whilst others will convey information over relatively short distances, e.g. from one level of the spinal cord to another.

The grey matter of the spinal cord is made up of nerve cell bodies, dendrites and unmyelinated neurons along with their associated neuroglia. The grey matter contains the association neurons which are involved in numerous body reflexes. Their function is to relay information from one neuron to another within the spinal cord. Structurally the grey matter forms columns within the spinal cord and when the spinal cord is viewed in cross section the grey matter forms characteristic shapes referred to as horns. These horns may be described according to their position within the spinal cord; thus the spinal cord may be said to contain anterior grey horns and posterior grey horns (Figure 2.22). The anterior grey horns are the areas associated with sensory activity.

The neurons of the peripheral nervous system enter and leave the spinal cord via specific roots called the posterior and anterior roots. Sensory neurons enter the spinal cord via the posterior root (also called the dorsal sensory root). The posterior root also contains the cell bodies of the peripheral sensory neurons. These are aggregated together to form an enlargement of the posterior root called the posterior root ganglion. The axons of the sensory neurons then continue along the posterior root into the spinal cord where they synapse with other neurons. Conversely, the peripheral motor neurons leave the spinal cord via the anterior root. The cell bodies of these motor neurons are situated within the anterior grey horns of the spinal cord and it is within these horns that they synapse with, and hence receive information from, other neurons. As a consequence of this the anterior grey horns are directly associated with motor activity and damage to these areas can result in severe motor impairment.

PROPRIOCEPTORS, REFLEXES, POSTURE AND COORDINATED MOVEMENT

Reflexes

In the context of exercise, movement and body control reflexes are used to:

(a) modify movement
(b) maintain posture
(c) prevent injury
(d) alter body metabolism in accordance with the demands of the exercise.

Whilst all are important, this section will concentrate upon the reflexes that directly affect the activity of skeletal muscle. Modifications to cardiac output, breathing and general metabolism are covered in later chapters.

Reflexes may be described as being innate reflexes if they require no learning or as conditioned reflexes if they require a learning process and hence some cortical activity. Typically, spinal reflexes tend to be innate whilst the more complex reflexes which require cortical processing are conditioned. Common reflexes involve a series of stages which may include the following:

1. A receptor or sense organ.
2. A sensory (afferent) neuron, which conveys information to the central nervous system.
3. The central nervous system, which may process the information and in so doing will commonly involve association neurons within the spinal cord and, in some cases, the brain. These association neurons can have either an inhibitory or an excitatory effect upon the neurons they synapse with.
4. Motor (efferent) neurons, which convey information from the central nervous system to muscle fibres.
5. Muscle fibres (grouped into functional motor units), which may be stimulated or inhibited from contracting by the reflex.

The stretch reflex

The basic stretch reflex (also called the myotatic reflex) provides an example of a relatively simple innate reflex which involves just two neurons whose synapse is situated within the spinal cord. Since only one synapse is involved, the stretch reflex is a monosynaptic reflex. Indeed, the basic stretch reflex is the only known monosynaptic reflex – all other reflexes involve more than two neurons and hence more than one synapse (such reflex arcs are therefore termed polysynaptic). The stretch reflex works in the following manner (Figure 2.23). When a muscle is stretched, the intrafusal fibres of the muscle spindle and the extrafusal fibres are both stretched in a similar manner. As a result of the stretching the muscle spindles send nerve impulses via

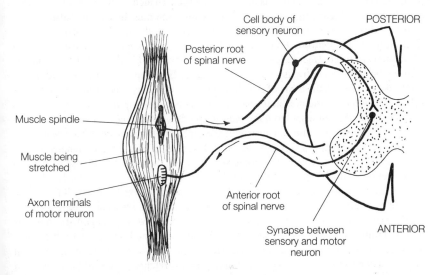

Figure 2.23 Illustrating the basic stretch reflex.

sensory neurons to the spinal cord (entering via the posterior root). Within the anterior horn of the grey matter of the spinal cord the sensory neurons synapse with alpha motor neurons which lead back out of the spinal cord via the anterior root and back into the muscle from which the sensory neurons originated. These alpha motor neurons innervate the extrafusal fibres of the muscle. In a stretch reflex the synapses between the sensory neurons and alpha motor neurons are excitatory and hence when the muscle spindles are stretched the excitatory impluses from the sensory neurons cause the alpha motor neurons to transmit impulses back into the muscle and, as a result, the extrafusal muscle fibres contract. This prevents further stretching of the muscle. Such reflexes operate continuously in the unconscious maintenance of muscle tone and posture. In this context they function to maintain the appropriate strength of static muscle contraction which is needed to resist external forces such as gravity. In reality the actual control and monitoring of such postural reflexes is somewhat more complex and usually involves areas of the brainstem as well as the spinal cord.

Alternatively, the stretch reflex may also operate on a more dynamic level. In this capacity it has a protective function whereby if a muscle is stretched suddenly the reflex contraction will inhibit further stretching and hence reduce the risk of the muscle being overstretched and damaged. The spindles within a muscle are sensitive to both the length and rate of stretch, which means that when a muscle is stretched the resulting reflex contraction will be of an appropriate strength to counteract the stretch. Stronger reflex contractions are therefore produced in response to rapid stretching near the muscle's maximum safe length.

Stretch reflexes are used in certain forms of neurological examinations to test for the correct functioning of the nervous system. Certain disorders and damage to the nervous system will result in an absence of the stretch reflex whilst other disorders may cause an excessive response. A common example of such a diagnostic reflex is the knee jerk reflex (patellar reflex). In this reflex the patellar tendon is tapped by the assessor. This causes the rectus femoris muscle (which is attached to the tendon) to be stretched. Hence the muscle spindles within the muscle send impulses to the spinal cord via sensory neurons. Within the spinal cord the sensory neurons synapse with alpha motor neurons that lead back into the rectus femoris; these will then stimulate various contractile (extrafusal) muscle fibres within the muscle to contract. Hence, the muscle contracts causing the knee to be extended (jerk forwards).

Whilst this forms the basis of the stretch reflex, in reality other neurons and other reflex arcs will be stimulated at the same time. This is a result of the sensory neurons which conduct the impulses from the muscle spindles synapsing with various neurons within the spinal cord and not just with the alpha motor neurons which lead back into the stretched muscle. These additional synapses will include synapses with inhibitory association neurons (interneurons) that will then in turn synapse with alpha motor neurons which innervate the muscle fibres of the antagonistic muscles (Figure 2.24). The inhibitory association neurons in this particular reflex arc will then have an inhibitory effect upon these motor neurons and, hence, when the muscle spindles (of the stretched muscle) send impulses to the spinal cord the antagonistic muscles will be inhibited from contracting. This response is termed 'reciprocal inhibition'. Since reciprocal inhibition inhibits the antagonist from contracting it has several important consequences. Firstly, the muscle being stretched may well have been put under stretch by its antagonistic muscle and therefore by inhibiting the antagonistic

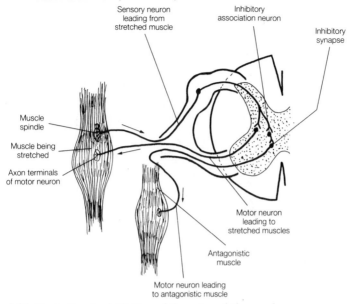

Figure 2.24 Illustrating the inhibition of the antagonistic muscles.

muscle from contracting the cause of the stretch may be removed. Secondly, if the muscle is to respond by contracting rapidly, its antagonist must relax in order to facilitate the movement. So, in the case of the knee jerk reflex, an initial stretching of the rectus femoris will cause a reflex contraction of the rectus femoris (a knee extensor) and a reflex inhibition of the knee flexors.

Additional reflex arcs and synapses within the spinal cord may include synapses between the sensory neurons from the muscle spindles and excitatory association neurons. These excitatory association neurons will then synapse with the alpha motor neurons that innervate the muscles that are synergistic to the one being stretched. These association neurons will have a stimulatory (excitatory) effect upon these motor neurons and thus, as the stretched muscle is stimulated to contract, the movement will be assisted by the reflex contraction of its synergists (Figure 2.25). Finally, the sensory neurons from the muscle spindles will also synapse with other neurons in the spinal cord, which will convey impulses up the spinal cord informing the motor centres of the central nervous system of the occurrence of the reflex response.

The tendon reflex

A function of the tendon reflex is to prevent the tendons and muscles from being overstretched and damaged. A muscle and its associated tendon may be placed under stretch by another force, or a tendon may be stretched when the muscle to which it is attached contracts forcefully. Both instances could cause an overstretching of the muscle and/or tendon and result in injury. The Golgi tendon organs are situated at the muscle–tendon junction, they detect when this region is being stretched. Stretching of the muscle–tendon region causes the Golgi tendon organs to send impulses

73

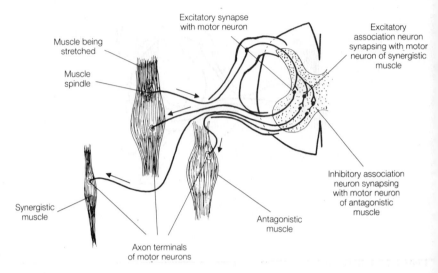

Figure 2.25 Illustrating innervation of the synergistic muscles.

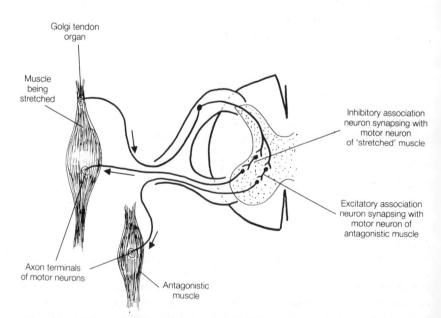

Figure 2.26 Illustrating the tendon reflex.

to the spinal cord via sensory neurons, which synapse with inhibitory association neurons within the grey matter of the spinal cord (Figure 2.26). These inhibitory association neurons then synapse with the alpha motor neurons that innervate the muscles's extrafusal fibres. The inhibitory effects of these synapses inhibit the motor neurons from transmitting impulses to the extrafusal fibres of the muscle thereby causing the extrafusal fibres to relax. This relaxation of the muscle will reduce the amount of stretch experienced at the muscle–tendon junction. The overall effect of this will be to reduce the risk of damage through overstretching of the muscle or tendon.

When a muscle contracts the force it exerts is conveyed through the tendon to the bone. When a muscle shortens the pull it exerts upon the tendon may cause the tendon to be stretched as its elasticity is taken up. Thus the tendon is stretched before movement of the bone occurs. An excessively forceful contraction of the muscle to which the tendon is attached could overstretch and damage the tendon. In practice this is usually prevented by the tendon reflex which reduces the strength of contraction, and an excessively strong and potentially damaging contraction is therefore inhibited.

In addition to the synapses already mentioned, the sensory neurons from the Golgi tendon organs will also synapse with excitatory association neurons that go on to synapse with the alpha motor neurons of the antagonistic muscles. In this way the antagonistic muscles will be stimulated to contract, further inhibiting the stretch that is put on the tendon. Finally, as with the stretch reflex, further synapses within the spinal cord may lead to information being passed up the spinal cord to the motor centres of the central nervous system giving information of the occurrence of such reflexes.

Reflexes and the control of movement

Almost any body movement, or the active movement of a body part, requires an extremely complex, coordinated integration of the activity of many muscles, their constituent motor units and the thousands of motor neurons which innervate them. During a body movement various skeletal muscles will be required to function in a variety of ways. For example, they may contract eccentrically, concentrically or isometrically, or they may be required to relax. Therefore, in order to achieve an effective movement the muscles need to be instructed to contract in the correct sequence with the appropriate recruitment of motor units. This requires nerve impulses of the correct strength to be directed along thousands of motor neurons in the correct temporal sequence.

Initially a complex coordinated movement may be considered to commence with a general command such as 'move leg' or 'pick up object' or 'write signature'. Such actions will require a specific set and sequence of nerve impulses. However, different occasions and different circumstances will require slight modifications to the movement and, hence, slight changes in the involvement of the muscles concerned. This will require modifications to the nerve impulses being sent to the motor neurons. Appropriate modifications to the impulses are achieved via the continuous monitoring of body position by the proprioceptors. This results in a continuous flow of sensory information being sent back to the central nervous system from the proprioceptors and other sense organs. The information being sent from these sense organs is then processed by the central nervous system and may be used to modify the command nerve impulses that are sent to the muscles. A movement will therefore be modified, according to the specific circumstances in which it is occurring.

An example of the way in which muscle spindles may bring about such appropriate adjustments in muscle contractions is illustrated on occasions when the muscles encounter an unexpected resistance or lack of resistance. When a motor unit is stimulated to contract, nerve impulses are sent via the alpha motor neurons to the extrafusal muscle fibres. At the same time nerve impulses are also sent via the gamma motor neurons to the intrafusal fibres of the muscle spindles. In this way both the extrafusal and intrafusal fibres are stimulated to contract. The sending of nerve impulses to both the extrafusal muscle fibres and the intrafusal muscle fibres of the muscle spindles is referred to as coactivation. When nerve impulses of a certain strength are sent to a muscle the muscle will be 'expected' to contract by a certain length. If, however, the muscle encounters a stronger resistance than expected, then it will shorten by less than the expected amount. Despite this the spindles within the muscle will shorten to their predetermined length and this will create a discrepancy between the length of the extrafusal and intrafusal fibres within the muscle. This difference is detected by the muscle spindles which inform the central nervous system of the discrepancy (via their sensory neurons). As a result of this new information, stronger impulses will then be sent to the muscle which will cause it to contract more forcefully to make up for the stronger than 'expected' resistance it is encountering.

Conversely, if the muscle encounters less resistance than 'expected' it will shorten by more than 'expected'. Again this discrepancy between its expected and actual length (as detected by the relative amounts of shortening of the extra-fusal and intrafusal fibres) will be detected by the muscle spindles and, as a result, the strength of motor nerve impulses will be reduced, thereby lessening the strength of contraction.

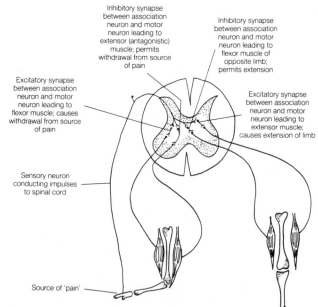

Figure 2.27 Illustrating the crossed extensor reflex.

The crossed entensor reflex

The crossed extensor reflex (Figure 2.27) provides an example of a somewhat more complex innate reflex, which occurs when pain is felt in one limb, as would occur if someone were to step on a sharp object, touch a hot object or sprain an ankle. When this happens there is a rapid reflex contraction of the flexor muscles in the limb experiencing the pain, which causes the limb to be rapidly withdrawn from the source of the pain. There is, at the same time, a rapid and forceful contraction of the extensor muscles of the opposite limb. In practice this means that if one was to step on a sharp object, then, at the same time as the leg experiencing the pain was rapidly withdrawn from the source of the pain, the opposite leg would be extended to support the weight of the body. A similar response would be seen if someone sprained an ankle or touched a hot object.

Reflexes and common body movements

Many body movements may be considered to be based upon complex reflexes. One example would be in the case of stumbling or tripping. If a person is to be physically balanced and stable, the centre of gravity must be positioned over their base: this is normally between the feet (Figure 2.28). When a person trips, the centre of gravity moves forward rapidly and, as a result, it may pass ahead of the feet. This causes the person to become unstable and liable to fall over. In response to the stumbling action and the instability of the body a complex reflex response occurs to rapidly move the leg(s) forward in order to prevent the person from falling. If the movement is rapid enough the feet will be moved so that the centre of gravity is once again directly above and the the person will regain his or her balance. At the same time as the legs move the arms may also be extended as a form of protection should the person be unable to regain his or her balance and fall.

As an extension of this, walking can be considered as a complex protective reflex which occurs when a person's centre of gravity passes ahead of his or her base, giving instability. Such actions may be automatically present in the form of reflexes,

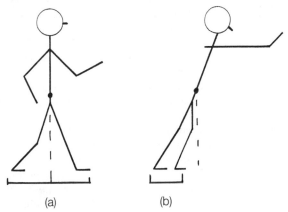

(a)   (b)

Figure 2.28 Illustrating the relationship between the centre of gravity and stability.

but as in the case of walking they need to be perfected through practice. Certain neurological disorders my result in a person being unable to perform these practised reflexes and hence lose the capacity to walk in a 'normal' manner.

When many complex movements, such as walking, are initially performed they require the individual to receive and process a large amount of sensory information in order to make the movements effective. Hence, when children first learn to walk they are hesitant and unsure since they have to make constant conscious adjustments to the movement. However, as the activity is practised synaptic changes may occur in the neural pathways involved in the activity and, as a result, the activity will require less conscious sensory information and will occur at a more subconscious level. Other complex movements such as writing and knitting also exhibit this capacity to be learned and performed at a subconscious level.

Reflexes and the maintenance of posture

The maintenance of posture requires many skeletal muscles to contract isometrically against gravity and other external forces. Body position is continuously monitored by the proprioceptors which send information via sensory neurons to the central nervous system. This enables the body to make slight adjustments to the strength of the muscle contractions. The movement of a limb, change in body position or alteration in the strength or direction of an external force will require an adjustment in the strength of contraction of the muscles that are used to maintain posture. These adjustments to the strength of isometric and/or slight isotonic contractions occur continuously at a subconscious level, enabling the automatic maintenance of posture and body position.

MUSCULAR TONE

Normally, the muscles of the body possess a certain amount of firmness or 'tone' even when they are essentially relaxed. This tone is, of course, increased during active contractions, such as when the muscles are maintaining the body's posture or influencing some body movement. This basic and persistent level of tone maintains the muscles in a state of 'readiness' and is attributable to both myogenic and neurogenic factors. The myogenic aspects refer to the residual firmness of the muscle and are primarily determined by the condition of the muscle fibres. This condition will be influenced by the intensity, type and frequency of contractions that the muscles regularly perform. It may therefore be considered as a 'training effect'. Disuse of a muscle for whatever reason will result in atrophy (hypotrophy) with a reduction in its size and strength; along with this there will be a loss of its myogenic firmness. Conversely, appropriate use of a muscle in activities such as work, excercise and therapy will help to develop and maintain the muscle's tone as well as its strength.

The neurogenic factors which influence muscle tone refer to the supply of low-intensity nerve impulses which the muscle receives. These low-level impulses keep the muscle in a state of slight contraction. This, again, maintains the muscle in a state of readiness and increases the 'resting' tone or firmness of the muscle. When required to maintain the body's posture the postural muscles of the body will receive stronger impulses which will increase their tone and firmness to an extent whereby they can resist external forces such as gravity. This may be described as their 'postural tone'.

If a muscle possesses too little tone it is described as being hypotonic, whereas the possession of too much muscle tone is referred to as hypertonicity. Certain disorders will result in muscles losing their neurogenic inputs and in such cases the muscle will become hypotonic. Flaccid paralysis is an example of hypotonicity. Conversely, some disorders result in the muscle receiving a constant supply of excitatory neurogenic inputs which are too strong. This may occur when there is an imbalance between the excitatory and inhibitory inputs. Certain conditions affecting the central nervous system can cause a reduction in the inhibitory inputs. An inadequate supply of inhibitory inputs results in an overstimulation of the muscles causing hypertonicity. Excessive muscle tone may be seen in cases of spasticity where the muscles possess an excessive firmness which causes them to resist movements during which they should relax and lengthen. This causes the limbs to have a degree of rigidity that impairs their movement and control. In addition, hypertonic conditions may result in an excessive response to certain reflexes owing to the overexcitability of the muscles. This is why specific reflex responses may be used in the diagnosis of certain conditions.

NEUROMUSCULAR DISEASES AND DISORDERS

Having described the basic physiology of the neuromuscular system it is now appropriate to describe briefly certain neuromuscular disorders that may be encountered by the therapist or exercise adviser. The diseases described in this section provide a variety of examples of conditions which should give the therapist or adviser a greater understanding of the problems they may encounter and the function of exercise in conjunction with the therapeutic practices associated with those diseases.

Multiple sclerosis (MS)

Multiple sclerosis (MS) is a disease of the central nervous system which is characterized by the progressive destruction of the myelin sheaths of the neurons. The disease specifically affects the neuroglia cells of the central nervous system. It is characterized by the appearance of patches of 'scar' tissue within the central nervous system. The patches of scar tissue are associated with the progressive disappearance of the oligodendrocytes which form the myelin sheaths and a progressive increase in the number of astrocytes. This results in an overall deterioration of the myelin sheaths in these areas and the formation of hardened patches or scars (sclerosis). These scarred areas may be found in both the brain and spinal cord. They may vary in size from less than 1 mm to over 5 mm and basically consist of connective tissue formed from the astrocytes which are far more abundant in these areas than in the non-MS sufferer. The destruction of the myelin sheaths affects the transmission of nerve impulses along the neurons and also leaves the nerve vulnerable to further damage. Multiple sclerosis symptoms may include temporary weakness, paralysis, numbness, tingling sensations in the extremities, double vision and tremors upon exertion. Sufferers may therefore become invalids. Multiple sclerosis may be an autoimmune disease which is initially caused by a virus. The disease is also characterized by periods of remission during which time the sufferer's physical condition may improve prior to further deterioration.

Poliomyelitis

Poliomyelitis, also called infantile paralysis, is caused by a virus which affects the central nervous system. Infection is caused by the ingestion of the virus which affects the motor cells of the anterior horn of the spinal cord. In an unaffected spinal cord the anterior horn contains cell bodies and dendrites, it is involved with the transmission of motor impulses from the central nervous system to the periphery and is therefore associated with motor activity. The polio virus destroys the cell bodies of the motor neurons and this results in a loss of the nerves which normally innervate the muscles (denervation). This, therefore, results in the denerved muscle fibres being unable to contract. The extent and seriousness of the disease will depend upon the number of motor units affected: if the number of fibres affected is relatively small this will cause muscular weakness; however, if a large number of fibres are affected substantial or complete paralysis of the muscle can result. In such cases the loss of the nerve supply, and hence the absence of nerve impulses that would normally stimulate the muscle fibres, will cause the muscle to atrophy.

Motor neuron disease

This is characterized by the degeneration of nerve cells within the anterior horn of the spinal cord followed by the degeneration of the peripheral motor neurons. As in the case of poliomyelitis, this denervation results in a loss of muscular function, paralysis and muscular atrophy. As the disease progresses there is a degeneration of the neurons in the brain from which the cranial nerves arise and, finally, a degeneration of the motor neurons of the cerebral cortex.

Parkinson's disease

This is a progressive disease of the motor cortex; it is caused by degeneration in the basal ganglia of the brain, primarily the substantia nigra. This degeneration results in a deficiency of the neurotransmitter dopamine. The basal ganglia consist of large masses of grey matter which regulate the subconscious contractions of skeletal muscles and aid in the control of conscious contractions. However, a deficiency in the neurotransmitter dopamine results in a general slowness of voluntary movement, a slow tremor at rest, postural deformities, a shuffling gait and muscular rigidity.

Myasthenia gravis

This is an autoimmune disease which results in antibodies from the body's own immune system 'attacking' the acetyl choline receptors at the neuromuscular junction. At an unaffected neuromuscular junction the transmission of a nerve impulse down the motor neuron causes the release of acetyl choline from the end of the neuron. The acetyl choline then crosses the gap between the neuron and muscle fibre and binds to specialized acetyl choline receptors on the muscle fibre. This initiates a series of events which ultimately result in the fibre contracting. However, in the case of myasthenia gravis the presence of antibodies at the acetyl choline receptor sites inhibits the binding of the neurotransmitter. This reduces the likelihood of the fibre contracting, and its overall effect upon the muscle is a reduction in the strength of contraction. As the disease progresses the neuromuscular junctions may become so severely affected that they cease to function effectively and, hence, muscular function is lost.

A stroke or cerebral vascular accident

A stroke may be caused by a blockage in a blood vessel leading to the brain. This will result in an area of the brain being deprived of oxygen. Alternatively, it may be caused by a cerebral vascular accident (CVA) such as a haemorrhage. Either of these events will cause the death of certain brain cells. Death of these cells may result in an impairment of normal motor activity through an imbalance of the excitatory and inhibitory impulses. Such imbalances may cause excessive muscular tone, as in the case of hypertonicity, or may result in flaccidity (hypotonicity) if the excitatory inputs are deficient. The effects of a stroke often include some degree of paralysis which commonly affects only one side of the body (hemiplegia).

Cerebral palsy

Cerebral palsy really refers to a group of motor disorders which are characterized by damage or maldevelopment of the brain, either prior to birth or during the first three years of life. It may affect the cortex of the brain, the basal ganglia of the cerebrum and/or the cerebellum. The maldevelopment or damage to these areas causes an impaired motor function and/or paralysis as well as severe learning difficulties for the child.

Epilepsy

The severity of epilepsy varies considerably amongst sufferers, ranging from its severest form (*grand mal*) to milder forms (*petit mal*). In its severest form the disorder is characterized by short recurrent attacks of motor and sensory malfunction. The sufferer is subject to bouts of irregular neural activity within the brain that cause the involuntary contraction of the skeletal muscles. This exhibits itself as an 'attack' where sufferers lose control of their motor activities during which time they may twitch, jerk and writhe violently. This may be preceded by a warning, such as flashes of light. The uncontrolled motor activity of the attack may be followed by coma. Milder forms of the disorder are characterized by a momentary loss of consciousness without convulsions. In such cases the cause is again inappropriate neural activity within the brain, which results in the suppression of normal waking functions.

Myopathies

Myopathies are diseases which primarily affect the muscle fibres. Such disorders may involve the degeneration of the fibres and include various specific muscular dystrophies such as Duchenne muscular dystrophy, which is genetically inherited and affects only boys. Such dystrophies cause muscular weakness, muscular deterioration and severe loss or impairment of normal muscular activities such as walking.

Peripheral nerve injury

This may occur as a result of a traumatic accident in which the nerve is severed. Owing to the lack of motor input to the muscle fibres they will not be able to contract (unless stimulated electrically by external sources) and, as a result, the muscle will atrophy. Damage to sensory neurons leading from the muscle will cause a loss of proprioceptive information and, as a result, this aspect of kinesthetic awareness and certain proprioceptive reflexes may be lost. A specific disease of the peripheral nervous system is Guillain Barre Syndrome. It is believed to be initiated by an infection and primarily affects the nerve roots leaving the spinal cord. The nerve roots become inflamed (polyneuritis), which inhibits the transmission of impulses along these neurons. As a result of the disease, muscular function may be impaired although a full recovery is possible.

Hypotonia, hypertonia and spasticity

As discussed earlier, hypotonia refers to the situation in which there is a substantially less than normal amount of muscle tone while hypertonia and hypertonic spasticity refer to conditions in which there is an excessive amount of muscle tone. Hypotonicity occurs when there are insufficient excitatory impulses reaching the muscle: this may be the result of neural damage in either the peripheral or central nervous systems, and causes flaccid muscles which will atrophy with disuse. Spina bifida is an example of a disorder in which damage to the central nervous system causes a loss of muscle function. In such cases the spinal cord is damaged thereby preventing the transmission of nerve impulses onto the motor neurons. Such damage usually occurs to the lumbar region of the spine and results in a loss of muscular activity of the legs (flaccid paralysis).

Alternatively, the flaccidity may be attributable to disorders within the muscle fibre itself or at the neuromuscular junction, as is the case with myasthenia gravis. Hypertonicity and spasticity occur when the muscle fibres receive an excessive amount of excitatory impulses. This may be caused by an imbalance between the normal excitatory and inhibitory inputs. If the inhibitory inputs are suppressed or absent then the unopposed excitatory inputs cause the muscle to maintain an excessive amount of tone and give the limbs a degree of rigidity. The hypertonicity of the muscle inhibits it from relaxing and lengthening, thereby preventing/inhibiting movements which require it to relax.

Ataxia

This is a general term that may be applied to a number of diseases or disorders which result in a failure of appropriate muscular contraction. This causes an awkwardness of movement which may refer to any muscle or group of muscles. However, specifically the term 'ataxia' is often used to describe 'difficulty in walking'. Proprioceptive ataxia is caused by disease of the sensory neurons which impairs the transmission of proprioceptive information to the central nervous system. Cerebellar ataxia is caused by damage to the cerebellum, which is involved with the control of motor function. Spastic ataxia results in stiff, rigid limbs; it is caused by abnormalities within the central nervous system and inhibits 'normal walking'.

Postviral fatigue syndromes

The term postviral fatigue syndromes (PVFS) is currently used to cover a group of diseases including myalgic encephalitis (ME). These diseases are not well understood but, owing to an apparent increase in their incidence, are now receiving more coverage. They are believed to have a viral origin and appear to affect people when they are in a state of general physical fatigue and stress. The link with stress is based upon research which indicates a suppression of the immune system under conditions of prolonged stress. This suppression will make the individual more susceptible to infection and less able to combat disease. Similarly, a person who is generally fatigued (referring to the fatigue experienced following weeks of overwork or repeated excessive amounts of overtraining or an inappropriate lifestyle, rather than the immediate fatigue experienced following a single bout of exercise) will also be more vulnerable to infection. In accordance with this, the diseases appear to be most prevalent amongst high achievers, especially those involved in stressful occupations and/or competitive sport. Furthermore, one of the suggested causes of the diseases is believed to be the participation in excessive amounts of exercise whilst suffering from a viral infection and/or in a general state of fatigue.

The diseases affect the muscles causing undue fatigue with the severity varying considerably. In a milder form they are manifested as a reduced capacity to exercise and compete. This is linked with an otherwise unexplained loss of fitness and the onset of fatigue at exercise intensities that the individual would previously have been able to sustain with relative ease. In a more severe form the diseases can cause severe fatigue and exhaustion during relatively mild forms of activity such as dressing. The diseases can also affect the nervous system causing depression. The treatment for the diseases usually includes rest and the cessation of exercise until the individual has recovered. A gradual increase in exercise participation may then be advocated with the intensity and volume of exercise increasing gradually over a period of weeks to months. The duration of these fatigue syndromes varies from a few weeks to a number of years. To date the exact physiology of these diseases remains a mystery and the precise details are likely to be complex, involving a number of factors. One factor that is currently being investigated is the viral suppression of mitochondrial activity, which, if proven, could go some way towards explaining the general reduction of the physical capacity of the muscles that is observed in sufferers of PVFS. However, other authorities on the subject suggest that the virus affects the central nervous system and that the site of 'fatigue' is within the brain.

EXERCISE AND REHABILITATION AFTER INJURY

Muscles, tendons and ligaments are frequently damaged in everyday activities such as stepping awkwardly down a step, colliding with an object or pulling a muscle during a sporting activity. Traumatic injury to muscles, tendons and ligaments often involves the tissue being overstretched and torn. In the case of muscle strains this may range in severity from the tearing of a few fibres to the complete rupture of virtually all fibres within the muscle. Damage to tendons and ligaments can again range from slight tissue damage to complete rupture.

Immediately following an injury to soft tissue, basic first aid procedures should be adopted. The precise nature of these will depend upon the severity of the injury and any complications. The first aid procedures will aim to minimize the extent of the injury and any internal bleeding. A common response to such injuries is to apply ice, compression and elevation (ICE) (unless more serious complications such as a fracture are also present). This is believed to reduce the internal bleeding and minimize the amount of scar tissue which, if excessive, can increase the time required for complete recovery.

All basic soft tissue injuries such as muscle strains, tendon strains and sprained ligaments will require a period of rest before the tissues are exercised. This will enable the healing process to commence and the ends of the wound to rejoin. The period of rest will depend upon the severity of the injury with slight muscle tears requiring 48 hours whilst a completely ruptured tendon will require weeks to regain the strength required for exercise.

Once the tissue has regained sufficient strength, exercise may be used to promote the healing process. Throughout the rehabilitation phase it should be well within the capacity of the injured tissue. Any slight overstretching will result in the weak tissue pulling apart and requiring further rest; therefore, care should be taken to strengthen the tissue with gentle exercise that does not place excessive strain or stretch on it. In general, muscles respond well and rapidly to light exercise that accelerates their recovery. Tendons and ligaments take longer to recover and in some cases may be permanently weakened. The use of additional support or strapping may be used to provide a joint with additional stability and reduce the risk of redamaging weakened ligaments. As the exercise rehabilitation programme progresses specific attention should be given to warming up the tissue either actively or passively prior to the exercise and to gently stretching the tissue. Muscles which heal short and those that are stiff are more vulnerable to damage.

Therefore, in summary, exercise can promote the recovery from an injury once the tissue has regained sufficient strength. The exercise should therefore place relatively slight demands on the tissue in order to promote the recovery process without risking further damage. As the tissue recovers the exercise loads can be gradually increased in order to assist with the regaining of the tissue's strength.

For details on the treatment of sport-specific injuries and related therapeutically based exercise programmes, see the recommended further reading.

3

Nutrition, energy and exercise metabolism

INTRODUCTION

The processes of growth, the repair of body tissues, muscle contraction and the general maintenance of the body in a healthy state all require energy. This energy is ultimately derived from food. Within the body the processes of digestion and metabolism convert the energy contained within food into a form that can be used by the body for the processes named above.

The amount of energy required by the body will vary depending upon the age of the individual, his or her state of health, the time of day and current state of activity/inactivity. Therefore, the body needs to be able to adjust the amount of energy that is available for various processes depending upon its current energy demands. For example, when moving from a state of rest to one of strenuous physical activity the energy expenditure of the individual may increase by up to tenfold. In addition, the supply of energy into the body is inconsistent. Energy enters the body in the form of food which is taken as meals or snacks. These are separated by periods of fasting that may last from a few minutes to many hours. These inconsistencies in the body's energy intake and energy expenditure mean that in the short term the body cannot depend upon increasing its energy intake immediately its energy expenditure increases; therefore, to ensure that the energy is available for increased activity when it is needed, the body carries its own reserves of energy. In practice, this means that when the body takes in food it stores any surplus energy. This can then be used between meals and/or during periods of high energy expenditure. The body stores the majority of this surplus energy as fat and carbohydrate (in the form of glycogen) which can then be broken down and utilized as an energy source when required.

Many of the metabolic changes that are observed before, during and after exercise are related to increasing the availability and effective utilization of these energy stores. The sections within this chapter will therefore briefly describe:

(a) aspects of energy intake (nutrition);
(b) the conversion of food energy into a form that the muscles can use during exercise;
(c) the use of different 'energy pathways' during exercise; and

(d) a number of metabolic responses that occur to facilitate the use of this energy before, during and after exercise.

EXERCISE NUTRITION

The topic of exercise and sports nutrition is vast and a number of key texts relating to the subject are listed at the end of the book. Similarly, the topic of 'exercise, diet and body weight' is also subject to much debate and is discussed in Chapter 8. Therefore this section will briefly present a number of key aspects of nutrition that are related to exercise and present a basis for understanding the implications of the energy pathways which are discussed later in this chapter.

THE COMPONENTS OF FOOD

Food is made up of:

1. Carbohydrate
   (a) simple sugars
   (b) complex carbohydrate
2. Fat
   (a) saturated fat
   (b) unsaturated fat
   (c) cholesterol
3. Protein
4. Vitamins
   (a) water soluble
   (b) fat soluble
5. Minerals
6. Water
7. Fibre
8. Other substances, including alcohol.

All these food components have an important role to play in health and exercise metabolism. Each will be discussed briefly in this context; for a more extensive coverage of the topic see the recommended further reading.

Carbohydrate

Carbohydrates are made up of carbon, hydrogen and oxygen. They range from simple sugars such as glucose and fructose to complex carbohydrates such as starch and glycogen. The complex carbohydrates are made up of many simple sugar units that are chemically bonded together to form large complex molecules. Simple sugars are contained within confectionery, fruit and many other common foods. Major sources of complex carbohydrate, in the form of starch, are potatoes, bread and pasta. When simple sugars or complex carbohydrates are eaten the processes of digestion and metabolism convert the sugar units into glucose. Some of this glucose will remain in the blood to be transported to, and taken up by, any cells that require it. Any excess glucose is taken up by the cells of the muscles or liver and converted into glycogen. Muscle glycogen and liver glycogen are similar to starch in that they are large complex molecules formed by combining many glucose units. Muscle glycogen provides a store of energy within the muscles that can be broken down into glucose units and used as an energy source when required. Liver glycogen also functions as an energy store which can be broken down into glucose units and released into the blood when the body needs more glucose. During prolonged forms of strenuous exercise this glucose may be used to supplement the muscle's own carbohydrate stores.

Fat

Several types of fat are found in the diet, including triglycerides, cholesterol, phospholipids, saturated fatty acids and unsaturated fatty acids. Fat is stored in the body as a source of energy, as well as providing insulation, being a major component of cell membranes and forming the structural basis of many important molecules such as the steroid hormones. Fat may be stored under the skin as subcutaneous fat, in specialized areas of fatty tissue (adipose tissue) or within the muscles. These stores of fat may be used as an energy source during times of low energy intake and/or high energy output. As an energy source triglycerides and fatty acids provide a major contribution to the energy requirements of the body. During exercise the release of body hormones such as adrenalin (epinephrine) will promote the breakdown and utilization of these fat stores.

Triglycerides are composed of fatty acids and glycerol in a ratio of 3:1, hence the name. Fatty acids may vary in size and structure and, chemically, may be classified as being saturated or unsaturated. These structural differences have implications for a 'healthy diet' with the unsaturated fats currently being preferred to the saturated varieties. Similarly, whilst cholesterol is an important fat, excessive amounts of cholesterol within the blood appear to be linked with an increased incidence of coronary heart disease. Fats are found in many common foods, especially in dairy products, oils and some meats. As an energy source fat is often used in combination with carbohydrate during exercise.

Protein

Protein is made up of amino acids. When a protein is eaten it is broken down by the process of digestion into its constituent amino acids. These are then absorbed into the blood stream and transported around the body to where they are needed. Amino acids are used as the 'building blocks' for constructing a person's own proteins, including those forming the structure of the muscle, enzymes which catalyze metabolic reactions and a number of hormones. Protein can be used as a source of energy but in the context of exercise it is usually of minor importance when compared with the contributions of carbohydrate and fat. Protein is, however, important for the repair of tissues and growth, both of which may be linked to exercise. Important sources of protein include meat, fish, eggs, soya and nuts.

Vitamins

Vitamins may be classified as being either water soluble (the B vitamins and vitamin C) or fat soluble (A, D, E and K). Vitamins fulfil a wide variety of key roles in many metabolic processes, including those of growth, repair and the energy pathways.

Minerals

The body requires a wide range of minerals which fulfil a wide variety of roles. Those of key importance in the context of exercise include:

- Iron (Fe), which forms part of the hemoglobin molecule found in red blood cells and is therefore important in the transportation of oxygen around the body.
- Calcium (Ca), used in the structure of bones and fulfils an important role in the process of muscle contraction.
- Phosphorus (P), used in the structure of bones.
- Sodium (Na), used in the transmission of nerve impulses.
- Potassium (K), used in the transmission of nerve impulses.

Water

Water is of vital importance to the body. It provides the fluid component of body fluids such as the blood and perspiration. It is therefore of key importance in the delivery of oxygen and nutrients around the body, the removal of waste products and the regulation of body temperature.

Fibre

Fibre or roughage is considered to be an important component of any healthy diet in preventing a number of gastrointestinal disorders.

Other substances, including alcohol

Other substances may be included in the diet in minor quantities and to some extent it is debatable as to whether they are 'food'. These include alcohol and caffeine, which are commonly ingested in most diets. In small doses their effect upon exercise metabolism is usually negligible, however they may be of concern in the context of health or the performance of the competitive athlete. In summary, these substances may have a beneficial or detrimental influence upon a person's physical capacity depending upon the individual, the type of exercise being undertaken and the quantity ingested.

DIETARY CONSIDERATIONS FOR EXERCISE

Current opinion is that the type of diet which is most appropriate for the exercising individual is the same as that which is generally recommended for health. This basically means that it should:

(a) be varied to ensure an intake of all essential nutrients;
(b) contain plenty of complex carbohydrates for energy;
(c) contain relatively little fat with an emphasis on the inclusion of unsaturated in preference to saturated fats;
(d) include appropriate amounts of protein, vitamins and minerals;
(e) include plenty of natural fibre;
(f) include plenty of fluids.

In practical terms this means a diet that contains:

(a) plenty of starch in the form of potatoes, bread and pasta;
(b) plenty of fresh fruit and vegetables, which will contain many of the essential vitamins and minerals required as well as starch;
(c) protein, which may be in the form of meat, fish, certain vegetables or dairy products.

The foods listed above will also contain some fat, with additional fat and sugar likely to be eaten in the form of spreads, cakes and confectionery, however, these may be omitted by those wishing to reduce this aspect of their diet. Overall, a person who is exercising regularly may need to eat more than one who is sedentary in order to achieve an energy balance, and to drink more fluid in order to maintain a fluid balance. However, beyond these slight adjustments no other alterations to the diet are considered necessary.

In terms of exercise one of the key aspects of nutrition is to maintain the body's stores of glycogen. As mentioned earlier, energy is stored as both glycogen and fat. However, whereas a person's fat stores are unlikely to be reduced to a level that inhibits exercise, it is possible for the glycogen stores to become depleted. If the glycogen stores do become depleted, leaving only fat as the available energy source, then this can dramatically reduce the capacity of the muscles to exercise. In physical terms glycogen depletion will make the individual feel weak and tired. Glycogen depletion can occur gradually over a period of days if the carbohydrate intake in the diet is insufficient to replace that which is being used. Alternatively, it can occur during prolonged endurance events and is commonly experienced by those running marathons. In this context glycogen depletion is referred to as 'hitting the wall' owing to the sudden onset of fatigue. Fat depletion is a long-term process, and whilst certain eating disorders may result in a person having very low stores of fat it is more often the case that a person's fat stores are somewhat larger than desirable, in which case the extra fat may inhibit their physical capacity by increasing their weight.

Adequate amounts of most vitamins and minerals will be eaten in a normal 'healthy' diet, although one mineral which may be deficient in some individuals is iron. An iron deficiency will reduce the physical capacity of individuals by limiting the amount of oxygen that they can transport in their blood. This will affect their aerobic capacity and may cause excessive tiredness and premature fatigue. Whilst these forms of anaemia occur in women and men they are more common amongst women due to a loss of blood during the menstrual cycle. In cases of anaemia a modification to the diet and/or iron supplements may be recommended.

The maintenance of body fluids is important prior to, during and after exercise since strenuous exercise will increase the loss of body fluid through perspiration. A significant loss of body fluid will reduce the capacity of the cardiovascular system and inhibit the body from regulating its temperature. This will result in an overall reduction in the individual's physical capacity, increase fatigue and in cases of severe dehydration, may cause permanent damage. Body fluid levels should therefore be maintained by regular intakes of water or similar fluids. The body can absorb approximately half a pint of fluid every half hour, replacement of this fluid becomes even more pertinent during hot weather when the rate of fluid loss during exercise can be far in excess of this. There is no value to be gained from depriving the body of water and in hot conditions it is advisable to drink before the onset of thirst. As a general indicator of appropriate body fluid levels the individual should be capable of producing copious amounts of dilute urine. Strong urine can indicate a state of fluid depletion which may be rectified by an increased intake of fluid.

ENERGY AND EXERCISE

If muscles are to work they need energy. This energy is obtained from the food consumed in the diet, with the principal energy sources being the carbohydrates and fats. Protein can also be utilized as a source of energy but its contribution during exercise is considered to be small relative to the other two components. The energy contained within food is used by the body to generate specific high-energy molecules that can be used in processes such as muscle contraction. The most important high-energy molecule that is synthesized by the body is adenosine triphosphate (ATP) and it is this molecule which muscles need in order to work. Millions of ATP molecules are used by the muscles during the process of muscular contraction. However, since ATP is a 'high-energy' molecule the body cannot store it in vast amounts. It is calculated that some muscles contain only enough ATP for approximately one second's worth of contraction. However, it must be in constant supply if the muscles are to work continuously and effectively. This constant supply is achieved via the body resynthesizing ATP as soon as it is used up: as the muscles use ATP, more molecules of ATP are produced thereby providing a continuous supply of this high-energy molecule and hence a continuous supply of usable energy for the working muscles.

The synthesis of ATP can be achieved via three metabolic systems or pathways:

1. The anaerobic alactic or phosphocreatine system
2. Anaerobic glycolysis or anaerobic lactic system
3. The aerobic system, which includes glycolysis (in the case of carbohydrates)

or beta-oxidation (in the case of fats), the Krebs cycle and the electron transport chain.

The use of these systems and their relative contribution in generating ATP during muscular work depends upon a number of factors, including the condition of the muscles, the intensity of the exercise, the availability of energy sources and the presence of metabolic waste products. Therefore, the three systems will initially be described separately and then their integration and usage will be discussed to illustrate their relative contribution during muscular activity.

It should also be realized that ATP is also used in a vast number of other metabolic processes within the body, not just muscle contraction. For example, it is used to provide the energy required in synthesis reactions of the body where molecules are constructed, in the ion pumps of the body which help to maintain the appropriate concentration of ions both inside and outside cells, and in any body reaction that requires energy. For such energy-requiring activities the synthesis of ATP will be similar to the processes described here (primarily using the aerobic system). However, in the context of this text it is necessary to concentrate upon the synthesis of ATP in the muscles. Since muscles require a lot of energy to perform their specialized function of contraction they need to have the capacity to synthesize large amounts of ATP. This is achieved through various physiological adaptations including an extensive blood supply and the presence of large numbers of specialized organelles such as mitochondria, which are the site of much of the ATP synthesis.

THE STRUCTURE OF ATP

Adenosine triphosphate is a complex molecule consisting of an adenosine unit with three inorganic phosphate molecules attached to it, hence the name (Figure 3.1).

The bond between the second and third phosphate groups is relatively unstable and can be broken to produce adenosine diphosphate (ADP) and inorganic phosphate (P_i). The energy released when this bond is broken can be harnessed and used in various metabolic activities of the body such as muscle contraction. In muscular contraction the high-energy ATP molecule is specifically linked to the process of cross-bridge cycling which is summarized below and illustrated in Figure 3.2:

1. A molecule of ATP becomes associated with the head of each myosin molecule (one ATP per myosin head).
2. The ATP molecule is converted into $ADP + P_i$ and the energy released 'charges' the myosin head causing it to change shape.
3. The ADP remains associated with the myosin head which becomes attached to a binding site on the actin molecule.
4. The ADP leaves the myosin head causing it to change shape, pulling the actin molecule past it.
5. Another ATP molecule becomes associated with the myosin which breaks away from the actin and is ready to repeat the process.

Since one ATP molecule is used up by each myosin head each time a new cross bridge is formed, the need for its rapid synthesis in large amounts can be appreciated.

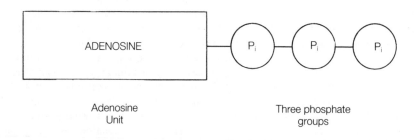

Adenosine
Unit

Three phosphate
groups

Figure 3.1 The structure of adenosine triphosphate (ATP).

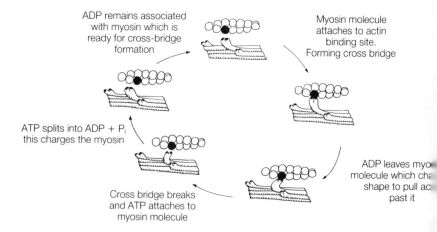

ADP remains associated
with myosin which is
ready for cross-bridge
formation

Myosin molecule
attaches to actin
binding site.
Forming cross bridge

ATP splits into ADP + P$_i$
this charges the myosin

ADP leaves myo
molecule which cha
shape to pull ac
past it

Cross bridge breaks
and ATP attaches to
myosin molecule

Figure 3.2 Illustrating the involvement of ATP in cross-bridge cycling.

Without the presence of ATP the process of cross-bridge cycling could not continue and hence the muscle would not be able to contract.

ATP SYNTHESIS

The synthesis of ATP involves the reforming of the bond between the second and third phosphates. This is part of a cyclic process with ATP being broken down into $ADP + P_i$ and then being resynthesized (Figure 3.3).

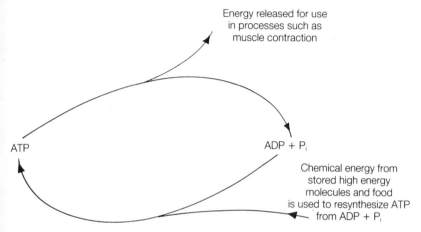

Figure 3.3 Illustrating the cyclic process of ATP breakdown and synthesis.

The energy for ATP resynthesis is derived from the energy contained within the food eaten, and the energy released from the breaking of the bond between the second and third phosphate groups is used to drive various metabolic reactions such as muscular contraction. Therefore, ATP provides the link between the energy contained in food and the energy used in muscle contraction and, in effect, it harnesses the energy stored within food in a way that can be used by muscles.

The next stage in understanding ATP synthesis is to study the various metabolic processes and pathways which cause the recombination of ADP and P_i and hence synthesize ATP. These have already been listed earlier in this section as:

1. The phosphocreatine system
2. Anaerobic glycolysis
3. The aerobic system (including glycolysis or beta-oxidation, the Krebs cycle and the electron transport chain.

THE ENERGY PATHWAYS

The phosphocreatine system

The phosphocreatine system is the simplest and most readily available method of

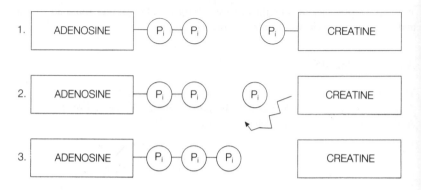

Figure 3.4 The phosphocreatine system.

resynthesizing ATP. The basic structure of phosphocreatine consists of an inorganic phosphate group (P_i) attached to a creatine molecule via a high-energy bond. When a muscle contracts the process of cross-bridge cycling causes the level of ATP in the muscle to fall whilst the amount of ADP + P_i in the muscle rises. This activates the phosphocreatine system and promotes a reaction between the phosphocreatine molecules and ADP. In this reaction the phosphocreatine molecules donate their phosphate groups and the energy associated with them to the ADP molecules, producing ATP and creatine (Figure 3.4).

The ATP generated from this reaction can then be used to continue to fuel the process of muscle contraction. The phosphocreatine system is a fairly uncomplicated process that is relatively quick and simple in metabolic terms. It provides a very readily available and easily accessible means of generating ATP when it is needed. Indeed, this system provides an almost instantaneous supply of ATP during the first few seconds of physical exertion. However, the muscles' stores of phosphocreatine are somewhat limited and become significantly depleted after only 5–6 seconds of intensive muscular activity. This means that for more prolonged forms of muscular activity, alternative energy pathways need to be employed.

Following intensive muscular activity the depleted phosphocreatine stores will need to be replenished. This is achieved by reversing the basic process during periods of low-intensity muscular work or rest. At this time the aerobic system (discussed later, page 96) produces excess amounts of ATP. Some of this excess ATP then reacts with the available creatine molecules. In this reaction the ATP molecules donate phosphate groups to the creatine molecules thereby resynthesizing phosphocreatine and ADP (Figure 3.5). In this way the stores are rapidly replenished, ready for the next bout of intensive muscular work.

Anaerobic glycolysis

Anaerobic glycolysis occurs in the fluid (cytoplasm) of the muscle cells. It involves the breakdown of glucose into pyruvic acid which, in the absence of oxygen, is then

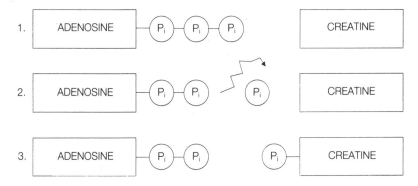

Figure 3.5 Illustrating the resynthesis of phosphocreatine.

converted into lactic acid. Hence the system is sometimes referred to as the anaerobic lactic system. This process will yield a total of two molecules of ATP for every molecule of glucose used. The starting point of glycolysis is often taken to be glucose, although in reality it could be a 'glucose unit' which is derived from the breakdown of glycogen (a polymer of glucose and the storage form of glucose in both the liver and the muscles). The breakdown of glucose to pyruvic acid also generates two pairs of hydrogen atoms which are picked up by the carrier molecule nicotinamide adenine dinucleotide (NAD) to form two molecules of $NADH_2$, the significance of which will be discussed later (p. 101) under the heading The electron transport chain.

The process of glycolysis involves approximately nine stages, each being controlled by specific enzymes. Overall each glucose molecule is eventually broken down into two molecules of pyruvic acid. During the process two molecules of ATP are used up but four are synthesized, therefore there is a net production of two ATP molecules. A more detailed description of glycolysis is illustrated in Figure 3.6.

At this point it should also be noted that the process of gycolysis also forms the first stage of the aerobic production of ATP. Both systems (anaerobic and aerobic) may be used concurrently but their relative contribution towards the production of ATP will depend upon the intensity of the muscular work being performed and the availability of oxygen within the muscle. If sufficient oxygen is available within the muscle then aerobic glycolysis will be the major energy pathway (the details of which are discussed later). If, however, there is insufficient oxygen present within the muscle or the demand for ATP is too large for it to be produced by the aerobic system alone, then anaerobic glycolysis will contribute towards the production of ATP. This will cause an accumulation of pyruvic acid which is then converted into lactic acid.

Being an acid, some of this lactic acid will dissociate into lactate and hydrogen ions (H^+). These hydrogen ions make the muscle more acidic (i.e. cause a fall in pH) and if there is a sufficient build-up of these hydrogen ions then fatigue ensues. This is felt by a burning, aching sensation in the muscles during intensive muscular work and, owing to the increased acidity, various functions associated with muscular contraction are inhibited. This includes the process of cross-bridge cycling and the production of ATP due to the inhibition of some enzymes involved in anaerobic

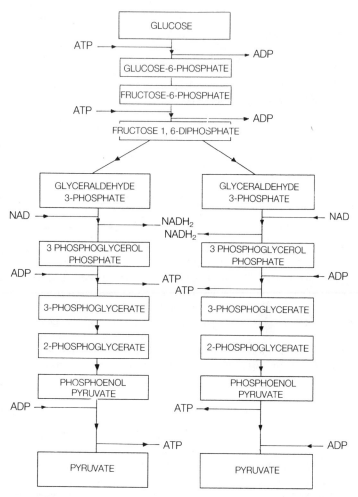

Figure 3.6 Glycolysis.

glycolysis, especially the enzyme phosphofructokinase. For this reason the anaerobic production of ATP cannot be used very extensively for prolonged periods of time; therefore the primary means of generating ATP is via the aerobic system, with the additional anaerobic lactic process being used to supplement the production of ATP during shorter bursts of more intensive muscular activity, when the supply of oxygen to the muscles limits the rate at which the aerobic process can function.

The aerobic production of ATP

The aerobic system provides the muscles with a continuous supply of ATP and, as the name implies, it requires oxygen. It is used under conditions of both rest and exercise. The system also uses both carbohydrate and fat, which means that its fuel reserves are far more extensive than those of the phosphocreatine system and unlike anaerobic glycolysis it does not produce fatigue-inducing lactic acid. This makes the aerobic system the primary source of ATP during low-intensity exercise and a significant contributor to the supply of ATP in more intensive activites, when it is used in combination with the two anaerobic systems.

The aerobic system may be divided up into three stages:

1. Glycolysis (in the case of glucose) or beta-oxidation (in the case of fats)
2. Krebs cycle, also called 'The citric acid cycle' or the 'tricarboxylic acid cycle' (TCA cycle).
3. The electron transport chain.

Glycolysis and beta-oxidation

Glycolysis The process of glycolysis was discussed earlier as a separate anaerobic system for the generation of ATP (Figure 3.6). However, if sufficient oxygen is available within the muscle the pyruvic acid that is produced by glycolysis is preferentially converted into acetyl coenzyme A and enters into the mitochondria (specialized organelles within the muscle) rather than being converted into lactic acid. This means that in the presence of oxygen ATP is produced without an accumulation of lactic acid and thus has the advantage of providing the energy for muscle contraction without causing fatigue. An additional advantage of the aerobic system is that the resultant acetyl coenzyme A can be further metabolized to produce even more ATP. Overall this means that far more energy is made available from the aerobic breakdown of glucose than via its anaerobic breakdown.

Key aspects of 'glycolysis' and its role within the aerobic system are as follows:

1. Glycolysis uses carbohydrate in the form of glucose or 'glucose units' which are derived from the breakdown of glycogen.
2. The first stage of carbohydrate metabolism is identical to that already discussed for anaerobic glycolysis. However, in the presence of adequate amounts of oxygen within the muscle the pyruvate is converted into an acetyl group and carbon dioxide is given off.
3. The acetyl groups react with molecules of coenzyme A to form acetyl coenzyme A, which then enter into the mitochondria of the cell. These combine with oxaloacetic acid to form citric acid (Figure 3.7). Citric acid is the starting molecule for the Krebs cycle, the second component of the aerobic system.
4. In the absence of adequate amounts of oxygen excess pyruvate is converted into lactic acid, the accumulation of which causes fatigue. This anaerobic breakdown of glucose into lactic acid can be referred to as the anaerobic lactate pathway.

Therefore it can be seen that the reliance upon the anaerobic lactate pathway depends upon the availability of oxygen within the muscle, with the aerobic system being used in preference whenever possible. Indeed, as will be discussed in the later sections, a major determinant of an individual's capacity to

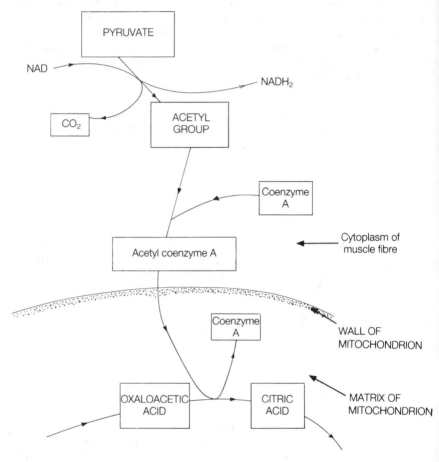

Figure 3.7 The conversion of pyruvate into acetyl coenzyme A and its entry into the mitochondrion.

perform prolonged forms of low-intensity muscular activity depends upon his or her ability to supply the muscles with oxygen. Furthermore, one of the major adaptations of the muscle to aerobic exercise is to increase the muscle's ability to use oxygen through increasing the capacity of the aerobic pathway within the muscle.

In summary, glycolysis results in the conversion of glucose molecules into pyruvic acid molecules (two pyruvic acid molecules for each glucose used) with a net gain of two ATP molecules per glucose used. The two pyruvic acid molecules can then be modified and enter into the mitochondria where they will be broken down further in a process that will ultimately produce more ATP.

Beta-oxidation As stated earlier, fat can also be metabolized aerobically to produce ATP; however, its initial metabolism is somewhat different to that of glucose. Fatty acids are a major energy source which the body utilizes both at rest and during exercise. Fatty acids consist of long chains of carbon atoms each of which has a number of hydrogen atoms attached to it. In order for fats to be used as an energy source they need to be broken down. Essentially the long chains of carbon atoms are broken down into small acetyl groups via a process called beta-oxidation. The acetyl groups then react with coenzyme A to produce acetyl coenzyme A which enters the mitochondria and participates in the Krebs cycle in the same way as the acetyl coenzyme A formed from glycolysis.

Krebs cycle

The Krebs cycle is named after the scientist (Hans Krebs) who carried out much of the original work into it. It is also known as the citric acid cycle or the tricarboxylic acid (TCA) cycle. The Krebs cycle occurs within the matrix of the mitochondria (Figure 3.8).

The Krebs cycle follows on from glycolysis or beta-oxidation, both of which result in acetyl coenzyme A entering the mitochondria. In the mitochondria coenzyme A breaks away from the acetyl group and moves back out of the mitochondria to collect another acetyl group, i.e. it acts as a carrier molecule which transports acetyl groups into the mitochondria. The acetyl groups left in the mitochondria combine with oxaloacetic acid to form citric acid. The Krebs cycle then consists of the sequential breakdown of citric acid back into oxaloacetic acid (Figure 3.9).

This breakdown process involves numerous enzyme-mediated steps and at various stages energy is released which may be gainfully used to synthesize ATP either directly or at a later stage. Upon completion of the cycle the oxaloacetic acid recombines with another acetyl group to once again form citric acid and hence the process is repeated in a cyclic manner.

During the Krebs cycle various products are produced, including ATP, carbon dioxide, pairs of hydrogen atoms and guanosine triphosphate (GTP). The carbon dioxide produced by the aerobic system (during the conversion of pyruvate into an acetyl group and during the Krebs cycle) diffuses out of the muscle fibre and eventually passes into the blood. In the blood the carbon dioxide is transported to the lungs

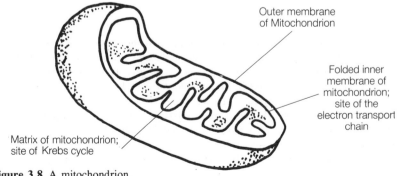

Outer membrane of Mitochondrion

Folded inner membrane of mitochondrion; site of the electron transport chain

Matrix of mitochondrion; site of Krebs cycle

Figure 3.8 A mitochondrion.

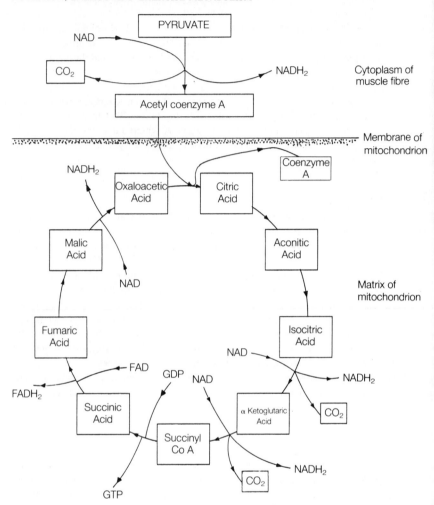

Figure 3.9 The Krebs cycle.

where it is exhaled. For each acetyl group (whether produced from glycolysis or beta-oxidation), two carbon dioxide molecules are produced in the Krebs cycle. For each pyruvic acid that is produced via glycolysis, one carbon dioxide molecule is produced in its conversion into an acetyl group and two are produced during the Krebs cycle. Since two pyruvic acid molecules are produced from each glucose molecule two carbon dioxide molecules are produced in the initial conversion of the two pyruvate molecules into the two acetyl groups. These are added to the two carbon dioxide molecules produced during each Krebs cycle, making a total production of six carbon dioxide molecules for each glucose molecule.

The Krebs cycle also results in the production of pairs of hydrogen atoms. These are picked up by two kinds of carrier molecules: nicotinamide adenine dinucleotide (NAD) and flavin adenine dinucleotide (FAD). These carriers are coenzymes which transport the hydrogen atoms to the next stage in the process (the electron transport chain). Hydrogen atoms are also produced during glycolysis and these are likewise picked up by NAD with two $NADH_2$ molecules being produced for each glucose molecule entering glycolysis. Later in the process, during its conversion into an acetyl group, pyruvic acid loses a further two hydrogen atoms and as a result two more $NADH_2$ molecules are produced for each initial glucose molecule. In each Krebs cycle four more pairs of hydrogen atoms are produced. This results in three molecules of $NADH_2$ and one of $FADH_2$. Since two molecules of acetyl coenzyme A are produced from each glucose molecule the cycle is repeated twice for each initial glucose molecule. Thus the Krebs cycle produces six $NADH_2$ and two $FADH_2$ molecules for each glucose molecule. Therefore, the breakdown of each glucose molecule in the processes of glycolysis, the conversion of pyruvate into acetyl coenzyme A and Krebs cycle produces a total of ten $NADH_2$ and two $FADH_2$ molecules.

Each Krebs cycle also produces one molecule of GTP, which can be considered to be equivalent to ATP as GTP reacts with ADP to produce ATP and GDP. So, for each glucose molecule, the Krebs cycle is considered to produce two ATP molecules (one per cycle). Thus, so far each glucose molecule which has entered the processes of glycolysis and the Krebs cycle has resulted in the net production of four molecules of ATP, ten of $NADH_2$, two of $FADH_2$ and six of carbon dioxide.

Each acetyl group which was produced from the breakdown of fat will undergo the same process in the Krebs cycle and hence will produce three $NADH_2$ molecules and one $FADH_2$. These hydrogen atoms are then transported by their carriers to the next stage of the process, 'the electron transport chain', during which some of the energy they contain is used to produce more ATP. Indeed, the majority of ATP molecules which are produced during the aerobic breakdown of glucose or fat are in fact produced during this third and final stage of the aerobic system.

The electron transport chain

This consists of a series of carrier molecules which are situated in the inner membrane of the mitochondria (see Figure 3.8). They are strategically organized to facilitate the passage of hydrogen atoms or electrons from one carrier to the next. At various stages in the transfer of the hydrogen atoms and electrons down the system energy becomes 'available' and this energy may be used to synthesize ATP from ADP and P_i (Figure 3.10). During the electron transport chain the hydrogen atoms are initially passed from NAD to FAD (bar, of course, those that were directly picked up by FAD from the Krebs cycle). This transfer produces one ATP molecule, and since each glucose unit produced ten $NADH_2$ a total of ten ATP molecules are produced at this stage. The next stage in the process involves the hydrogen atoms being passed from FAD to coenzyme Q (also known as ubiquinone). At this point the hydrogen atoms dissociate into hydrogen ions (H^+) and electrons (e^-). The electrons are then passed from ubiquinone along a series of cytochrome carriers: cytochrome b, cytochrome c, cytochtome a and cytochrome a_3. During the transfer from cytochrome b to cytochrome c and from cytochrome a to cytochrome a_3, ATP

101

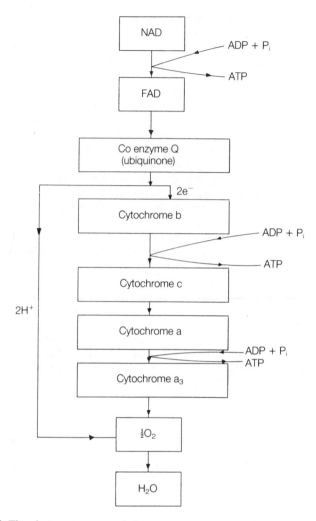

Figure 3.10 The electron transport chain.

is produced. So for each glucose unit (which produced ten $NADH_2$ molecules and two $FADH_2$) a further 24 ATP molecules are produced. Thus, for each glucose molecule a total of 34 ATP molecules are produced in the electron transport chain: three for each of the ten $NADH_2$ and two for each of the two $FADH_2$. In summary, therefore, each molecule of glucose which is broken down via the aerobic system produces a total of 38 ATP: two from glycolysis, two from the Krebs cycle and 34 from the electron transport chain (see Figure 3.11 for details).

The final electron acceptor in the electron transport chain is oxygen, which reacts with the electrons and hydrogen ions to produce water. The rate at which the whole

Process	Products per glucose unit		Net production of ATP after electron transport chain
Glycolysis	2 ATP	$\longrightarrow$	2 ATP
	2 NADH$_2$	$\longrightarrow$	6 ATP
Formation of acetyl coenzyme	2 NADH$_2$	$\longrightarrow$	6 ATP
Krebs cycle	2 GTP	$\longrightarrow$	2 ATP
	6 NADH$_2$	$\longrightarrow$	18 ATP
	2 FADH$_2$	$\longrightarrow$	4 ATP
Total			38 ATP
Summary equation	$C_6H_{12}O_6 + 6 O_2 \longrightarrow 6 CO_2 + 6 H_2O$ Glucose Oxygen Carbon Water dioxide		

Figure 3.11 Table summarizing the production of ATP from the aerobic system.

system can work largely depends upon the availability of oxygen. In effect an inadequate supply of oxygen can be visualized as causing a 'bottleneck' in the system much like a traffic jam. This means that even if the process of glycolysis is accelerated to produce more ATP, the pyruvate can only enter into the Krebs cycle at the rate determined by the supply of oxygen. Therefore, if glycolysis is greatly accelerated (as occurs during strenuous muscular activity) much of the excess pyruvate will not be able to enter the Krebs cycle. Instead it starts to accumulate and is converted into lactic acid. The build-up of lactic acid then makes the muscles more acidic and hence causes fatigue.

THE USE OF THE ENERGY PATHWAYS DURING EXERCISE

The two anaerobic systems (phosphocreatine and anaerobic glycolysis) tend to be used either in the early stages of muscular activity before the aerobic system has had a chance to respond to the increased demands for ATP, or during very intensive periods of muscular activity when the aerobic system is unable to generate ATP at a fast

Substrate	Energy yield per litre of oxygen (Kcal)	Energy yield per gram of substrate (Kcal)
Glucose	5.05	4.02
Fat	4.74	8.98

Figure 3.12 Table summarizing the ATP yields from glucose and fat.

enough rate to meet the demands of the muscles. Therefore, the anaerobic systems may be considered to supplement the supply of ATP that is constantly produced by the aerobic system. In reality, therefore, it is not just a matter of turning the systems on or off or switching from one to the another, but of the systems being used together with the relevant pathways and metabolic reactions being phased in and out.

During exercise the relative contribution of each pathway towards the production of ATP depends upon:

(a) the intensity of the exercise;
(b) the state of various physiological factors; and
(c) the body's capacity to cope with the demands of the activity.

In terms of energy yield (ATP production) per unit of oxygen, glucose is a more economical energy store than fat (Figure 3.12). If, however, fat and glucose are compared in terms of energy yield (ATP production) per unit of weight then 1 gram of fat produces more energy (ATP) than 1 gram of glucose. Hence, in terms of weight fat may be considered to be more economical. These ideas can be expanded upon when further considering the energy stores and ATP production; that is, it is advantageous to store fat because, per unit of energy, it weighs less and can provide energy at an adequate rate when working at low intensities. However, fat cannot be utilized as rapidly as carbohydrate and requires the use of more oxygen (which is a limiting factor during muscular activity of a high intensity). This means that during most forms of physical activity a combination of fat and carbohydrate (glucose or glycogen) is used, with a greater proportion of carbohydrate being used as the intensity of the exercise increases.

Under conditions of strenuous muscular activity the amount of oxygen available in the muscles becomes inadequate to supply ATP at the required rate via the aerobic system. The muscles, therefore, utilize the anaerobic pathways to supplement the production of ATP. At this point it should be noted that the phosphocreatine system is also used in the initial stages of muscular activity since there may be a slight delay between the commencement of more strenuous muscular activity and the increased activity of the aerobic system. The phosphocreatine system will therefore be used to provide additional ATP until the aerobic system has increased its ATP production to cope sufficiently with the new increased rate of demand (if it can).

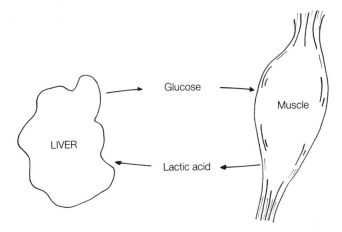

Figure 3.13 The Cori cycle.

During strenuous physical activity some of the lactic acid produced will diffuse out of the muscles into the blood. It will then be transported via the blood to the liver where it will be converted back into glucose. This glucose will then be released back into the blood and transported to the exercising muscles for use as an energy source. The overall process of producing lactic acid from glucose and then converting it back into glucose is called the Cori cycle (Figure 3.13). The Cori cycle is of significant importance during prolonged periods of exercise as it helps to prevent fatigue by, firstly, reducing the amount of lactic acid and, secondly, sustaining the body's glycogen stores.

Following strenuous muscular activity during which the anaerobic systems have been used, the aerobic system operates to facilitate recovery from the exercise. After a bout of exercise the aerobic system will produce excess ATP which can be utilized to resynthesize the phosphocreatine stores and reduce the amount of lactic acid that will have accumulated. This is often referred to as 'repaying the oxygen debt' and explains why people continue to breathe hard and have a heart rate that is higher than their resting rate for some time after they have ceased the exercise.

PHYSIOLOGICAL RESPONSES BEFORE, DURING AND AFTER EXERCISE

When changing from a state of rest to one of physical activity there is an increase in the amount of energy that is needed by the muscles. This will result in an increased production of metabolic waste products such as carbon dioxide and heat. In order to facilitate the increased use of energy, to prevent a rapid build-up of waste products and to maintain body temperature within acceptable limits, a number of physiological responses occur before, during and after exercise. These may be considered under the following headings:

1. Pulmonary responses
2. Cardiovascular responses
3. Hormonal responses

Pulmonary responses

The lungs provide the site of gaseous exchange between the air and the cardiovascular system. Within the lungs the inhaled air that is high in oxygen oxygenates the blood whilst the blood releases carbon dioxide into the lungs. This is then breathed out with the exhaled air. Air which is inhaled contains approximately 79% nitrogen, 21% oxygen and small traces of other gases such as carbon dioxide. Exhaled air typically contains 79% nitrogen, 16% oxygen, 4% carbon dioxide and small traces of other gases. Whilst the precise amounts of oxygen and carbon dioxide in expired air will vary depending upon the individual and their state of activity, the important points to note are the decrease in oxygen with a corresponding, although not always exact, increase in carbon dioxide. The oxygen consumption and production of carbon dioxide are a direct result of the activity of the aerobic energy pathway that is used to generate the ATP that is required for muscle contraction. In terms of volume, a person at rest may use about 0.5 litres of oxygen per minute and produce a similar amount of carbon dioxide.

The energy demands of most forms of exercise will result in an increase in the activity of the aerobic pathway. This will therefore increase the muscles' need for oxygen and their production of carbon dioxide. During strenuous forms of exercise a person's oxygen consumption can rise to over 3.5 litres per minute and in excess of 5 litres in élite endurance athletes. To supply the muscles' demand for more oxygen, both the rate and depth of breathing are increased. At rest a person's breathing rate may be 12 times per minute and the volume of each breath approximately 0.5 litres. This results in a 'pulmonary ventilation' of 6 litres per minute ($12 \times 0.5 = 6.0$). During strenuous exercise there is a significant increase in these respiratory parameters. The rate of breathing may increase to 45 breaths per minute whilst the volume of air inhaled with each breath may increase to 3 litres. This produces a pulmonary ventilation of 135 litres per minute. The precise values for pulmonary ventilation will depend upon the individual, his or her lung capacity and the intensity of the exercise. In basic terms this increase in pulmonary ventilation substantially increases the amount of oxygen getting into the lungs and the amount of carbon dioxide that is removed from the lungs. This, therefore, facilitates the oxygenation of the blood (which then transports the oxygen to the muscles) and the removal from the body of the carbon dioxide that the blood has transported from the muscles.

An increase in pulmonary ventilation may be observed before, during and after exercise. The slight increase that may occur before exercise is an 'anticipatory response' which helps to prepare the body for the exercise. These preparatory changes in pulmonary ventilation are stimulated by the activity of the sympathetic nervous system and sympathetic hormones such as adrenalin (epinephrine). Once physical activity has commenced these neural and hormonal inputs will continue to promote pulmonary ventilation with the strength of their stimulation depending upon:

- the acidity of the blood and cerebrospinal fluid
- carbon dioxide production
- oxygen consumption
- heat production
- joint movement.

All these factors are related to an increase in muscular activity which increases oxygen consumption, carbon dioxide production and heat production. An increase in carbon dioxide production will also result in an increase in the acidity of the blood and cerebrospinal fluid owing to the reaction between the carbon dioxide and the water of the body fluids which produces carbonic acid:

$$\underset{\substack{\text{Carbon-}\\\text{dioxide}}}{CO_2} + \underset{\text{Water}}{H_2O} \longrightarrow \underset{\substack{\text{Carbonic}\\\text{acid}}}{H_2CO_3}$$

Strenuous exercise will also result in the production of lactic acid which will make the blood and cerebrospinal fluid even more acidic, thereby further increasing pulmonary ventilation. The pulmonary response to exercise is therefore in proportion to its intensity. Other factors, such as heat production and joint movement, which also influence pulmonary ventilation, are also likely to occur in proportion to the exercise intensity.

Upon completion of a bout of exercise the body does not immediately return to its resting state because, during the exercise, there may have been an accumulation of waste products and heat, along with a depletion of energy stores and oxygen. For these reasons the pulmonary ventilation may remain elevated until these factors have been restored to their resting levels, which will usually occur within a few minutes of the end of the exercise but will again depend upon the type, intensity and duration of the exercise as well as the fitness of the participant.

Cardiovascular responses

The function of the cardiovascular system is to transport the blood around the body. The heart acts as a pump, the contraction of which moves the blood through the blood vessels. The heart is made of cardiac muscle and consists of two parts: a left side and a right side. Each side is divided into two chambers: an atria which receives blood from either the body or the lungs and a ventricle which pumps blood to either the body or the lungs. In a normal heart the blood cannot pass directly from one side to another and the two sides of the heart contract together in synchrony. At rest the heart may beat approximately 72 times per minute. At rest each side of the heart will eject approximately 70 ml of blood each time it contracts. Blood ejected from the right side of the heart is transported via the pulmonary arteries to the lungs where it is oxygenated and gives up its carbon dioxide (Figure 3.14). It then returns to the left side of the heart. The left side of the heart then pumps the oxygenated blood to the muscles and other parts of the body. As the blood passes through tissues and organs, such as the muscles, it will give up its oxygen and collect waste products such as carbon dioxide. This 'deoxygenated' blood then returns to the right side of the heart to be pumped back to the lungs and the cycle is repeated.

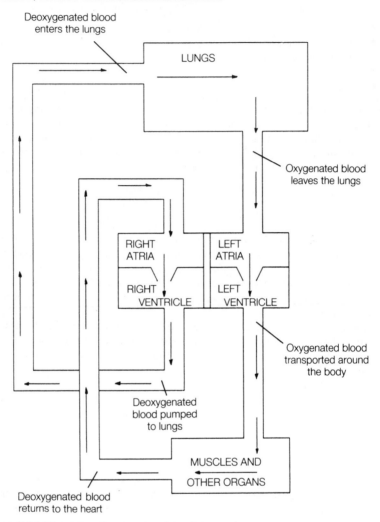

Figure 3.14 Diagrammatic representation of the cardiorespiratory system.

The frequency with which the heart contracts is known as the heart rate (HR) – in beats per minute (bpm) – while the amount of blood ejected by each side of the heart with each beat is called the stroke volume (SV). Together these parameters determine the amount of blood which is ejected by each side of the heart each minute, this is called the cardiac output (CO). The cardiac output of an individual will depend upon a number of factors, including their age, gender, size and current state of activity. Typical resting values for an adult would be as follows:

$$72 \times 70 = 5040$$

(bpm)	(ml per beat)	(ml per minute)
Heart rate	Stroke volume	Cardiac output

So for an adult a typical resting cardiac output would be in the region of 5 litres per minute.

To supply muscles with more oxygen during exercise the cardiovascular system has to increase its delivery of oxygenated blood to the muscles. This will also facilitate the removal of waste products and assist with the process of thermoregulation, as the blood takes away heat from the active muscles. An overall increase in the supply of blood and, hence, oxygen to the muscles is achieved via:

(a) an increase in cardiac output;
(b) changes in the circulation of blood around the body.

An increase in cardiac output occurs through a combination of an increase in heart rate and stroke volume, both of which increase in proportion to the intensity of the exercise. During intensive forms of exercise the heart rate may increase to around 180 bpm whilst the stroke volume may increase to 140 ml per beat. This will result in a cardiac output of approximately 25 litres per minute.

In addition to an overall increase in the cardiac output during exercise, the distribution of blood around the body can also be adjusted. This is achieved via the vasodilation of blood vessels which supply the exercising muscles and the vasoconstriction of blood vessels that lead to other areas such as the gut. This results in an increased proportion of blood going to the muscles which are a 'priority' area during exercise, whilst organs that are not very active during exercise receive a smaller proportion of the blood supply. Furthermore, the increased blood supply to the muscles will also increase their supply of important energy sources such as glucose and fat.

Prior to exercise there may be an 'anticipatory' rise in heart rate, with slight changes in the circulation. More substantial changes in cardiac output and circulation occur during exercise and are brought about by:

- neural influences
- hormones
- intrinsic factors.

The neural influences refer to an increase in the activity of the sympathetic nervous system along with a decrease in the activity of the parasympathetic nervous system. This has the effect of increasing the heart rate and stroke volume as well as effecting the dilation or constriction of appropriate blood vessels.

The hormonal changes primarily refer to an increased secretion of the sympathetic hormones adrenalin and noradrenalin (epinephrine and norepinephrine) into the blood stream. These hormones bring about similar effects to those of the sympathetic nervous system.

The intrinsic factors affecting cardiac output relate to a stretch reflex within the heart. During exercise blood returns to the heart at a faster rate, which causes an increased filling of the chambers of the heart and causes the walls of the heart to be stretched. This stretching results in a more forceful contraction of the heart so that more blood is ejected with each beat. Within the circulation intrinsic factors include changes in the acidity, carbon dioxide and oxygen levels within the blood, which will induce the vasodilation of blood vessels within the exercising muscles.

During strenuous exercise there may be an accumulation of metabolic waste products within the body and an oxygen debt may occur. For these reasons the cardiac output is likely to remain above its resting level for some time after the exercise has ceased. During this 'recovery period' the enhanced blood supply to the muscles will help to repay the oxygen debt and remove any waste products. Thus the cardiovascular responses to exercise will continue until the levels of acidity, carbon dioxide, oxygen and temperature have been restored to an appropriate level.

The most significant influences on cardiac output and circulation are:

- the acidity of the blood and cerebrospinal fluid
- carbon dioxide production
- oxygen consumption
- heat production.

From this it can be seen that between them the pulmonary and cardiovascular responses of the body increase the supply of blood, oxygen and other nutrients to the exercising muscles. They also enhance the removal of metabolic waste products that would induce premature fatigue. It can also be seen that factors which stimulate the pulmonary and cardiovascular responses are similar and that the extent of their responses are in proportion to the intensity of the exercise.

Hormonal responses

The hormonal changes observed before, during and after exercise are complex. The precise nature of such changes depends upon the type of exercise, the intensity of the exercise, the duration of the exercise and the fitness of the individual. In summary, the majority of these changes are associated with:

(a) increasing the supply of nutrients and oxygen to the muscle;
(b) removing metabolic waste products; and
(c) promoting the repair and growth of tissue after the exercise, which will include promoting the general improvements in the condition of the muscles and other associated tissues that occur with regular exercise.

Almost all the hormones of the body affect or are affected by exercise in some way. Very often their actions are interrelated, making the topic of exercise endocrinology complex. Therefore, only a brief summary of the effects of a few key hormones are given.

Adrenalin and noradrenalin (epinephrine and norepinephrine)

The secretion of these hormones from the adrenal medulla of the adrenal glands increases both prior to and during exercise. They stimulate a number of pulmonary and cardiovascular responses that promote an increase in the supply of blood and oxygen to the exercising muscles. They also stimulate the release of glucose from the liver and fatty acids from adipose tissue. In summary, they therefore enhance the supply of energy to the muscles as well as promote its utilization and the removal of waste products.

110

Growth hormone

The secretion of this hormone increases during exercise. It has a number of effects upon the body, including promoting the release of fat for use as an energy source and the repair/growth of tissues after exercise.

Testosterone

Testosterone is an anabolic (growth-promoting) hormone as well as being androgenic (promoting the male secondary sexual characteristics). In the context of exercise its primary role is in the growth and repair of tissues following a bout of exercise. Anabolic steroids mimic both the androgenic and anabolic effects of testosterone, which causes them to be used by participants in a number of sports to enhance their athletic performance.

Cortisol

This hormone promotes the production of glucose from other metabolites via a process called gluconeogenesis. This additional glucose is a significant source of energy during prolonged forms of exercise. On a long-term basis excessive over-training may result in the overproduction of cortisol. This produces an imbalance between it and other hormones. The suggested effects of such an imbalance include suppression of the immune system which makes those who overtrain more vulnerable to minor infections such as colds and flu.

Erythropoetin

This hormone promotes the production of red blood cells. It is therefore produced in response to exercise and enhances the oxygen-carrying capacity of the blood.

Summary

In summary, when moving from a state of rest to a state of exercise there is an increase in the energy requirements of muscles. This increase is proportional to the intensity of the exercise. In response to increased energy needs, a number of pulmonary, cardiovascular and hormonal changes occur within the body. These changes increase the muscles' supply of oxygen and nutrients such as glucose and fat. They will also facilitate the removal of metabolic products such as carbon dioxide, lactic acid and heat (accumulation of which causes premature fatigue). Since these responses take time to come into full effect they have implications for considerations such as gradually increasing the exercise intensity during an exercise session and, similarly, gradually reducing its intensity at the end of the session. These considerations are discussed more fully in the section 'Warming up and cooling down' on page 122.

THE CAUSES OF FATIGUE

Physiological fatigue may be considered to be a state in which the maintenance of a certain intensity of exercise is inhibited or prevented. There are many suggested causes of fatigue, several of which may act simultaneously to produce the overall sensation and inhibit muscle contraction. The causes of fatigue may be considered under four headings:

1. The depletion of energy stores
2. The accumulation of inhibitory metabolic waste products
3. Dehydration
4. Neurological fatigue

Although these factors are listed separately, they are often interrelated and will frequently occur simultaneously.

The depletion of energy stores

During extremely intensive short-duration muscular activity, such as weight training and sprinting, it is possible for the muscle's stores of ATP and phosphocreatine to become depleted. However, they are rapidly replenished and even in these forms of activity they are generally considered to be of secondary importance in causing fatigue when compared with the effects of an accumulation of metabolic waste products such as lactic acid.

During physical activity that is sustained for several minutes it is usual for both fat and carbohydrate (in the form of glucose or glycogen) to be used as an energy source. If the duration of the activity is in excess of 90 minutes it is possible for the glycogen stores of the body to be significantly reduced. This 'glycogen depletion', with its consequent lowering of blood glucose levels, will result in the muscles being deprived of this important energy source and thus making them more dependent upon fat. Unfortunately, fat cannot be used to generate ATP at a very rapid rate which means that the rate of supply of ATP to the muscles slows down. This greatly inhibits their capacity to contract, and induces a situation – commonly experienced by marathon runners near the end of a race – termed 'hitting the wall'. Whilst glycogen depletion is less likely during exercise of a shorter duration, a diet that is deficient in carbohydrate may cause a steady depletion of the glycogen stores over a period of days and this form of fatigue can then occur with exercise that is sustained for less than 90 minutes.

The accumulation of inhibitory metabolic waste products

During very strenuous muscular activity ATP is produced via the anaerobic pathways. This supplements the aerobic production of ATP which may not be producing ATP at a fast enough rate for the demands of the muscle. If substantial amounts of ATP are produced via anaerobic glycolysis there will be an accumulation of lactic acid making the muscle more acidic. The increase in acidity has an inhibitory effect upon a number of the processes that lead to muscle contraction.

1. The production of glycolysis can be inhibited, thereby inhibiting further production of ATP. The increase in acidity is specifically thought to inhibit the enzyme phosphofructokinase which controls one of the key stages of glycolysis.
2. The contractile process of cross-bridge cycling can be inhibited. Here the increase in acidity may inhibit the release of calcium ions from the sarcoplasmic reticulum and/or their binding to the troponin molecule.

The increase in acidity will also be detected as a burning sensation or pain within the muscles. This is a relatively short-term form of fatigue as the level of lactic acid will fall rapidly upon cessation of the exercise and will return to its resting levels within a few minutes.

Dehydration

During prolonged forms of exercise the body may sweat profusely in order to regulate its temperature. The hotter and more humid the environment the greater the sweat loss is likely to be. If fluid is not replaced during exercise the participant can rapidly become dehydrated. This reduction in fluid volume will affect the efficiency of the cardiovascular system, reducing its capacity to supply the muscles with oxygen. This may therefore contribute towards other forms of fatigue. If the state of dehydration persists then the participant may stop sweating in order to conserve body fluids. This will reduce the body's ability to lose heat and may rapidly lead to overheating (hyperthermia). If body temperatue rises to a few degrees above its optimum, many metabolic reactions will be impaired due to the sensitivity of enzymes to temperature. In extreme cases dehydration can lead to collapse, which if not treated may be fatal. Thus a state of semi-dehydration will reduce the capacity of the body to exercise and cause a form of general fatigue. Dehydration may be prevented or reduced by a regular intake of fluids before, during and after exercise. Half a pint every half hour in hot conditions is recommended by many authorities.

Neurological causes

Possible neurological causes of fatigue include the depletion of acetyl choline at the neuromuscular junction and/or neurotransmitter at synapses. In this context it has also been suggested that fatigue could occur within the central nervous system. The precise physiological nature of central nervous system fatigue is complex but may be significant in prolonged forms of exercise. Repeated use of the joints may also contribute towards a general feeling of fatigue during endurance type activity.

A note of caution

In addition to the causes of fatigue outlined in this section a general feeling of fatigue is also associated with certain disorders such as post-viral fatigue syndrome and anaemia. Fatigue may also occur when the body is combating a minor disease such as a cold or 'flu and in these circumstances it would be unwise to exercise. Therefore, although certain types of fatigue (normally short term) are naturally associated with strenuous exercise, the participants and their supervisors should be wary of other types that are of a more general nature and could indicate a disorder or illness. It should also be stressed at this point that severe fatigue or exhaustion is often unnecessary during an exercise session. In many cases an exercise intensity that induces mild fatigue will be sufficient to stimulate the desired benefits: the condition of exhaustion is often only an occasional necessity to those involved in competitive sport.

4

The principles of exercise
and fitness training

EXERCISE PRINCIPLES AND TERMINOLOGY

When discussing the effects of exercise upon the body and suggesting appropriate exercises, certain principles need to be considered. With some slight modification these principles are appropriate for anyone participating in exercise, ranging from the myocardial infarction patient or stroke victim to the athlete rehabilitating from a strained muscle. These principles may be discussed under the following headings:

1. The training effect
2. Overload
3. Specificity
4. Intensity
5. Duration
6. Frequency
7. Recovery
8. Progression
9. Reversibility

The principles are applicable in a variety of conditions and circumstances, including the applied activity-related situations used by the occupational therapist and the exercise areas which may be available to nurses, physiotherapists and other specialists whether in the hospital setting, the home or the gymnasium.

The training effect

Appropriate forms of exercise provide a stimulus for the body to improve its physical capacity. If an appropriate form of exercise is repeated often enough it will promote long-term adaptations to the exercise: this is called the 'training effect'. The type of adaptations, and hence the training effect induced by exercise, are very specific to that form of exercise. For example:

(a) strengthening exercises will stimulate the muscles and tendons to adapt by becoming stronger;

(b) aerobic exercises will stimulate an improvement in the cardiovascular system via changes in the condition of the heart, blood vessels and even the muscles themselves;

(c) stretching exercises produce a training effect that can be observed as improvements in an individual's flexibility/mobility.

Training effects may be observed within days or weeks of commencing an exercise programme. The rapidity and extent of improvement will depend upon a number of factors, including the nature of the exercises being undertaken and the condition of the participant.

Overload

Overload refers to the principle that in order to stimulate an improvement in the physical condition of the body, it must experience a suitable amount of physical stress – that is, it must experience certain physical stresses that are greater than those it would normally encounter during everyday life. Practically speaking, this means that in order to improve an individual's flexibility at a joint, the muscles and tendons associated with that joint must be stretched in an appropriate manner. This stretch may be achieved by the individual or with the assistance of another person or external object. However, the overall effect will be the same, i.e. moving the joint/limb beyond the range of motion it would normally encounter in everyday life.

The principle of overload can also be illustrated in the development or maintenance of muscular strength. In order for a muscle to maintain its current level of strength it must be used. If it is not used it will lose its strength and may atrophy: this is most clearly illustrated when a limb is immobilized and put in a cast, as in the case of a broken leg. For a muscle or group of muscles to improve their strength they need to be used more intensively than normal. This could be achieved with the use of weights or by exercising the muscles against the resistance of the person's own body weight. Overload is therefore an important prerequisite for improving the strength of muscles. Within this context the exact nature of the exercises that are needed to improve strength will depend upon the physical condition of the individual.

To promote improvements in the cardiovascular system it is again essential to apply the principle of overload. For cardiovascular fitness, overload refers to making the cardiovascular system work harder, increasing the body's demand for oxygen and raising the heart rate to an appropriate level (the details of which are discussed in a later section).

Specificity

The specificity of an exercise or exercise programme refers to a number of exercise-related factors.

1. The improvements in physical condition are only observed in the parts of the body that are being exercised and hence receiving overload. For example, arm exercises will not improve the strength of the leg muscles and, similarly,

exercising the right side of the body will not improve the condition of the left.

2. The type of training effects produced by the exercise are specific to that type of exercise. In practical terms this means that in order to develop muscular strength, strengthening exercises need to be done and these need to place an appropriate amount of overload on the muscles. Similarly, for the development of cardiovascular fitness, exercises that place overload on the cardiovascular system need to be undertaken. Therefore, when planning an exercise programme it should be remembered that strengthening exercises will not improve flexibility and, similarly, flexibility exercises will not improve cardiovascular fitness. However, it should also be noted at this point that many forms of physical activity will in fact use a combination of strength, flexibility and cardiovascular fitness. They will therefore have the effect of physically stressing the body in a number of different ways and may have an effect upon all three aspects of fitness. This is especially true in the case of activity-based exercises such as swimming or remedial gymnastics.

3. Specificity also refers to the way in which muscles are used. Exercising them through a limited range of motion – for instance, doing biceps curls from a fully extended elbow to one that is flexed at 90 degrees – may well improve the strength of the biceps through this particular range of motion, but may not have such a substantial effect upon their strength through the range of motion from 90 degrees to the position where the elbow is fully flexed. Specificity also refers to the sequence in which the muscles are used to produce a particular movement. Hence, to improve a particular movement the muscles need to be used and exercised by performing the full movement, although alternative forms of movement/exercises may assist in the improvement of the action, as will be seen in a later section.

Intensity

Intensity refers to the degree of difficulty of the exercise. In terms of strengthening exercises, lifting a light object or pushing against a slight resistance would be considered as a 'low-intensity' exercise. Conversely, lifting a heavy object or pushing against a large resistance would be considered as a high-intensity exercise. Similarly, the concept of intensity can also be applied to stamina exercises. For instance, walking, swimming or cycling at a relatively slow, easy pace would be considered as low intensity, whereas running, cycling or swimming at a fast pace, where the individual really has to work hard, would be considered as high intensity.

In this context it is also possible to apply the concept of 'relative exercise intensity' to how difficult someone finds an exercise. To illustrate this by example, a fit individual may be able to cycle at 15 mph and find that pace relatively easy and comfortable. It would therefore be perceived as being of low intensity. However, an unfit individual cycling with that person is likely to find the same speed rather fast and may have to work hard to keep up. This will cause the unfit individual to perceive the exercise as one of 'high intensity'. Thus, it can be seen that the perceived intensity of an exercise will depend upon the relative fitness of the individual. This example helps to emphasize the point that it is important that any form of exercise is pitched at the appropriate intensity for the individual concerned since the same exercise may be too easy for some and too difficult for others. In summary, any exercise programme needs to be 'personalized' to ensure that it is appropriate for the participant.

Duration, repetitions and sets

The duration of an exercise refers to how long it lasts. This is closely linked to its intensity since high-intensity exercises cannot be maintained for as long a duration as low-intensity exercises. A simple example would be that of cycling where an individual may only be able to sprint (high intensity) for a few seconds before becoming fatigued and having to slow down. However, if they pedal at a slower pace (low intensity) they may be able to continue the exercise for a far greater duration. Duration tends to be recorded in terms of time or even distance. When performing stretching exercises an individual may be advised to hold a stretched position for a duration of 15 seconds or, when swimming, they may be advised to swim continuously for a duration of 20 minutes. Conversely, in the latter example the duration of the swim could be prescribed as 30 lengths.

In some forms of exercise repetitions are more applicable than duration; for example, asking someone to step up and down on a step or when lifting weights. In such cases it may be appropriate to recommend that an exercise is repeated twenty times rather than suggesting that it should be continued for a duration of, say, 30 seconds. Both duration and repetitions can be used to determine the length of time spent on the exercise, but in practical terms it is often easier to count repetitions.

Some forms of exercise need to be of a fairly high intensity if they are to be effective, and this is especially so for strengthening exercises. This means that the duration of the exercise will be relatively short, i.e. only relatively few repetitions will be achieved before fatigue ensues and the participant needs to rest. Since a single short bout of a particular exercise is unlikely to convey any substantial benefits to the participant the exercise bout will need to be repeated. This is achieved by incorporating 'sets' into an exercise session – that is, the participant will complete a number of specified repetitions of one exercise (one set), rest and then repeat the exercise. For example, if someone was to step up and down on a step 30 times, rest, repeat the exercise, rest and then repeat the exercise again this would be described as three sets of 30 repetitions. Strengthening, mobility and stamina exercise sessions may all be organized in this manner to optimize their effectiveness.

Frequency

Frequency refers to how often an individual performs an exercise session – for example, three times a week or twice a day. The frequency of an exercise session will depend upon numerous factors, including the content of the session, the condition of the individual and his or her other commitments (including other sessions of physical activity).

Recovery

Recovery can refer to the rest periods taken within an exercise session, or to the rest interval between exercise sessions. Both are important. In exercise sessions which include repeated bouts (sets) of relatively high-intensity exercise the recovery periods are required to allow the body to remove waste products from the muscles and restore itself to a condition that will enable it to repeat the exercise. The exact nature and duration of the recovery period will depend upon the nature of the exercise session and the condition of the participant. Recovery within an exercise session may be passive or active.

1. A 'passive' recovery will take the form of a complete rest.
2. An 'active' recovery may take the form of a period of relatively low-intensity exercise that is sufficiently easy to enable the body to recover. Alternatively, it could take the form of a different exercise; for example, during a strength training session participants may exercise the muscles of their upper body and allow those muscles to recover while they exercise their leg muscles, after which they may again exercise the muscles of their upper body. This form of recovery maximizes the amount of time spent exercising within a session.

Recovery between exercise sessions is also important. As a general rule, the more intensive the exercise the longer the recovery period. Relatively low-intensity exercise may be repeated daily whilst high-intensity exercise can put sufficient stresses upon the body such that it may need 48 hours in which to recover. Repeating the exercise session before the body has fully recovered is likely to result in the rapid onset of fatigue and may therefore reduce the effectiveness of the session. Repeatedly exercising without adequate recovery can lead to overfatigue. This will reduce the body's physical capacity rather than increasing it, and may lead to overuse injuries.

Progression

When the body is subjected to an appropriate physical overload it will respond by making adaptations to the physical demands being placed upon it. If the exercise is of an appropriate type, intensity, duration and frequency, distinct physical improvements will occur. These improvements in physical condition will mean that the individual will become more able to cope with the same type of exercise and will begin to find it easier and, as a result, the same exercise session will begin to have less of an 'overload' effect. However, overload must be maintained if an individual is to continue to improve, and thus the exercise session needs to be altered so that it once again places an appropriate amount of overload upon the individual. This is referred to as progression. Progression or a 'progressive overload' can be achieved via a number of alterations to an exercise programme. However, it is important that any progression is gradual, since if it is too rapid the individual's body will find the new level of overload too demanding. Too much overload will reduce the benefits of the exercise and in some cases may even be detrimental, as can happen when an individual tries to do too much. For example, an individual can strain a muscle when trying to lift a weight that is too heavy, or can develop an overuse injury if sessions

119

that are too long are performed repeatedly. Overuse injuries can also occur if the frequency of sessions is increased to the extent that the body does not have enough time to recover between the bouts of exercise. However, on a positive note, applying a steady gradual progressive overload that is within the capabilities of the participant will prevent such occurrences.

In practice, progression can be achieved by manipulating one or more variables in the exercise programme. For example, it may be achieved by altering the intensity, as would be the case if someone were to walk faster or lift heavier weights. Alternatively, the duration of the exercise can be increased by lengthening the time spent exercising and/or the number of repetitions or sets included in the session. Further means of applying progression include increasing the frequency of the exercise, reducing the amount of recovery or adding extra exercises or different exercise sessions into an individuals programme (this would have the added advantage of providing variety in the programme). In summary, progression may be achieved by altering one or a combination of factors with the exact means of progression depending upon the individual circumstances. Examples of progression are given in each of the sections that describe the different forms of exercise.

Reversibility

Reversibility refers to the fact that if a body part or system, such as a muscle or the cardiovascular system, is not used, or the amount of work it performs is substantially reduced for a period of days or weeks, then its physical capacity will decline. In simple terms this means that if someone stops exercising for a prolonged period of time the physical capacity of that person will be diminished. In the case of strengthening exercises, if an individual stops exercising his or her muscles the muscles will become weaker. Similar effects can also be observed with the flexibility and stamina aspects of fitness. The rate of reversibility will depend upon the individual and his or her physical condition. However, since a noticeable reversal in physical condition will not manifest itself for a number of days, or even weeks in some cases, the relatively short duration required to produce a full recovery from an exercise session (perhaps a few days) will not cause a person's physical capacity to decline.

THE BENEFITS OF PLANNED EXERCISE PROGRAMMES AND MONITORING

The aims of an exercise programme may be complex. An exercise programme may be undertaken to improve the physical condition of individuals, to maintain their current condition or to minimize the decline of their condition. In addition, an exercise programme may also convey numerous psychological and/or sociological benefits. Regardless of the kind of exercise programme being embarked upon, it should be designed with specific short-term and long-term goals which may or may not be revealed to the paticipant. Short-term goals are usually set over a period of 6 to 8 weeks and provide the participant with something to aim for. They also give the programme a point of focus, rather than it being a series of exercise sessions with no apparent direction. Setting out the next few weeks' exercise sessions in a written format helps to clarify the programme for both the participant and the therapist. This may have the added psychological benefits of demonstrating the direction and progression of the programme to the participant.

Quite often it is useful to commence an exercise programme by conducting an assessment of the participant's current physical condition. This may take the form of:

(a) measuring mobility at different joints;
(b) assessing the response of the heart and cardiovascular system to exercise;
(c) assessing the strength of particular muscles.

Assessments that are undertaken in an objective and quantitative manner can provide very valuable information that may be used immediately or referred to at a later date. The information collected during an assessment may be used to:

(a) design the initial programme;
(b) provide a means of monitoring the effectiveness of the exercise programme;
(c) modify a programme when necessary.

The overall effect should be to produce a programme which includes appropriate levels of intensity, duration, frequency and overload. It should therefore be far more effective than a random series of exercise sessions which may also lack appropriate specificity and progression. A more detailed coverage of the uses and benefits of physiological assessments is presented later in this chapter.

Most exercise programmes will need to be set out over a period of about 6 to 8 weeks since this is the duration over which some distinct improvements may be expected. However, within this time span the programme should be dynamic and subject to any changes felt necessary by the professional. For example, such changes may be necessary if the individual finds the exercise programme too easy. Alternatively, a complication such as 'flu or other illness may require the programme to be modified and made easier in the weeks immediately following the illness. Modifications may also be precipitated by such factors as personal likes or dislikes of a certain exercise session and the motivation of the participant.

INDIVIDUALIZING EXERCISE PROGRAMMES

To enable the most benefit to be derived from an exercise programme it needs to be specific to the individual's personal condition, needs, likes and dislikes. The exact content of a programme will depend upon the physical condition of the person and what he or she is seeking to achieve. An exercise programme for a 55 year old who is rehabilitating after a heart attack will be different from that of a 22 year old who is recovering from a broken leg. In addition, the likes and dislikes of individuals influence motivation and are important, especially when they may be asked to undertake some of a programme unsupervised: if people dislike their prescribed programme they are less likely to adhere to it. It is, of course, not always possible to give someone a programme that is 'enjoyable' but where options and alternatives are available these should be discussed with the participant. The ease of personal access to exercise facilities, such as a gym or swimming pool, may also have some bearing upon the precise content of a programme.

A major consideration when personalizing an exercise programme is the current physical capabilities of the participant. This may be assessed using standardized tests for flexibility, strength, stamina and muscular endurance. The methods use to evaluate each of these aspects of physical capacity are described separately in the chapters associated with each component of fitness. In addition to the practical advantages of 'knowing someone's physical capabilities' when designing an exercise programme, physical assessments and monitoring also have a psychological value. By individualizing a programme, assessing and monitoring it in this manner, the programme is seen to be specific to that individual and the personal aspect of the process is enhanced.

WARMING UP AND COOLING DOWN

Warming up and cooling down are both very important aspects of any exercise session and should not be neglected. Warming up refers to a preparatory phase at the beginning of an exercise session. It generally involves a short period of low-intensity exercise which prepares the body for the more strenuous aspects of the session. It also has an important role in reducing the risk of injury that could happen if over-exertion occurred without the person being physically prepared for the exercise. Cooling down refers to a short period of time at the end of an exercise session. The cooling-down phase, again, tends to involve a short period of low-intensity exercise which gradually returns the body to its 'resting state'. The cooling-down phase is believed to reduce the risk of muscular soreness which may occur the day after an exercise session and reduce the risk of fainting or collapse after such a session.

Warming up

Any exercise session should always commence with a period of warm-up. In some cases it may take the form of a distinct series of preparatory exercises whilst in other sessions it will simply involve performing the activity at a relatively low intensity before gradually increasing the intensity to the desired level. A warming-up period is important for the following reasons:

1. It prepares the body for the physical exertion that follows. This optimizes the participants' physical condition enabling them to cope more easily with the activity. It also enables them to get the most benefit from the session.
2. It may refamiliarize the participants with the content of the session, especially if the warm-up includes specific movements that will be used in the main part of the session.
3. It reduces the risk of injury (cold muscles do not stretch very easily) and it reduces the risk of premature fatigue which can occur if the cardiovascular system is unprepared for strenuous activity.
4. It reduces the risk of unnecessary stress being placed upon the heart.

A typical warm-up may involve some gentle 'loosening exercises', followed by a few minutes of low-intensity aerobic activity and then a series of preparatory stretching exercises. This may last for approximately 5 to 10 minutes depending upon the intensity of the session which follows. During the warm-up the participant may wear additional clothing to ensure that the overall body and muscle temperature is elevated sufficiently. The loosening exercises at the start of the warm-up may include activities such as 'heel raises' and 'shoulder circling' (see Chapter 5 for details of specific loosening exercises). These are gentle activities which begin to prepare the body for exercise and are especially important if the participant has been inactive for a while – for instance, if he or she has just got out of a car or has been sitting at a desk for some time.

The aerobic exercise may involve low-intensity activities such as cycling slowly on an exercise cycle, walking around the room or some modified exercise for those unable to walk. This has the effect of increasing the heart rate, diverting blood to the exercising muscles and raising the overall temperature of the muscles. Thus the supply of oxygen to the muscles is increased and the heart is prepared for more strenuous activity.

The stretching exercises provide the final phase of warm-up and ensure that the muscles and tendons are prepared for the exercise. An important reason for doing stretching exercises is to prevent the muscles and tendons from being overstretched during the session. Such a warm-up will also prepare the joints for physical activity, preventing or minimizing any joint problems.

In some cases the final stage of the warm-up will include doing part of the exercise session at a low intensity. For example, if the session involved the use of weights a person may do a few repetitions of very light weights as part of the final warm-up, or, if the session involved cycling on an exercise cycle, the person may spend the first few minutes pedalling against a very light resistance.

The physiological effects of a warm-up are as follows;

1. Cold muscles, tendons and connective tissue do not stretch very easily. Stretching without a warm-up is therefore unlikely to produce the best effects. Warming up also relaxes the body and muscles, which further allows them to be stretched effectively. It is also believed that cold muscles and tendons are more prone to damage since they are more likely to tear when cold.

2. In the case of aerobic type exercises, a warm-up prepares the heart, cardio-vascular system and muscles for the activity. A warm-up increases the heart rate gradually. Research has shown that if the participant attempts to perform a strenuous form of activity without an adequate warm-up it may cause cardiac arrythmia (irregular activity of the heart), even in those without heart disease.

3. A warm-up also causes the blood to be diverted to the exercising muscles. This is achieved by getting the blood vessels leading to the working muscles to dilate (enlarge) whilst those leading to other parts of the body which are not involved in the exercise, such as those leading to the gut, constrict. In this way the blood is diverted towards 'priority' areas such as the muscles which require an increased supply of oxygen during bouts of exercise.

4. Attempting to exercise strenuously without a warm-up may result in the muscles having to work without an adequate supply of oxygen. This forces them to

use anaerobic processes to supplement their production of ATP. As a consequence, lactic acid accumulates and the muscles may become prematurely fatigued at an exercise intensity that they may have been quite capable of sustaining had they been warmed up beforehand.

5. A warm-up increases the temperature of the body. This increase in temperature facilitates and speeds up many of the processes associated with exercise metabolism. It increases the rate of nerve impulse transmission, the rate of oxygen delivery to the muscles and the speed of the reactions associated with the production of ATP. Therefore, in this context, a warm-up may be said to optimize the condition of the body, preparing it for the strenuous physical activity to follow.

6. In the case of strength exercises a similar argument to those listed above may be applied, whereby a warm-up prepares the muscles for the physical demands of the exercise by increasing their temperature. This increases the rate of the metabolic reactions used in the production of ATP and reduces the risk of their being damaged through overstretching when cold.

Cooling down

A cool-down involves a short period of time at the end of an exercise session during which the physical activity of the body is gradually reduced to almost its resting level. A cool-down therefore often involves a period of low-intensity aerobic exercise which is gradually reduced, followed by a few gentle stretching exercises. This has a number of effects:

1. The gentle aerobic activity helps to get rid of any metabolic waste products which may have accumulated during the exercise session. Various research studies have demonstrated that this form of active recovery is better in achieving this than a passive recovery where the participant stops exercising suddenly at the end of each session. The benefits of an active recovery are believed to be related to the muscles continuing to receive a more extensive supply of oxygenated blood which will also assist with the removal of metabolic waste products.

2. The cool-down assists the general functioning of the cardiovascular system. During exercise the blood is pumped around the body by the action of the heart. However, the blood is assisted in its return to the heart (venous return) by the active contraction of the working skeletal muscles. If a person stops exercising suddenly the heart continues to beat fast sending blood around the body, but because the exercise has ceased the blood is no longer assisted in its return to the heart. It is suggested that this is one of the reasons why people sometimes feel faint immediately after exercise. During a cool-down the heart rate is gradually lowered to its resting level and the venous return continues to be assisted by the actively contracting muscles, thereby preventing this problem.

A few minutes after the end of a cool-down the participant's heart rate is unlikely to be completely at its resting level but should be within about 30 beats of what it was before the exercise session started. This will, of course, be influenced by the overall physical condition of the individual and any medication that he or she may be taking. It may also be influenced by the content of the session, with more demanding sessions requiring a more extensive cool-down.

The cool-down period also provides the opportunity for the inclusion of additional stretching exercises, which may be desirable especially if they were not included as part of the main session. The inclusion of stretching exercises within the cool-down period not only helps to gradually lower the activity level of the body at the end of the session but it may also prevent stiffness the following day. The cool-down period is also likely to be a time when the body is warm, making the muscles receptive to stretching. The most effective stretching can therefore be performed at this time.

CONSIDERATIONS FOR SAFE EXERCISE SESSIONS

If an exercise programme is to provide an effective form of therapy, certain factors need to be considered in order to ensure the general safety and 'well being' of the participant. These include;

1. Warming up and cooling down
2. Appropriate clothing and footwear
3. Correct exercise technique
4. Appropriate progression
5. Safety of the equipment and the exercise environment
6. Food and drink.

Warming up and cooling down

The importance of a warm-up and cool-down were discussed extensively in the previous section. In summary, a lack of warm-up may:

(a) result in premature fatigue;
(b) increase the risk of ruptures and strains;
(c) increase the risk of overuse injuries such as tendonitis.

The benefits of a cool-down have also been discussed and in summary include:

(a) gradually returning a number of metabolic and physiological processes to their resting state;
(b) reducing the risk of post-exercise dizziness or fainting;
(c) reducing the risk of post-exercise soreness.

Appropriate clothing and footwear

In any exercise situation the clothing worn needs to be appropriate. In general terms it needs to permit movement and provide adequate warmth whilst facilitating the loss of excess heat. However, clothing should not be so loose that it may get caught in the equipment being used: this is especially important when using exercise machines such as cycle ergometers or multigyms. Throughout an exercise session the participants should be comfortably warm: i.e. there is no value in making the participant sweat excessively. Therefore, the participants may need to alter what they wear during a session. It is usual to commence a session with a number of layers, some of which may be removed after the warm-up or at appropriate intervals as the participants feel necessary.

Appropriate footwear is very important in weight-bearing activities. Inappropriate footwear, or lack of footwear, may result in excessive stresses being placed upon the muscles, bones and joints during the activity. Therefore, footwear with adequate cushioning is most desirable. In this context comfort and protection are the key factors. Even if working indoors, shoes will protect participants' feet from grit, abrasions and infection to which they may otherwise be susceptible.

Correct exercise technique

In recent years there has been much concern over safety during certain forms of exercise and specific exercises. This stems from the belief that certain exercises, if performed incorrectly, could result in minor injuries to some people. This concern covers all forms of exercises, including those used to develop flexibility, strength and muscular endurance. For this reason it is important that the participants are always shown the correct technique for all the exercises included in their programme. Demonstrating the exercises is often more informative than describing it, since the participants may visualize an exercise differently to that being described by the therapist. This could result in participants performing an inappropriate and potentially unsafe exercise when unsupervised. Supervision of an exercise session is especially important during the initial stages of the programme when the participants may be unsure of the exercises prescribed. Such factors will be discussed in depth in the section on flexibility and strength training and, where appropriate, with each specific exercise. Inappropriate techniques may result in strained muscles and back pain, as well as being less effective in developing the participants' physical condition.

Appropriate progression

In any exercise programme it is important that the participants progress steadily. As an individual's physical condition improves this provides positive motivation which may cause him or her to wish to progress more rapidly than is desirable. It should be remembered that any form of exercise, however beneficial, places certain physical stresses upon the body. The body needs time to adapt to these stresses and if progression is too rapid, overuse injuries may result. For example, in strength training the force which the muscles produce is conveyed to the bones via the tendons. It is generally considered that the tendons take longer than the muscles to adapt to the stresses of strength training. Therefore, if participants progress rapidly at the speed that is dictated by the increased strength of their muscles they may exceed the capabilities of their tendons, which adapt more slowly. This may result in the tendons being overstressed causing injuries such as tendonitis or in extreme cases rupture. It is therefore up to the adviser to design an exercise programme which is progressive, and which the participants see as being progressive, yet does not cause them to progress too rapidly. This element of gradual progression needs to include the duration, intensity and frequency of the exercise as well as the gradual introduction of new forms of exercise.

Safety of the equipment and the exercise environment

Safety of the equipment refers to a multitude of factors, most of which will be highlighted by the manufacturer. These will include regular servicing, oiling of certain moving parts, ensuring that weights are securely fixed by collars and that the participants cannot hurt themselves upon moving parts. Other safety factors include the use of mats for floor exercises such as sit-ups and the use of the correct keys (not makeshift alternatives) when using multigym type equipment.

A further concern is the safety of the environment itself. Apparatus which is poorly arranged may cause the users to bump into it and hurt themselves. It is also important that apparatus is not left lying around the exercise room in dangerous positions for someone to trip over. Such safety considerations should be strictly applied and become even more important if the room is crowded.

Food and drink

As a general rule it is not advisable to eat within one hour of exercising or to exercise within three hours of a substantial meal. This is largely attributable to the discomfort caused by a full stomach. The recent ingestion of food may also cause nausea in some cases, as well as place an additional strain upon the body. However, liquids should be readily available and taken at liberty since it is undesirable for the participant to become dehydrated. Dehydration will cause unnecessary fatigue, discomfort, or a lack of concentration and will therefore reduce the effectiveness of the session. Whether the adviser permits liquids into the exercise area or recommends that they be consumed elsewhere will depend upon the circumstances, but for safety reasons glass, etc., should not be brought into an exercise area where it is at risk of being broken.

WHEN NOT TO EXERCISE

It is widely established that appropriate exercise in the form of therapy or recreation can convey numerous benefits to many people. However, there are occasions when it is inadvisable to exercise. For example, it is unwise for anyone to exercise whilst suffering with basic viral infections such as influenza. Indeed, there is a misconception amongst many individuals who believe that a hard exercise session will enable them to 'sweat it out' and accelerate their recovery. Medical evidence would suggest that this could be rather hazardous. Certain incidents suggest that if a person infected with a virus attempts to exercise the virus may cause a greater amount of inflammation and even permanent damage to body tissues. Of greatest concern in this context is the possibility of the virus affecting the heart and causing pericarditis, which may result in permanent damage to the heart. Other studies have also shown that there is an increased incidence of cardiac arrythmia in those exercising with a virus even if they have no other apparent cardiac disorders and are otherwise healthy. A further cause for concern are postviral fatigue syndromes including myalgic encephalitis (ME). The cause of these disorders is currently unclear, however certain evidence would suggest that there is a viral link and that people are most susceptible if they are physically fatigued and/or in a state of physical or mental stress. In this context it is therefore inadvisable to exercise when suffering from a viral infection since it may increase the individual's risk of contracting ME or a similar syndrome.

A further factor to consider when recommending that someone should not exercise is the presence of specific injuries. Whilst exercise may provide a useful form of rehabilitation if undertaken at the correct time, certain exercises performed at the wrong time may themselves aggravate an injury. Thus the timing of the inclusion of certain exercises into a programme is of importance. For instance, if the participant is suffering from tendonitis then it may be advisable to stop or minimize any form of exercise which places stress upon that tendon until the condition improves sufficiently to permit exercise without pain or subsequent soreness. A typical example would be in the case of jogging and tendonitis of the achilles tendon. In this case an alternative form of exercise, such as swimming, may be pursued until the inflammation is sufficiently reduced. Therefore, in the case of tendon injuries exercise should be undertaken with caution and progression should be gradual.

Basic muscle injuries such as simple partial ruptures tend to respond well to exercise after an initial rest of approximately 48 hours. Gentle exercise at this time appears to enhance the healing process, but if commenced prior to this may aggravate the injury by damaging the weak tissues. Once exercise has been introduced into a rehabilitation programme the intensity, duration and frequency of the exercise should be increased very gradually in accordance with the limitations imposed by the injury. Exceeding these limitations is likely to aggravate the injury and therefore the emphasis should be on working within the individual's capabilities and not at the limit.

In practical terms the question may not simply be whether to exercise or not but whether a form of exercise is appropriate for an individual at that particular time. For example, circumstances may suggest that an individual should stop doing one form of exercise and take up an alternative. This could occur at any stage of an exercise programme and may involve a change in the intensity of the exercise. Additionally, it should also be remembered that what is beneficial to one individual may not be beneficial to another, once again emphasizing the importance of personalizing exercise programmes. For instance, a blind individual who has no other disabilities will be capable of exercising as hard as an individual with sight. Indeed, there are many blind individuals who actively train and compete in sports such as athletics. However, an individual rehabilitating after a coronary heart attack will require a very different level of exercise intensity. Therefore, there are certain individuals who have specific conditions that will make their participation in certain forms of exercise inadvisable.

EXERCISE AND MEDICATION

Certain forms of medication may also preclude an individual from exercising. It is therefore important that the therapist be aware of any drugs that the participant is taking and of any implications that these may have. This information should be gained directly from the participant's medical practitioner or an appropriately qualified specialist.

Beta-blockers provide an example of drugs which reduce the heart rate: when a person taking beta-blockers exercises, the heart rate is maintained at a low level. In such cases it is therefore inappropriate to refer to their heart rate training zone (see Aerobic or activity-based exercises, page 243) as their appropriate exercise heart rate is likely to be well below the heart rate training zone of an individual who is not on such medication. In such cases exercising to a level of perceived exertion is usually more applicable. This may involve exercising at an intensity which makes the individual 'slightly breathless', but no harder. Alternatively, a more quantitative assessment of an individual's perceived exertion may be utilized, such as the 'Borg scale' (see the Borg scale of perceived exertion, page 245).

In certain contexts exercise has been shown to enhance the effectiveness of medication. For example, in a number of studies it has been demonstrated to aid the reduction of moderately high blood pressure. In some situations it has also been found to reduce the amount of medication required by the individual. For instance, in the case of diabetes mellitus it has been shown that exercise can increase the body's sensitivity to insulin thereby reducing the amount required by insulin-dependent diabetics.

THE EFFECTS OF DIFFERENT TYPES OF EXERCISE

All forms of exercise will involve all the major aspects of fitness to a greater or lesser extent. These include muscular strength, suppleness, cardiovascular fitness and muscular endurance. Therefore, the common grouping of exercises into flexibility, strength and aerobic exercises tends to refer to the major effects of the exercises, though this is not always their sole effect. For example, a particular exercise may have the primary objective of increasing hip mobility, but it may also enhance the strength of the muscles around that joint. Similarly, press-ups are primarily prescribed to enhance arm and shoulder strength, yet they may also enhance the strength/ endurance of the abdominal muscles which have to work as fixators throughout the exercise. The situation becomes even more complex when the exercise sesssion is activity based, as in the case of swimming or gymnastics. Such activities will have many effects upon numerous aspects of fitness (flexibility, strength, endurance and cardiovascular fitness) and different parts of the body.

A further aspect to be considered is the effect of exercise upon proprioception, kinasthetic awareness and the learning of motor skills. Learning to control the lowering of a weight on a multigym or pedalling a cycle ergometer can provide great benefits for those with motor learning difficulties; in addition to which the psychological and sociological benefits of exercise should not be overlooked. Many individuals derive great benefits and much pleasure from the participation in exercise, be it in the context of therapy, a social activity or a competitive sport. Indeed, sport for the disabled is increasingly popular with more and more disabled individuals training and competing in sport for the enjoyment they derive from it. Therefore, the reasons for embarking upon an exercise programme and its content should be considered very carefully in the light of the multiplicity of effects it can have upon the individual.

PHYSIOLOGICAL ASSESSMENTS AND THE EVALUATION OF PHYSICAL CAPACITY

Reasons for conducting a physiological assessment

A physiological assessment can provide the therapist with much valuable information, and some of the reasons for conducting such an assessment are given below.

1. It provides information on the participant's current physical condition which may then be used to devise suitable exercise loads and personalize an exercise programme according to requirements. In this context an initial assessment prior to the commencement of an exercise programme is often advisable. Later assessments may be used to modify the programme.
2. It provides some initial data for comparison so that an exercise programme can be monitored and improvements quantitatively measured. This enables the adviser to see whether the programme is suitable and effective. It also provides positive feedback and motivation for the participant.
3. An assessment can provide an individual with an indication of his or her current physical condition by comparing their results to standardized 'norms' for the population.
4. A comprehensive assessment which includes clinical tests may detect problems associated with health such as hypertension or atherosclerosis. The subject may then be cleared for exercise, or an exercise programme may be modified and devised according to any detected problems.
5. The assessment session may provide a focus which will enable the assessor and assessed to discuss aspects of exercise, health and, where appropriate, the reasons for incorporating exercise into the treatment/rehabilitation programme.
6. An assessment may be used as a short-term goal, giving the participant an objective to aim for and providing a focus within the programme.

The exact content of a physiological assessment will depend upon the condition of the participant and the aims of the exercise programme. The content of an assessment needs to be specific to the 'training effects' of the programme and also needs to be appropriate for the physical capacity of the participant. Exhaustive tests are clearly unsuitable and inadvisable for some individuals, but may be appropriate for others. For additional information refer to the list of recommended further reading.

Physiological assessments prior to an exercise programme

Prior to the commencement of any exercise programme it is usually advisable for the participant to undergo some form of physiological assessment and/or thorough medical check-up. This applies to virtually all individuals but the extent and nature of the assessment will vary considerably depending upon age, medical history and current level of participation in physical activity. For some individuals it may involve a series of simple questions and physical tests which will provide the therapist with appropriate background knowledge of the participant's current physical condition. This basic information may then be used, along with any available medical records, to devise a suitable exercise programme.

Examples of the type of tests that may be administered by the therapist are described in later chapters on the different components of 'fitness'. Basic flexibility measures are likely to involve the use of a goniometer, simple strength tests may use a dynamometer and an aerobic capacity assessment could involve a submaximal cycle ergometer test. Although these basic tests may be suitable for virtually all individuals it is often desirable for the participants to get medical clearance to exercise before undertaking such tests. This is especially so for participants who are over 40 and have not undertaken any form of regular, vigorous exercise for some time. It also applies to those who are suffering from specific medical conditions, such as recovering from a heart attack. In such cases a more extensive physical evaluation will typically include an assessment of the participant's blood pressure and, in some cases, an exercise ECG. These will obviously be performed by specialists in the field; however, the information provided by such tests will be of value to the therapist in designing the individual's exercise programme. Specific medical conditions may also require special considerations and information concerning these aspects should also be obtained by the therapist from appropriate sources.

An initial physiological assessment may be undertaken for a number of reasons and, depending upon its content and the way in which it is administered, it can provide important information for both the assessor and the assessed. Some authorities suggest that in an ideal situation it may be desirable for everyone to undergo a regular, extensive physiological asessment including a stress test with an exercise ECG. However, whilst such procedures may be desirable, they are in practice often expensive and time consuming and the facilities are not always available. In addition, the cost and extensiveness of the tests may discourage potential participants. Therefore a balance needs to be obtained between the most extensive form of assessments available and what is practically feasible. In practice, a physiological assessment may be multistage, with only a percentage of the participants proceeding to each stage. An example is given below.

Stage 1

A basic lifestyle questionnaire which seeks to gain information about current levels of physical activity, medical disorders and what medication the participant is currently taking. Other information concerning smoking habits, stress, whether there is a history of coronary heart disease (CHD) in the family, diet and age are also important. The questionnaire should provide the therapist with information on the participant, risk factors which may be present and preliminary information about the participant's capabilities and expectations. Such a questionnaire may also be used to discover the forms of exercise the participant might enjoy doing.

Stage 2

The initial questionnaire may be followed by an evaluation of blood pressure if this information is not already available. This should be performed by a suitably qualified individual and if it should reveal hypertension, additional care should be taken when the individual undertakes certain forms of exercise. As a further precaution, if the assessor is not medically trained and assesses someone with blood pressure values of around 165/95, then the assessor may prefer not to conduct any further exercise tests on the individual until appropriate assurances have been obtained from the participant's medical specialist. High blood pressure will not normally preclude a person from all forms of exercise but may preclude him or her from some (especially isometric work). This is also likely to require a reduction in the intensity of any activities. In the case of the initial assessment the assessor may simply evaluate the individual's aerobic fitness using very light exercise intensities that would be substantially less than those used for a person with normal blood pressure.

Stage 3

A basic physical assessment of aspects of the participant's physical capacity. This may include a submaximal assessment of the individual's aerobic capacity and/or flexibility measures and/or strength tests and/or coordination tests. The results of these tests may then be used directly in prescribing the exercise loads which will be incorporated into the resulting exercise programme.

Other factors which may be assessed include an evaluation of body composition, lung function tests and an assessment of blood lipids. However, the relevance of each of these will depend upon the individual being assessed. If the participant does exhibit a number of health risk factors such as smoking, obesity and hypertension then a more extensive exercise stress test may be desirable if it has not already been administered.

Stage 4

Exercise stress test with electrocardiogram (ECG). This will be conducted by a specialist who will then liaise with the therapist over the condition of the participant and the exercises that may be appropriate.

Summary

In summary, assessment procedures may be multistage with only those individuals revealing a high number of risk factors in the basic assessment being recommended for more comprehensive tests. Basic tests of aerobic fitness, flexibility and strength are likely to be conducted by the therapist. The more specialist tests such as the measurement of exercise ECGs, $\dot{V}O_2$ max and 'onset of blood lactate accumulation' (OBLA) will be undertaken by appropriate specialists. However, since the therapist may well encounter individuals who have had these tests the rationale behind them is briefly outlined at the end of this chapter.

Repeated physiological assessments and monitoring

Once a participant has spent a number of weeks on an exercise programme it may be useful to reassess his or her physical fitness. Repeat assessments may be conducted every 6 to 12 weeks if desired and can be useful for a number of reasons:

1. They may act as a short-term or intermediate goal for the participant.
2. They provide information upon whether the exercise programme has been effective.
3. The data from such assessments may be used to modify the exercise programme.
4. The data may provide positive feedback for the participant.

Exercise stress testing

One reason for doing an exercise stress test is that although individuals with chronic heart disease (CHD) will quite often exhibit a normal resting ECG, abnormal ECGs occur when they are exercising at relatively high intensities. However, it has to be said that even this test will not detect all CHD sufferers: it is suggested that 25% of CHD sufferers will still exhibit a normal ECG whilst exercising. However, on the positive side it can detect about 75% of those with CHD and hence appropriate precautions may be taken with their exercise programmes. If an abnormal ECG is detected, then the individual may then undergo further tests after which he or she may or may not be cleared to exercise.

The information obtained from such tests may also be used by the specialist to inform the therapist of the level of exercise intensity that would be suitable for the participant. Thus the specialist may stipulate specific exercise intensity guidelines based upon the responses of the participant's heart during exercise.

$\dot{V}O_2$ max and OBLA tests

These tests are usually only of significance to those competing in competitive sports for which aerobic fitness and muscular endurance are key factors. $\dot{V}O_2$ max refers to the maximum amount of oxygen that a person can utilize. It is usually measured in litres of oxygen per minute or millilitres of oxygen per kilogram of bodyweight per minute. The measurement of $\dot{V}O_2$ max requires sophisticated apparatus that can measure oxygen consumption, carbon dioxide production and a number of other factors. It is therefore usually conducted in a laboratory setting using an ergometer that is appropriate to the participant's sport, such as a treadmill, cycle ergometer, rowing or canoeing ergometer. During the assessment the participant is required to exercise at an intensity that produces exhaustion, during which time the individual's oxygen consumption is measured. In general, there is a good correlation between an individual's $\dot{V}O_2$ max and his or her capacity to perform endurance exercise. In basic terms this means that the higher a person's $\dot{V}O_2$ max, the fitter that person is for aerobically based sport. This makes $\dot{V}O_2$ max an important component of fitness.

However, the correlation between $\dot{V}O_2$ max and performance is not perfect and other factors will contribute towards a person's aerobic fitness. One of these factors is the intensity of exercise that can be performed without an accumulation of lactic acid. Since it is the accumulation of lactic acid that is a major cause of fatigue, the greater the intensity of exercise that can be performed without this occurring is clearly important. For example, if there are two runners with the same $\dot{V}O_2$ max but one can run faster before lactic acid begins to accumulate (onset of blood lactate accumulation: OBLA) then that runner should be able to run faster than the other in endurance events. In practical terms this could mean that runner A has an OBLA at a speed of 18 km/h while runner B has an OBLA at 19 km/h. If both were to run at 18.5 km/h runner A would exceed the OBLA and hence would fatigue while runner B would remain below the OBLA and would be able to maintain the pace. In practice, OBLA is important in many endurance sports including running, cycling, canoeing, rowing and swimming.

Recent research would suggest that a number of illnesses can significantly reduce the $\dot{V}O_2$ max and OBLA of competitive sportspeople and therefore the measurement of these parameters may be relevant in monitoring participants for illlness as well as evaluating the effectiveness of their training. For details on how to perform $\dot{V}O_2$ max and OBLA tests see the recommended further reading.

5

Mobility and flexibility exercises

THE IMPORTANCE OF JOINT MOBILITY OR FLEXIBILITY

The terms mobility and flexibility are used interchangeably by some authorities and yet may convey different meanings when used by others. Some authorities use the term mobility to refer to active movement and flexibility to refer to passive movement at a joint. However, the use of such terms tends to be inconsistent in the literature and therefore in this text no distinction will be made between them.

In general the joints of young children are extremely flexible but as people get older they can lose their flexibility through the ageing process, lack of use, injury and medical disorders. Throughout life even the most basic body movements require a degree of joint mobility and if joint mobility is diminished for whatever reason then the range of movement possible at that joint will be restricted. A reduction in the amount of movement permissible at a joint may make certain movements or activities more difficult, and in some cases beyond the capabilities of the individual. This may impede an individual's capacity to be independent and mobile, to undertake activities such as housework and gardening or even to perform basic reaching movements. In an exercise context it may significantly reduce a person's potential by inhibiting key movements. A lack of joint mobility can also make an individual more vulnerable to injury during physical exertion and more prone to 'stiffness' following sporting or household activities. Therefore, the development and maintenance of joint flexibility are important if the individual is to be able to perform many basic movements and activities with ease and without discomfort during or after the activity. For the therapist, the amount of flexibility needed by the patients will depend upon their intended lifestyle. Some individuals will desire basic levels of flexibility that will permit them to move freely and accomplish basic household tasks. Others will desire a far greater degree of flexibility that will enable them to participate successfully in a sporting activity. Whilst the development of this sports-related flexibility may primarily be the role of the coach, it is often the therapist who initiates stretching activities to improve flexibility after an injury.

In many cases joint mobility is diminished due to underuse. This occurs when a joint is not regularly exercised through its full range of movement. In such cases joint flexibility may be enhanced by basic stretching routines that help to restore a fuller range of movement at the joint. This will make movements of the joint easier and also make such movements less likely to cause discomfort. In other instances an injury, or the effects of a disease, may complicate the situation, in which case a programme of stretching exercises needs to take such complicating factors into consideration. In basic terms, when trying to develop joint mobility the therapist should be wary of any exercise that causes pain. Pain is a warning of potential damage and, unless such movements are specifically prescribed by the individual's medical specialist as an integral part of a rehabilitation programme, they should be avoided.

THE DETERMINANTS OF JOINT MOBILITY OR FLEXIBILITY

A person's flexibility or mobility refers to the amount of movement available at a joint or over a range of joints. Each joint of the body is structured to permit certain kinds of movement whilst preventing others. This has the overall effect of enabling effective movement and at the same time providing stability. For instance, the structure of the knee joint permits flexion and extension movements in one plane but largely inhibits all other movements. In contrast to this, joints such as the hip and shoulder have a structure that permits a far greater variation of movement including flexion and extension in various planes, abduction and adduction, rotation and circumduction.

The amount of movement permissible at a joint depends upon a number of factors. These include:

1. The shape of the bones
2. The joint capsule and the ligaments
3. The muscles and the tendons associated with the joint.

In general, each joint permits specific types of movement which are characteristic of that joint and common to virtually everyone. For example, all 'normal' knee joints move in the same manner, as do all hips. These gross movements are largely determined by the general structure of the joint. However, when studied in detail it is apparent that some individuals have more mobility at a particular joint or joints than others. This is because there is a certain amount of variation between different individuals in the exact structure of their joints. This variation in joint structure, and hence mobility, may be due to any of the factors listed above including the exact shape of the bones, the position and length of the tendons and the structure of the muscles and tendons associated with the joint.

When attempting to develop an individual's flexibility it is appropriate to try to alter some of the factors associated with the joint but inadvisable to affect others. For instance, the shapes of the bones at the joint are inherent to the individual and exercise programmes should not seek to alter them. Similarly, structures such as the ligaments and joint capsule, which play an important role in providing joint stability, should not be altered through exercise. The ligaments are structured and situated so as to permit movement in the 'desired' plane(s) of motion but restrict movement in undesired plane(s). In the case of the knee the lateral, medial and cruciate ligaments permit the natural flexion and extension of the knee but restrict undesirable twisting or sideways movements. If ligaments are overstretched (as in the case of a sprained ankle) the joint loses its stability which makes it less effective and more vulnerable to further damage. The structures which flexibility exercises seek to stretch are the muscles and, to some extent, the tendons associated with the muscles. Muscles and tendons which are 'short' or 'tight' will restrict movement at a joint. By lengthening them and reducing their 'tightness', mobility or the potential for movement will be increased. Appropriate mobility or 'loosening' exercises are also reported to convey other benefits to the joint such as promoting the production of synovial fluid, thereby helping to lubricate the joint, and some stretching exercises will also help to stengthen the muscles associated with the joint. Finally, a programme of stretching exercises may also be utilized as a means of relaxation for the individual. Indeed, stretching exercises are often used as a means of combating 'stress' in many individuals from a wide variety of backgrounds.

In summary, flexibility exercises aim to improve the lubrication of the joint and enhance joint mobility. This is achieved by lengthening the connective tissue within the muscles and tendons that are associated with the joint (Figure 5.1). The diverse physical, social and psychological benefits conveyed by flexibility exercises means that they may be utilized by the therapist when treating a variety of conditions.

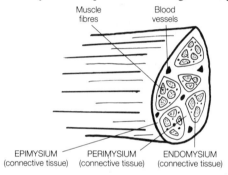

Figure 5.1 Illustrating the connective tissue situated within a muscle.

However, whilst flexibility exercises may form the major component of a therapy programme designed to improve joint mobility they are unlikely to be the only component. Indeed, such exercises should be used in conjunction with other forms of therapy such as joint manipulation and 'accessory glides' which are commonly used by therapists in this context.

SAFETY AND EFFECTIVE FLEXIBILITY EXERCISES

Flexibility exercises seek to retain and/or improve a person's flexibility by stretching the *muscles* rather than joint structures, such as the ligaments, which provide stability. It is therefore important that the *joints* are stretched correctly, and this is achieved by employing the correct stretching technique and ensuring that the joints are only stretched when they are in the correct alignment. To be effective, stretching exercises need to be of the correct type, which usually means gentle loosening exercises and prolonged static stretching rather than vigorous ballistic stretching movements.

There are many misconceptions over how to stretch the muscles and tendons. In general, vigorous ballistic stretching should be avoided since it has been demonstrated to convey a risk of injury and be a less effective form of stretching. The risk of injury to the joint during ballistic stretching is due to the dynamic nature of the exercises, during which the momentum of the movement can force the joint beyond its safe limits. This can damage the ligaments, tendons and muscles associated with the joint. In addition to the safety aspects, ballistic stretching has been demonstrated to be less effective than static stretching. This, again, is due to the ballistic nature of the movement which initiates the muscle's 'stretch reflex' (see section on The stretch reflex, p. 71). The overall effect of the stretch reflex causes the muscle fibres to contract, and hence the muscle tenses. This prevents the connective tissue within the muscle from being effectively stretched and lengthened. In comparison, static stretches permit a more effective lengthening of the connective tissue by holding the stretch for a prolonged duration and thereby inhibiting the stretch reflex (see section on The stretch reflex, (p. 71) and Golgi tendon organs (p. 73)). However, it must also be realized that not all static stretches are necessarily safe, and static stretches that are incorrectly performed convey a risk of injury. The safety of a static stretch primarily relates to the alignment of the joint as it is being stretched: an incorrect alignment may result in an overstretching of the ligaments; a correct alignment results in a safe and effective static stretch. Details of such precautions are given with each of the exercises presented later in this chapter.

Loosening exercises involve slow, controlled movements that will mobilize a joint and enhance its range of movement. Provided that all loosening exercises are performed at a slow, controlled speed they will not overstretch or damage the joint.

Warm-up is also a factor concerning the safety and effectiveness of stretching exercises. Warm muscles and joints stretch more easily than cold ones and this means that stretching after a warm-up will be safer and more effective. The warm-up prior to a session of stretching exercises may be active or passive. An active warm-up may be in the form of gentle exercise that elevates the muscle temperature while a passive warm-up could involve the application of heat, such as a heat lamp, warm towels or a bath. In some cases an active warm-up will be preferable as it can be more effective in raising the temperature of deep muscles. In practice both can be effective and the choice of warm-up is likely to depend upon the condition of the participant.

THE EFFECTS OF FLEXIBILITY EXERCISES

The aim of flexibility exercises is to increase or maintain the range of movement a person has at a joint or over a range of joints. This needs to be achieved without the joint losing any of its stability. In a carefully designed programme the musculature around a joint may also be strengthened with appropriate exercises. This will provide the joint with a greater degree of stability and an increased capacity for movement. The development of joint flexibility should not be at the expense of overstretching the ligaments and therefore flexibility exercises should concentrate on increasing the length of the muscles. This is primarily achieved through a lengthening of the connective tissue which extends throughout the muscles and forms the connections to the bones. In addition, it is suggested by some authorities that stretching will lengthen the muscle fibres by increasing the number of sarcomeres in the fibres. This is difficult to assess objectively and is therefore an area of debate. It is also reported that appropriate mobility exercises can promote the production of synovial fluid at a joint and thereby enhance its lubrication. This will have implications in the treatment of specific joint disorders.

THE JOINTS OF THE BODY

Central to the topic of flexibility and mobility exercises are the joints of the body. It is therefore essential for the therapist who is seeking to maintain or develop an individual's flexibility to have a good understanding of the joints of the body. Such an understanding will provide the therapist with a greater insight into the objectives of the exercises and the limitations that are placed upon individuals by their basic anatomy and physiology. This knowledge should also enhance the therapist's ability to devise effective and safe stretching programmes for the individuals with whom they work.

The human body contains over 200 joints or articulations. These may be classified according to their structure and/or the amount of movement that is permissible at the joint. The joints of the body may therefore be classified as follows:

Classified by permissible movement
1. Synarthrodial (no movement)
2. Amphiarthrodial (slight movement)
3. Diarthrodial (freely moveable)

Classified by structure
1. Fibrous
   (a) Suture
   (b) Syndesmosis
   (c) Gomphosis
2. Cartilaginous
   (a) Synchondrosis
   (b) Symphysis
3. Synovial
   (a) Ball and socket
   (b) Hinge
   (c) Gliding
   (d) Condyloid or ellipsoidal
   (e) Saddle
   (f) Pivot.

Fibrous joints may be synarthrodial or amphiarthrodial; similarly, cartilagenous joints may be synarthrodial or amphiarthrodial. Synovial joints are diarthrodial. The following section on joint structures and joint actions will use both forms of classification depending upon which is most appropriate.

139

Synarthrodial joints

These joints permit no movement, examples of which include the fibrous sutures of the skull and the cartilagenous epiphyseal plates. The sutures of the skull are formed by bones which have irregular jagged edges that fit together and are held firmly in place by fibrous tissue. Other types of synarthrodial joints are the synchondroses. These are cartilagenous joints which include the epiphyseal plates and the connection between the first rib and sternum. An epiphyseal plate is an area of hyaline cartilage which is found between the epiphysis and diaphysis of a growing bone. Like other synarthrodial joints this joint permits no movement in normal circumstances; however, a severe blow may cause it to be damaged and the cartilage to move. This can result in growth deformities unless corrected. During the normal course of growth and development the hyaline cartilage of an epiphyseal plate is eventually replaced by bone, and this replacement is complete upon the cessation of growth. Therefore, this type of joint is only present in those who have not reached full physical maturity.

Amphiarthrodial joints

These joints permit a very limited amount of movement between the bones. Amphi-arthrodial joints may be fibrous or cartilagenous. Examples of fibrous joints, where the bones are connected to each other via fibrous tissue, are the mid and interior tibiofibular joints and the articulations between the shafts of the radius and ulna. These fibrous joints are classified by structure as syndesmoses. In cartilagenous amphiarthrodial joints the bones are separated by a disc of fibrocartilage. Examples of this type of joint include the symphysis pubis of the pelvis and the joints of the vertebral column.

Diarthrodial joints

These joints permit movement in certain directions, with the exact extent and direction of movement depending upon the shape of the bones and other factors such as the muscles and ligaments associated with the joint. Synovial joints are diarthrodial and will be discussed in some depth later in this section.

Fibrous joints

Fibrous joints permit little or no movement and, as the name would imply, the bones are held together by fibrous tissue and there is no joint capsule. Fibrous joints may be subclassified as being sutures, syndesmoses or gomphoses. A suture is a synarthrotic joint where the ends of the bones are held firmly together by fibrous connective tissue, examples of which are the sutures of the skull. Gomphoses are also synarthrotic, having a peg and socket structure with examples including the articulations between the teeth and jaw bones (maxilla and mandible). Syndesmoses are fibrous joints which permit

140

a small amount of movement and are therefore functionally classified as amphi-arthrotic. Like the synarthrotic fibrous joints (sutures) the bones are connected by fibrous tissue but are not held together quite as tightly thereby permitting a small amount of movement. Examples of syndesmoses include the articulations between the radius and ulna and between the tibia and fibula.

Cartilagenous joints

As the name would imply, the structure of cartilagenous joints involves the bones being held together by cartilage. Cartilagenous joints that permit no movement (synarthrodial) are classified structurally as synchondroses whilst those that permit a small amount of movement (amphiarthrodial) are classified structurally as symphyses. Examples of synchondroses include the epiphyseal plate and the articulation between the first rib and sternum, while examples of symphyses include the joints between the vertebrae, both of which were discussed earlier under the headings of Synarthrodial joints and Amphiarthrodial joints.

Synovial joints

In the context of exercise therapy the joints which concern the therapist in the development of movement are primarily the diarthrodial joints of the body and the amphiarthrodial joints of the vertebral column. Diarthrodial (freely movable) joints are structurally classified as synovial joints because of the presence of synovial fluid within a joint capsule. Synovial joints possess certain characteristics including:

    (a) space between the articulating bones called the synovial cavity;
    (b) presence of synovial fluid within the synovial cavity, which lubricates the joint;
    (c) joint capsule;
    (d) articular cartilage covering the articulating ends of the bones;
    (e) synovial membrane which secretes the synovial fluid.

The generalised structure of a synovial joint is illustrated in Figure 5.2.

    A synovial joint possesses a joint cavity which is enclosed by a ligamentous capsule. This is lined with a synovial membrane which secretes synovial fluid into the cavity and provides lubrication for the joint. The articulating ends of the bones which form a syno-vial joint are covered with a smooth hard-wearing cartilage (articular cartilage). This is usually hyaline cartilage but in a few cases it is made of fibrocartilage. Also asso-ciated with synovial joints are ligaments which provide the joint with strengthening and stability. The ligaments permit movement in the desired directions but restrict move-ments that would damage the joint or make it unstable. Other structures associated with synovial joints are the bursae. These are fluid-filled sacs which prevent excessive friction and damage to tissues around the joint. The bursae are situated between moving struc-tures and the joint itself. They therefore prevent a muscle or tendon from being damaged and worn as it continually rubs past the joint. Synovial joints may also contain discs of fibrocartilage within them. These discs are known as menisci and provide the joint with additional stability as in the case of the lateral and medial menisci of the knee.

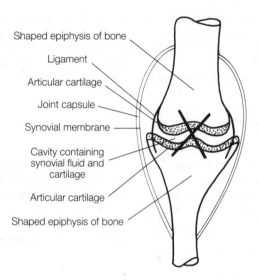

Shaped epiphysis of bone

Ligament

Articular cartilage

Joint capsule

Synovial membrane

Cavity containing synovial fluid and cartilage

Articular cartilage

Shaped epiphysis of bone

Figure 5.2 Illustrating the generalized structure of a synovial joint.

There is a great deal of variation in the precise structure of the synovial joints of the body. They are therefore subclassified according to their function and the amount of movement they permit. The basic types of synovial joint are:

1. Ball and Socket
2. Hinge
3. Gliding
4. Condyloid
5. Saddle
6. Pivot.

Whilst these joints are classified according to their structure and the major movements they permit, it should be noted that in some cases other slight movements may also be possible. For instance, although the knee and elbow are primarily considered as hinge joints, a slight amount of rotation is possible. Therefore such categorizations are to some extent generalizations.

Ball-and-socket joints

The ball-shaped end of one bone fits into a socket formed by the other bone(s) of the joint. This kind of joint (Figure 5.3) permits an extensive amount of movement in many planes including flexion, extension, abduction, adduction, rotation and circumduction. Examples of these joints are the hip and shoulder.

Hinge joints

This name can be slightly misleading as the joint does not have a pin extending

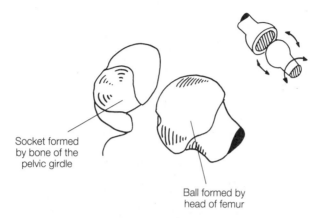

Socket formed
by bone of the
pelvic girdle

Ball formed by
head of femur

Figure 5.3 Illustrating the structure of a ball-and-socket joint.

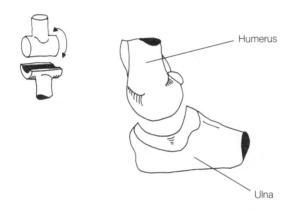

Humerus

Ulna

Figure 5.4 Illustrating the structure of a hinge joint.

through it (as in the case of a true hinge). However, like a hinge these joints primarily permit movement in just one plane. The structure of a hinge joint (Figure 5.4) involves the convex surface of one bone fitting into the concave surface of another. Examples of hinge joints include the knee joint, elbow joint and the first and second joints of the phalanges which permit the flexion and extension movements of the fingers and toes.

Gliding joints

Gliding joints (Figure 5.5) permit a limited amount of movement in many directions as the bones slide past each other. Examples of gliding joints include those between the tarsals of the foot, the carpals of the hand and that between the sternum and clavicle.

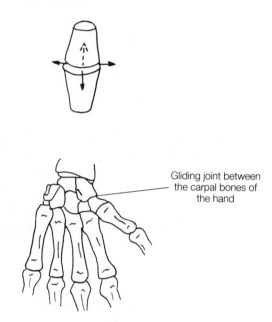

Figure 5.5 Illustrating the structure of a gliding joint.

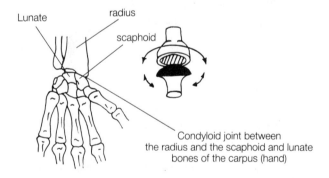

Figure 5.6 Illustrating the structure of a condyloid or ellipsoidal joint.

Condyloid or ellipsoidal joints

The structure of a condyloid or ellipsoidal joint (Figure 5.6) includes a shallow elliptical cavity in one bone into which fits an oval or ellipsoid-shaped head (condyle) of another bone. An example of a condyloid joint is the wrist, where the structure of the joint enables extension/flexion, abduction/adduction and circumduction movements. Examples of such joints include the wrist and the metacarpal/phalangeal joints btween the fingers and the metacarpals of the hand.

144

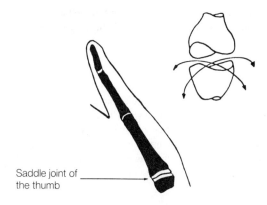

Figure 5.7 Illustrating the structure of a saddle joint.

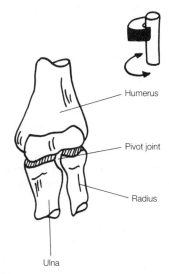

Figure 5.8 Illustrating the structure of a pivot joint.

Saddle joints

The carpometacarpal joint of the thumb provides the one example of a saddle joint (Figure 5.7). The bones are shaped much like a saddle being convex in one direction and concave in another. The shape of the bones permits a considerable range of movement including flexion, extension, abduction, adduction and circumduction.

Pivot joints

The structure of a pivot joint (Figure 5.8) consists of a hole (fossa) in one bone into which fits the boney process of another. Pivot joints enable rotations to occur, an

145

example being the ulna and radius where the rounded head of the radius rotates within a concave notch of the ulna. This enables the rotation of the forearm.

Sesamoid bones

The exact functions of some sesamoid bones remain unclear and they may serve a number of specific functions with respect to movement. In general they are found within the tendons of some muscles where they alter the angle of pull of the muscles. This can make the action of the muscle more efficient. An example of a sesamoid bone is the patella (knee cap), which is situated within the patellar tendon. The positioning of the patella also provides the knee joint with a degree of physical protection against blows.

THE ASSESSMENT AND MONITORING OF JOINT MOBILITY

The objective assessment and monitoring of a person's flexibility may fulfil many functions. An initial assessment may reveal immmobility at specific joints and hence indicate joints which may need to be exercised. An initial assessment will also provide an objective measure of the amount of mobility a person possesses at specific joints. These measurements can then be compared with subsequent measurements, thereby enabling a person's joint mobility to be objectively monitored. If desired, these measurements may be used to provide positive feedback to the participant as well as informing the therapist/adviser of the effectiveness of the exercise programme.

When assessing a person it is essential that the methods of measurement are standardized along with the conditions under which the measurements are taken. For example, the assessor may choose to measure the participant's mobility after he or she has performed an exercise session and is already warm. If this is so then all comparative measurements should be taken following a similar session since the participant is likely to be more flexible after a session than before it. Ideally, the same time of day should be used since most people are far less flexible first thing in the morning. The room in which the assessment takes place should also be comfortably warm; if the person is cold then he or she is liable to be less flexible. A few preparatory stretches may also be advisable and should be encouraged before all assessment sessions since this could have a substantial effect upon the results.

The instrument commonly used to measure joint mobility is the clinical goniometer, which can be used to assess movement at virtually any joint. The instrument is placed on the body part that is to be moved, the dial is set to zero, the limb is moved (either actively or passively depending upon which aspects of mobility are being measured) and the assessor records the degree of movement that has been measured by the instrument. There are several variations on the goniometer but all are basically simple to use and an assessor may become proficient in their use with relatively little practice. An illustration of the use of a goniometer is given in Figure 5.9, showing the measurement of shoulder abduction.

Alternative methods for assessing flexibility involve standardized tests such as the sit and reach test or back hyperextension test. These are less applicable in the clinical

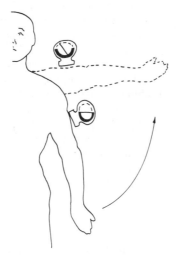

Figure 5.9 Illustrating the use of a goniometer.

setting since they tend to measure movements over a range of joints and, as such, are therefore less specific in the readings they produce.

All individuals vary in their level of flexiblity due to certain inherited factors. This applies to both their current level of joint mobility and their potential to improve. Therefore, although norms may be applied in the assessment of joint movement the key issue is likely to be the monitoring of an individual and a comparison between that person's current scores and previous ones. When monitoring, careful measurement is important and a comprehensive set of records should be kept for each individual. In this context the use of appropriate movement terminology will aid in the communication of such records between therapists and when comparing or discussing the results.

TYPES OF FLEXIBILITY EXERCISES

General introduction

As with most forms of movement, different vocabularies may be used by different authorities. In this text flexibility exercises will be considered under three headings:

1. Static stretching
2. Ballistic stretching
3. Loosening exercises.

Of these three types the static stretching and loosening exercises are advocated by this text. Concerns regarding the use of ballistic stretching are discussed later.

Flexibility exercises may be undertaken either as a separate session designed specifically to develop/maintain joint mobility or they may be incorporated into a more diverse session designed to develop a number of aspects of physical capacity. Such sessions will therefore involve other activities, together with the flexibility exercises that are often included as part of the warm-up phase of an exercise session. The inclusion of flexibility exercises into a warm-up is strongly recommended since not only will they develop flexibility but they are likely to enhance the effectiveness of the session and reduce any risk of injury which may occur if the muscles are unprepared for strenuous activity. During the initial stages of a warm-up gentle loosening exercises are strongly recommended to mobilize the joints and prepare the body for activity. At this time gentle static stretches are also effective, provided that the stretches are gentle and not forced. Once the muscles have warmed up a greater degree of stretch may be applied by repeating the static stretches in a more concerted manner.

Sessions which include flexibility work may have the following format:

1. Flexibility specific session:
   (a) possible passive warm-up (if an active warm-up is not to be included later);
   (b) gentle loosening exercises;
   (c) gentle static stretching;
   (d) active warm-up to elevate muscle temperature (if this is being used rather than a passive warm-up);
   (e) intensive stretching exercises: this forms the major content of the session;
   (f) gentle loosening exercises to cool down.
2. Flexibility as an element within another session:
   (a) gentle loosening exercises;
   (b) gentle static stretching;
   (c) active warm-up to elevate muscle temperature and prepare the body for the activity;
   (d) further loosening and static stretching;
   (e) major content of the session, which may be aerobic, strength or activity based, or a combination, during which phase additional flexibility exercises may be incorporated to provide a recovery from the strenuous elements of the session as well as being of value in their own right;
   (f) cool-down, which should include flexibility exercises.

Static stretching

Static stretching involves a joint being slowly stretched with the stretched position being held for a number of seconds. Static stretching exercises may be considered under three subheadings: active or non-assisted stretching, passive or assisted stretching and proprioceptive neuromuscular facilitation.

Active or non-assisted stretching

In active or non-assisted stretching the stretch on a relaxed muscle is achieved through the active contraction of the participant's own muscles (with the stretched muscle being antagonistic to those contracting and therefore, by definition, being relaxed and lengthened during the stretch). Active stretching may also help to develop the strength of the muscles used to cause the stretch.

Passive or assisted stretching

In this form of stretching the stretch on a muscle is achieved with the assistance of some external force or object. For instance, the therapist or adviser may apply a gentle force which stretches a muscle further than participants could achieve on their own. Alternatively, a stationary object such as a wall may be used to increase the amount of stretch that is possible. Another way of increasing the amount of stretch is by having the participants assist the stretch, as is the case when they use their arms to pull their legs further into a stretched position and hold them in a position that they would be unable to do without the assistance of their arms. It is usually possible to achieve a greater degree of stretch with passive/assisted stretching than with active/non-assisted stretching.

Proprioceptive neuromuscular facilitation

This, known as PNF, is a more advanced form of stretching which may be used to develop muscular strength as well as flexibility. PNF works on the basis that a muscle may be stretched further if it first undergoes a maximal static contraction. PNF may be active or passive, the difference between the two will be discussed, together with the exercises, later in this chapter.

The physiology of static stretching

Static stretching has been demonstrated to be a most effective way of improving mobility at a joint, and because it is static it does not convey the risks associated with ballistic stretching, which are discussed later in this section. During a static stretching exercise a muscle is stretched to the point where the participant can feel the stretch and perhaps even slight discomfort but not sufficient to cause pain. The stretch applied to the muscle will result in the muscle spindles (see proprioceptors) detecting the stretch and sending signals to the central nervous system via sensory neurons. This will result in impulses being sent back to the muscle from the central nervous system, causing some of the muscle fibres to contract. This causes a certain amount of tension to develop within the muscle, preventing it from being stretched further. However, if the stretch is held for at least 6 seconds the Golgi organs (other proprioceptors situated at the muscle–tendon junction) send signals to the central nervous system which inhibit this stretch reflex. Thus after about 6 to 10 seconds the tension in the muscle is reduced and the muscle may be stretched a little further without pain or risk of damage. This process may then be repeated a number of times to produce an effective stretch on the muscle and, more specifically, on the connective tissue situated within the muscle. In this way the connective tissue between the muscle fibres, and in some cases the tendons, is effectively stretched thereby increasing the range of movement that is permissible at the joint.

In practice, for effective static stretching the following sequence of events and considerations should be adhered to:

1. The muscles should be warmed up and relaxed.
2. They should be slowly moved to the point of stretch (to minimize the stretch reflex).
3. They should be held in the stretched position for at least 15 seconds (for effective stretching and to inhibit the stretch reflex).
4. The stretch should then be slowly increased.
5. Steps 3 and 4 should be repeated a number of times before allowing the limb back to its resting state.
6. The participant should try to relax and keep the stretched muscles as relaxed as possible throughout the exercise.
7. The therapist should talk to the participant throughout the exercise to try to ensure that he or she remains relaxed and does not tense up the muscles.
8. The stretch must not be forced: it is therefore important for the participant to inform the therapist of the amount of stretch being experienced.
9. When the therapist is applying a force to assist the stretch care must be taken not to overstretch the muscles.

Thus a key aspect of static stretching is the holding of the end position which enables the initial stretch reflex to be inhibited. The stretch reflex is also one of the reasons why vigorous ballistic stretching is not recommended as a means of developing joint mobility.

Static vs ballistic stretching

Ballistic stretching involves a 'bouncing action' and, as such, involves a limb being moved rapidly through its full range of motion towards the full extent of the joint's permissible movement. For a number of reasons ballistic stretching is not only less effective than static stretching but also conveys a risk of injury.

1. The connective tissue within a muscle is more effectively stretched if it is held in the stretched position (as with static stretching) rather than being quickly stretched.
2. In ballistic stretching the momentum of the moving limb may cause the joint to be forced beyond its normal and safe range of motion. This can cause the muscles and associated joint structures to be overstretched and damaged. The slow nature of static stretching prevents the movement from exceeding the safe limits of the joint.
3. During ballistic stretching the muscle spindles, which react to both the rate and extent of a stretch, initiate a strong stretch reflex. This will cause the muscle fibres to contract and shorten. However, the momentum of the limb may force the muscle to continue to be stretched against its attempted contraction. This conflict may result in damage to the muscles or tendons.
4. During a ballistic movement the stretch reflex is likely to be initiated before

the limb reaches the limits of the joint's normal range of motion. Even a gentle bouncing action may be sufficient to initiate a basic stretch reflex and cause a musle muscle to 'tense up'. This will prevent the connective tissue from being effectively stretched and the joint from reaching its maximum range of movement.

Therefore, in general, ballistic stretching is not advised as a means of developing joint mobility and/or increasing the length of the muscles. However, whilst ballistic stretching is inadvisable, it does not mean that all stretching or mobility exercises have to be static. Loosening exercises are an alternative form of stretching that may be safely used to complement static stretches. Unlike ballistic stretches which use vigorous movements, the movements used for loosening exercises are slow and controlled. In some cases it will also be performed well within the subject's range of static flexibility.

Loosening exercises

Loosening exercises form an important aspect of flexibility work. They often involve slow, controlled circumduction movements at joints such as the ankle, hip, wrist and shoulder. Like static stretching they may also be active/non-assisted or passive/assisted. In the case of assisted loosening exercises the assistance comes from either the participant or the therapist. For example, a greater range of movement may be produced at the ankle joint if the movement is assisted with the hands. Such loosening exercises may be used as part of a warming-up process prior to static stretching or some other form of activity.

Another form of loosening exercise may involve gentle swinging actions of the arms or legs. These are similar to the ballistic actions condemned in the previous section; however, it should be emphasized that these loosening exercises should be performed well within a participant's normal range of motion for that joint and participants should not attempt to increase their range of motion by swinging close to their normal range of static flexibility. It should also be emphasized that these loosening exercises should be performed in a controlled 'gentle' manner and should not be fast or vigorous. Gently swinging the leg from the hip provides an example of such actions which are performed as a 'loosening' activity within a session rather than as a specific attempt to give a permanent increase in mobility at a specific joint.

GENERAL CONSIDERATIONS FOR STRETCHING EXERCISES AND STRETCHING ROUTINES

When performing flexibility exercises it is important that the joints involved are stretched through their 'normal' range of movement and not out of their normal alignment. Stretching a joint in a 'unnatural' alignment can overstretch the ligaments of the joint making it less stable. In all cases of static stretching the stretched position should be reached in a slow and controlled manner, without jerking or bouncing. The stretched position should then be held for a minimum of 6 to 15 seconds, after which the stretch should be gently extended and held for at least a further 6 seconds. This process may then be repeated two or three times for each stretch. Each stretching exercise may then be repeated a number of times on each joint. During the initial exercise sessions the static stretches should be held for a minimum of 6 to 10 seconds, but as the participant becomes more familiar with the exercises the stretches may be held for a longer period of time, extending up to a minute for each stretch.

Loosening exercises should be conducted in a slow and controlled manner. The emphasis of these exercises is on a slow, gentle stretch and the exercises should not force the joint. Each exercise should be performed about six times on each limb and, where appropriate, should be repeated in both directions, i.e. clockwise and anti-clockwise. The specific factors to be considered with each exercise will be presented with details of the exercise later in this chapter.

The stretching exercises presented in this section represent a comprehensive selection which may be used to stretch most of the major muscle groups of the body and, hence, develop the mobility of most of the major joints of the body. However, the therapist may apply modifications to those exercises, depending on circumstances and the joints on which he or she wishes to concentrate. The number of flexibility exercises used in a session, the duration for which the stretches are held and the number of repetitions of each exercise will depend upon individual circumstances. Factors such as the amount of time available and the condition of the participant will have a major influence in dictating the precise design of the session.

Some muscles extend over more than one joint and to achieve an effective stretch on these muscles the position of both joints should be considered. Examples of such muscles include the gastrocnemius and members of the hamstring group. If the stretches are being used as part of a warm-up prior to some other activity then time may dictate that each static stretch will be held for just 6 seconds and repeated just once or twice. If, however, the stretches are being used to specifically develop or maintain joint movements then a more extensive stretching routine will be undertaken, with each static stretch being held for a longer period and repeated several times. Throughout such a session the participant should keep warm, and therefore the exercises may be interspersed with other activities as well as attention being paid to the clothing worn.

Therapists or advisers may select any number of stretches from those presented in this chapter according to the aims of the session. They may choose to concentrate upon specific joints or they may wish to stretch all the major joints. With practice and experience it is also possible for a therapist to modify certain stretches according to individual needs, and thus an extensive repertoire of stretching exercises may be developed. There are a number of exercises that may be used to stretch the muscles associated with any particular joint, and the choice of which variation of stretch is most effective for, or applicable to, the individual must be left to the professional judgement of the therapist. Since people vary in their anatomical make-up, some individuals may find one particular exercise very effective for stretching a muscle group, such as the hamstrings, whilst another individual may prefer a variation of that exercise. Therefore, the overall stretching routine will be developed through the experience and knowledge of the therapist in conjunction with the participant's own perception of the ease and effectiveness of the exercises.

In order to ensure that the participant performs all the desired stretches at each session it is usual to produce a list or chart of the exercises which may be ticked as each one is completed. In this way no stretch is likely to be forgotten. Progression should also be included in the exercise programme, and recording the time for which each stretch should be held, together with the type and number of stretches included in each session, will help to demonstrate progression to the participant. This will also aid the therapist in ensuring that the progression within the programme is steady and logical rather than random. Regular monitoring at four- to six-week intervals may also provide positive feedback for both the participant and assessor, informing them of the effectiveness of the exercises. As with all forms of exercise, flexibility work needs to be frequent. Ideally a stretching routine should be repeated at least once every day. Therefore, the participants should be encouraged to perform the routine or at least some of it every day, even if the therapist is unable to see them so frequently.

EXAMPLES OF STATIC STRETCHING EXERCISES

When undertaking any of the exercises presented in this section it should be remembered that the stretched position should be reached slowly and then held. These exercises are a combination of active and passive exercises, many of which may be modified into an assisted form if the therapist so wishes. With such assisted stretches good communication is required between the participant and therapist if the correct amount of stretch is to be achieved. Also, while certain exercises are reported to stretch the same muscle groups, the participants may find some exercises more effective than others and that the different stretches may be effective in different regions of the same muscle group. For instance, while stretches 10 and 11 are both designed to stretch the muscles of the hamstring group, the participant may find that stretch 10 causes more stretch at the distal end of the muscle group near the knee with stretch 11 being more effective at the proximal end near the hip joint. The precise effectiveness and region of stretch will vary between individuals because of each person's unique anatomical make-up.

1. *Achilles and soleus stretch* (Figure 5.10). Stand with one foot approximately 3 feet behind the other, then flex the knee of the back leg whilst keeping the

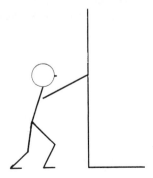

Figure 5.10

153

foot flat on the floor (this exercise will stretch the achilles tendon and the soleus muscle of the back leg). During the exercise the knee of the front leg will also have to be flexed slightly and a support such as a wall or table may be used for balance. Hold the stretch for the desired duration and repeat on both legs.

2. *Gastrocnemius stretch* (Figure 5.11). Stand approximately 3 feet away from a support such as a wall. Place the hands on the wall for support then take a step back with one foot. Place the sole of the back foot flat on the floor and keep the knee of the back leg fully extended. To achieve this the knee of the front leg will need to be flexed slightly. Stretch should be felt in the gastrocnemius: if it is not then try moving further away from the wall and/or tilting the hips forwards towards the wall. Hold the stretch for the desired duration and repeat on both legs.

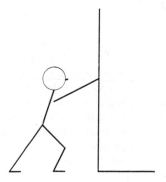

Figure 5.11

3. *Hip flexor stretch* (Figure 5.12). Kneel on one knee as illustrated, then move the hips forwards slowly until stretch is felt in the hip flexors of the back leg. When doing the stretch the participant should place the hands on the floor to provide stability and should keep the front knee over the front foot. Hold the stretch for the desired duration and repeat on both legs.

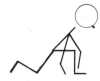

Figure 5.12

4. *Adductor stretch 1* (Figure 5.13). Stand with the feet apart, approximately 18 inches wider than shoulder width, then outwardly rotate one leg so that one foot is facing forwards whilst the rotated one faces to the side. Keep the forward facing foot flat on the ground and the corresponding knee extended. Then flex the knee of the sideways facing foot and gently lower the body until stretch is felt in the adductor muscles of the extended leg. When flexing the knee and lowering the body it may be necessary to move the feet further apart for comfort and further adjustments to foot positioning may be needed to attain the ideal position with the flexed knee being positioned directly above the outwardly rotated foot. Hold the stretch for the desired duration and repeat on both legs.

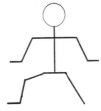

Figure 5.13

5. *Adductor stretch 2* (Figure 5.14). This is performed in a seated position. The participant sits as illustrated with the soles of the feet touching and the elbows resting gently on the thighs. This may produce an initial stretch which may be enhanced by the participant pushing down on the thighs with the elbows.

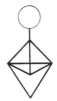

Figure 5.14

6. *Hamstring stretch 1* (Figure 5.15). This is most likely to be performed as an assisted stretch. The participant should lie on his or her back and flex one hip raising the leg whilst keeping the knee extended. Alternatively, the therapist may raise the leg. The leg should then be eased forward by further flexion of the hip until the point of resistance or slight discomfort is reached. Stretch should be felt in the hamstrings and the position should be held for the desired duration before lowering the limb. When performing this stretch with the aid of a therapist good communication is required between the participant and therapist to ensure that the correct amount of stretch is applied. The participant

may be able to perform this stretch without the aid of a therapist by using an aid such as a short piece of rope or clothing which is looped around the foot and pulled on in order to achieve the stretch. An advancement of this stretch is described in the section on PNF later in this chapter.

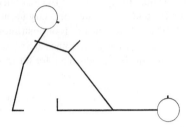

Figure 5.15

7. *Hamstring stretch 2* (Figure 5.16). Place one foot on an elevated object that is approximately 2 feet high (a chair will usually suffice). Keep the knee of the elevated leg extended and place the hands on the thigh of the elevated leg. Flex forwards from the hips, trying to keep the back straight, and slide the hands down towards the ankles of the elevated leg, without curving the back too much. The stretch should be felt in the muscles of the hamstring group. If the stretch is felt directly behind the knee rather than in the main body of the muscles then the knee should be flexed slightly and the stretch repeated with a slightly flexed knee, which should produce the desired stretch in the muscles.

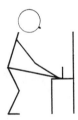

Figure 5.16

8. *Hamstring stretch 3* (Figure 5.17). This is a variation of stretch 7 and i performed from a kneeling position on the floor. The participant kneels or one knee and extends the other leg in front of them. The participant then place the hands on the thigh of the extended leg. From this position, they flex a the hips and slowly slide the hands down the extended leg towards the foot In performing this stretch the participant should attempt to keep the back straigh in order to ensure that the stretch occurs in the hamstrings and does not stres the back.

Figure 5.17

9. *Hamstring stretch 4* (Figure 5.18). This is a variation on stretch 7 and is performed from a seated position on the floor. When performing this stretch both legs may be extended, or one may be flexed with the foot positioned next to the knee of the extended leg. As with the other variations of the hamstring stretch the emphasis is on stretching the hamstrings without putting stress on the back. This may be ensured by keeping the back relatively straight and bending from the hips.

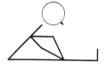

Figure 5.18

10. *Hamstring stretch 5* (Figure 5.19). Place a pile of books or mats on the floor, stand behind them and then bend down to place the hands flat on the books or mats. The knees should now be flexed; then, whilst keeping the hands flat on the pile, slowly try to extend the knees. This should produce a gentle stretch in the hamstrings. If the participant can fully extend the knees whilst keeping the hands on the mats or books, then the exercise should be tried with a smaller pile or even with the hands flat on the floor. Whilst appearing to be similar this exercise is preferable to the more traditional 'Stand and touch the toes' exercise. This is because in this preferred version the muscles are being stretched by the action of other muscle groups rather than the movement being

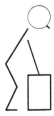

Figure 5.19

caused by gravity, as is the case when 'touching the toes'. Indeed the 'touching the toes' exercise is now commonly avoided by many authorities because it may put unwanted strain on the back of some individuals.

11. *Hamstring stretch 6* (Figure 5.20). The participant should lie on their back, with their head resting gently on the floor. Flex the knee and hip of one leg, bringing the knee up towards the chest. Grasp the knee with both hands and gently pull the knee towards the chest, keeping the other leg fully extended and flat on the floor. Stretch should be felt in the hamstrings.

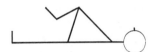

Figure 5.20

12. *Quadriceps stretch* (Figure 5.21). Stand on one leg whilst fully flexing the knee of the other leg. Grasp the ankle of the flexed leg with the hand and hold it close to the buttock ensuring that the knee is in the correct alignment and is not twisted or rotated. To apply additional stretch the participant should extend the hip joint whilst continuing to hold onto the ankle. To do this, the participant will need to lean forward slightly in order to maintain balance. This should produce a stretch in the quadriceps muscles. Since the quadriceps extend over two joints the hip must be extended and the knee flexed if an effective stretch is to be achieved over the whole muscle group.

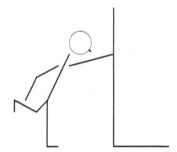

Figure 5.21

13. *Back stretch* (Figure 5.22). The participant should lie on their back on the floor in a relaxed position. Then try to push the lower back into the floor and hold the position for a few seconds. This is a general back exercise which may

help to reduce or prevent certain forms of back pain. It may also help to develop the strength of the back muscles as well as back mobility.

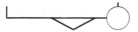

Figure 5.22

14. *Upper back and shoulder stretch* (Figure 5.23). Kneel on the floor as illustrated, stretching the arms out in front of the head and placing the hands on the floor. Note that when performing this stretch the participant should not sit back on the heels but should lean forwards. The hands should then be moved forwards along the ground until the 'stretched' position is reached. Stretch should be experienced in the upper back and shoulders.

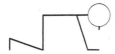

Figure 5.23

15. *Lower back and hip stretch* (Figure 5.24). The participant should lie on their back in a relaxed position. When stretching the left side the left arm should be abducted at right angles to the body with the palm touching the floor. The left knee should then be flexed at 90 degrees and the left foot crossed over the right knee. The left leg is then grasped by the right hand and pulled across the right leg in an adduction movement. The left knee should be eased across until stretch is felt down the lateral side of the left hip and lower back. The stretch may be enhanced by turning the head to the left whilst performing the stretch. In order to stretch the right hip and right side the positions need to be reversed.

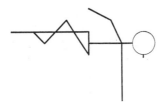

Figure 5.24

16. *Abductor stretch* (Figure 5.25). To stretch the left abductor muscles the participant sits on the floor and crosses the left leg over the right, placing the left foot just to the right of the right knee. The participant then turns the body to the left as far as it will go and places the right elbow on the lateral side of the left knee (the lateral side being the side which is furthest from the midline of the body when standing in the anatomical position). The participant then uses the right elbow to push the left knee further to the right until stretch is experienced in the abductor muscles down the left side of the body. As with the previous stretch the positions need to be reversed in order to stretch the muscles down the right side of the body.

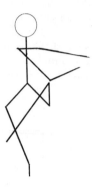

Figure 5.25

17. *Side stretch* (Figure 5.26). To stretch the left side of the body the participant abducts or flexes the left arm so that it is raised above the head, and turns the palm of the hand so that it comfortably faces inwards. They then laterally flex to the right, and stretch should be felt down the left side of the body. The position should then be held for the desired duration and the positions reversed in order to produce the stretch on the right side of the body.

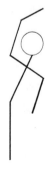

Figure 5.26

18. *Shoulder and arm stretch 1* (Figure 5.27). The hands should be clasped in front of the body and then the shoulders flexed to raise the arms above the head. The hands should remain clasped together and, if possible, the shoulders should reach a position of hyperflexion whereby the hands are positioned behind the frontal plane of the body. Stretch should be encountered in the shoulders and arms. This stretch may easily be assisted by the therapist.

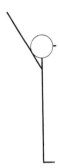

Figure 5.27

19. *Shoulder and arm stretch 2* (Figure 5.28). This is a variation of stretch 18. The participant lies face down with the arms extended above the head. Clasp the hands together and then try to raise the hands off the floor. During the exercise the participant should attempt to get the hands as high as possible whilst keeping the elbows extended and chin on the floor. This should produce stretch in the arms and shoulders.

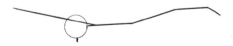

Figure 5.28

20. *Shoulder and arm stretch 3* (Figure 5.29). The participant flexes one elbow and adducts the arm across in front of the body in an attempt to touch the opposite shoulder blade. Additional stretch may be achieved by pushing up on the elbow of the stretched shoulder with the hand of the opposite arm.

Figure 5.29

21. *Shoulder and arm stretch 4* (Figure 5.30). Firstly, the shoulder is fully flexed until the arm is in a vertical position. The elbow is then flexed so that the lower arm extends down the back and the hand can touch the spine. The participant should attempt to reach as far down the spine as possible. This should produce some stretch in the shoulder and arm. The stretch may be enhanced by placing the hand of the opposite arm on the elbow of the 'stretched' arm and pushing downwards. This produces a greater amount of stretch in the arm and shoulder regions.

Figure 5.30

22. *Shoulder and arm stretch 5* (Figure 5.31). One arm is flexed at the elbow so that it is positioned behind the back and the back of the hand touches the opposite shoulder blade. The arm is therefore positioned so that it is reaching up the back. The participant then attempts to reach as high up the back as they can. This produces an initial amount of stretch. The hand of the opposite arm is then placed under the elbow of the stretched arm and pushed upwards, thus applying more stretch. The position should then be held for the desired duration.

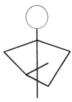

Figure 5.31

23. *Shoulder and arm stretch 6* (Figure 5.32). This is a combination of stretches 21 and 22. One arm performs stretch 21 such that it is reaching down the back whilst the other arm performs stretch 22 such that it is reaching up the

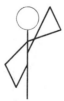

Figure 5.32

back. The participant then attempts to get the hands to touch. If this can be done then an attempt should be made to clasp the hands together and apply additional stretch by pulling with the appropriate arm.

24. *Shoulder and arm stretch 7* (Figure 5.33). Both shoulders are flexed so that the arms are extended in front of the body. The hands are linked together by linking the fingers with the palms touching. Whilst keeping the fingers linked the palms are then turned outwards so that they face forwards, away from the body. In order to do this it will be necessary to flex the elbows. The hands are then pushed away from the body by extending the elbows. The arms may also be raised or lowered in order to alter the stretch. This exercise produces a stretch in the arms and the shoulder region.

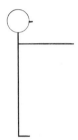

Figure 5.33

25. *Shoulder, arm and chest stretch 1* (Figure 5.34). The participant stands facing a wall or similar fixed object with one arm abducted so that the hand is at shoulder height with the palm touching the wall. The body is then turned away from the wall and away from the abducted arm whilst keeping the palm of the hand flat against the wall and the arm parallel to the wall. This will produce stretch in the shoulder of the abducted arm.

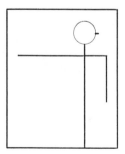

Figure 5.34

26. *Shoulder, arm and chest stretch 2* (Figure 5.35). This is a variation of stretch 25 and requires the assistance of the therapist. The participant stands in the anatomical position and then abducts both arms to shoulder height. The

therapist stands behind the participant and grasps both wrists. The therapist then gently eases back the participant's arms keeping the hands at shoulder height until appropriate stretch is felt in the shoulders. With this stretch some individuals with very good shoulder mobility may be able to get their arms to cross behind their back whilst others with less shoulder mobility may be able to get their arms only just past the frontal plane.

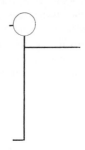

Figure 5.35

27. *Neck lateral flexion* (Figure 5.36). The neck is laterally flexed to one side to produce stretch on the opposing side. During this stretch the shoulders should be kept down and level to maximize the stretch.

Figure 5.36

28. *Neck flexion and extension* (Figure 5.37). The neck is slowly flexed forward so that the chin rests on the chest and the position is held for a number of seconds. The neck is then slowly extended so that the head tilts back and this position is also held for a number of seconds, after which the exercise may be repeated.

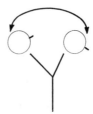

Figure 5.37

29. *Extension of the spine* (Figure 5.38). Extension or hyperextension stretching of the spine may be achieved with the following exercise, which can also be used to develop the strength of the back muscles. If this exercise causes pain or excessive discomfort it should not be continued. The participant lies face down and places the hands behind the head or clasps them behind the back. The participant then attempts to raise the chest off the floor by hyperextending the back. This position should only be held for a few seconds and, because of the muscle strength required, not everyone will be able to perform it.

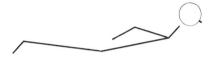

Figure 5.38

30. *Forward flexion of the spine* (Figure 5.39). Some degree of stretching of the spine will be achieved in the flexion of the back during hamstring stretches 7, 8, 9 and 10, although in these exercises the emphasis is on ensuring that the stretch is in the hamstrings and that there is no excessive strain on the back. This exercise is specific for the back. The participant sits on the floor and brings the knees up to the chest. The arms are then wrapped around the knees and the head is put on the knees forming a tightly tucked position which should be held for a number of seconds. As an advancement on the exercise the participant may then roll gently onto the back and rock forwards and backwards 6 to 12 times. This should only be done on a well-cushioned mat or other suitable surface. This latter variation is clearly not entirely a static stretch since movement is involved, although the spine itself is being held in a static position.

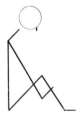

Figure 5.39

31. *Spinal rotation* (Figure 5.40). Spinal rotation will be incorporated into exercises 15 and 16. However, as a specific spinal rotation exercise the participant should stand with the feet about shoulder width apart, and should then slowly twist the upper body (rotate in the transverse plane) as far as it will go whilst keeping the feet firmly positioned on the floor. The head should lead

the rotation and greater stretch may be achieved if the arms are raised to shoulder height and are used to enhance the rotation of the spine.

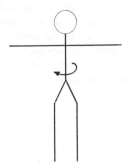

Figure 5.40

32. *General stretch* (Figure 5.41). This simple stretch involves the participant lying on the back on the floor with the feet together and the arms extended above the head. The participant then tries to extend the body as much as possible, making it as long as possible. This may be held for 5 to 10 seconds and is typical of a general stretch which someone may perform naturally first thing in the morning or after being in a constricted position for some time. It is often a useful stretch to conclude a flexibility session.

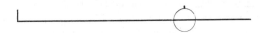

Figure 5.41

EXAMPLES OF LOOSENING EXERCISES

The loosening exercises presented in this section should be performed in a slow and controlled manner. In all the exercises (bar the leg and arm swings, exercises 7 and 8) the emphasis of the exercise should be upon easing the joint through its maximum range of movement. Where applicable, all rotation and circumduction movements should be performed in both clockwise and anticlockwise directions. All the loosening exercises described here may be performed in an active or assisted manner. The assisted versions may have the advantage of producing a greater range of movement at the joint whilst the active versions may have desired benefits upon improving muscle tone and muscular strength at the joint. It is therefore up to the therapist to decide which is most appropriate for the individuals with whom they are working.

1. *Ankle circumduction* (Figure 5.42). The participant sits on the floor or a seat and slowly circles one foot in a clockwise direction. The movement should be slow and the emphasis should be upon trying to make the circle as large

as possible. The movement should then be repeated in an anticlockwise direction before performing the exercise on the other ankle. This exercise may be active or passive and assisted with either the participant or therapist using hands to assist the movement. The movement should be repeated 6 to 12 times in each direction for each ankle.

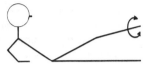

Figure 5.42

2. *Wrist circumduction* (Figure 5.43). This exercise for the wrists is equivalent to that previously described for the ankles. Whilst keeping the forearm relatively still the wrist should be slowly circumducted in a clockwise direction, trying to circumscribe as large a circle as possible. The movement should be performed 6 to 12 times in both directions for both wrists. Again, the exercise may be active or passive and assisted depending upon the requirements of the participant.

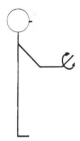

Figure 5.43

3. *Shoulder circumduction* (Figure 5.44). The participant stands or sits in a position which will not impede the arm movements. In this exercise both shoulders

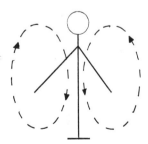

Figure 5.44

167

may be exercised at the same time with one arm mirroring the movements of the other. The movement is a circumduction of the shoulders during which the arms attempt to circumscribe as large a circle as possible. During the movement the arms should be brought in front of the body so that they cross, and the movement should be repeated 6 to 12 times in both directions for both shoulders.

4. *Hip circumduction* (Figure 5.45). For this exercise the participant should hold on to a support for balance. The participant stands on one leg and flexes the hip and knee of the other leg, raising the knee until it is approximately at the same height as the hip. The circumduction movement then moves the knee towards the midline of the body and then away in a circular movement. During this movement the amount of flexion upon the knee will vary. The movement should be repeated 6 to 12 times in each direction for each hip.

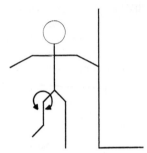

Figure 5.45

5. *Heel raises* (Figure 5.46). The participant stands with the feet approximately shoulder width apart. Both heels are then raised off the ground, putting the weight over the balls of the feet. The heels are then slowly lowered back down to the ground and the movement repeated. The exercise may be repeated 10 to 20 times or more if it is being used as a loosening exercise prior to some other activity such as jogging.

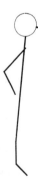

Figure 5.46

6. *Shoulder shrugs (shoulder elevation and depression)* (Figure 5.47). In this exercise the participant starts with the shoulders in a comfortable and relaxed position. The shoulders are then elevated as high as possible (keeping the arms in a relaxed position by the sides). This position should be held for about 5 seconds and then the shoulders should be lowered (shoulder depression) as far as they can go, once again holding the position for about 5 seconds. The exercise may be repeated about six times. A similar exercise could involve a more continuous movement of the shoulders without holding the end positions, or even clockwise and anticlockwise rotations of the shoulder joints (in the sagittal plane) with the arms kept by the sides.

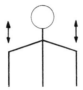

Figure 5.47

7. *Arm swings (together and in opposite directions)* (Figure 5.48). This exercise is similar to the shoulder circumduction exercise (no. 3) previously described. However, in this exercise the arms are primarily moved in the sagittal plane in a circular motion (if the participant is viewed from the side). Initially this exercise may be performed using one arm at a time, with the movement being repeated in both clockwise and anticlockwise directions 6 to 12 times. The exercise may also be performed with both arms working together in the same direction (mirroring each other's movements) and finally it may be performed with the arms moving in opposite directions, which will require a greater degree of coordination.

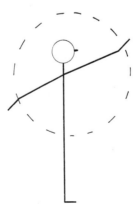

Figure 5.48

8. *Leg swings* (Figure 5.49). This is a dynamic exercise and therefore it must be emphasized that the leg swings should be gentle and performed well within the participant's normal range of static flexibility. It is also advisable that it only be performed after appropriate static hamstring flexibility exercises have been used to stretch out the muscles. The participant stands on one leg using a support for balance. The other leg is then gently swung back and forth in a relaxed manner with the extent of the movement being well within the participant's range of static flexibility in both directions. During the swinging movement the knee may be naturally flexed. The movement may be repeated 6 to 12 times for each leg.

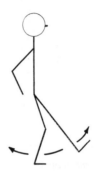

Figure 5.49

9. *Spinal and hip rotation* (Figure 5.50). The participant stands with the feet approximately shoulder width apart. The participant then rotates the upper body in a circular motion (in the transverse plane). The extent of the movement may be enhanced by using the hips in a similar rotatory action. The movement should be performed slowly and repeated 6 to 12 times in both clockwise and anticlockwise directions.

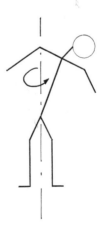

Figure 5.50

PROPRIOCEPTIVE NEUROMUSCULAR FACILITATION

Proprioceptive neuromuscular facilitation (PNF) is an advanced form of stretching which also has the added advantage of developing the strength of some of the muscles that are associated with the joint being exercised. PNF works upon the basis that a muscle can be stretched further if it has first undergone a maximum isometric contraction. The basis of PNF is illustrated using an example of a hamstring stretching exercise (Figure 5.51); however, it can easily be applied to a number of the other static stretching exercises described earlier in this chapter. PNF should only be performed after an extensive warm-up (which should elevate the muscle temperature) and a series of preliminary static stretches upon the muscles which are to be stretched using PNF. Like all forms of exercise PNF should be introduced slowly with a gradual increase in duration, repetitions and frequency. PNF stretching may be considered under two headings:

1. Active PNF
2. Passive PNF.

Most PNF exercises require the assistance of a therapist or helper, however in some cases the exercise may be modified so that a stretching aid, such as a rope or towel, may be used instead. It may be unwise to use PNF stretching routines with those individuals who suffer from high blood pressure, since PNF involves a degree of isometric muscular contraction and these individuals are generally advised to avoid isometric exercises.

Active PNF

PNF stretching for the hamstrings (Figure 5.51). The participant lies on his or her back in a relaxed position. One leg is then elevated (by flexing the hip joint) as high as possible, keeping the knee extended. At this point the restriction on further hip flexion should be due to the stretch on the hamstrings. The therapist then holds the limb in this position for 10 seconds. It may be easiest for the therapist to support the limb with his or her shoulder, as this is the best position for the therapist to resist

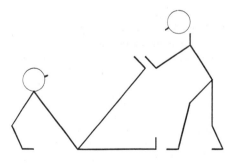

Figure 5.51

the contraction of the leg which occurs during the next phase. This will almost certainly be the best position if the participant is relatively strong; however, with a weaker participant the therapist may find it sufficient to resist the movement using hands and arms. The participant then contracts the hamstrings as fully as possible, trying to push the leg down whilst the therapist holds it in position. This maximal isometric contraction is maintained for a full 10 seconds. The participant then relaxes and tries to raise the leg as high as possible (by flexing the hip joint): this should result in the leg being moved further than it was at the start of the exercise. (This form of PNF is called 'active' because, at this point, it is the participant who actively moves the leg during this phase of the exercise, using the active contraction of his or her own muscles.) Once the position of maximum stretch is again reached, the process is repeated. An active PNF exercise may therefore include a number of cycles, the stages of which are indicated below:

1. The participant elevates the leg to the stretched position.
2. The stretched position is held for 10 seconds.
3. The participant performs a 10 second maximal isometric contraction. The contraction is resisted by either the therapist or a stretching aid.
4. The participant relaxes and then elevates the leg further to the stretched position.
5. Stages 2, 3 and 4 are repeated for the desired number of cycles.

Each cycle may be repeated three or four times before the leg is lowered and the process repeated upon the other leg. The exercise may be repeated on each leg a number of times. However, as mentioned earlier, progression up to this level of repetitions and duration should be gradual.

Should the participant want to perform the exercise without the aid of an assistant, then a towel or similar object may be looped over the foot and the ends held by the participant. This may then provide the resistive force during the contraction phase. As stated earlier, a number of the static stretching exercises previously described may be modified to incorporate aspects of PNF.

Passive PNF

Passive PNF is very similar to active PNF. However, they differ during just one phase of the process. With passive PNF it is the therapist who moves the limb to its point of maximum stretch rather than the participant moving it through the active contraction of his or her own muscles. The process should therefore include the following stages:

1. The therapist elevates the participant's leg until the participant states that an appropriate amount of stretch can be felt.
2. The stretched position is held for 10 seconds.
3. The participant then performs a maximal isometric contraction for 10 seconds (the same as for active PNF). The contraction is resisted by either the therapist or a stretching aid.

4. The participant relaxes and the therapist elevates the leg further until the participant states that an appropriate amount of stretch has been achieved.
5. Stages 2, 3 and 4 may be repeated for the desired number of cycles.

This version of PNF obviously requires good communication between the therapist and participant if the correct amount of stretch is to be applied. This method may be more effective than the active form but the therapist may consider active PNF to be preferable because of the opportunity for the participants to exercise other muscles (in producing the movement in active PNF). As with active PNF the use of stretching aids such as towels may make it possible for the participant to perform the exercise without the aid of a therapist.

Finally it should again be emphasized that PNF is a more intensive form of stretching than the simple static and loosening exercises described earlier. It should therefore be undertaken with caution and introduced gradually with particular attention being paid to warm-up.

6

Exercises for the development of muscular tone and strength

THE IMPORTANCE OF MUSCULAR STRENGTH

The skeletal muscles of the body fulfil many functions. They initiate the movement of the body and body parts; they regulate movements which are being caused by external forces; they prevent unwanted movements; and they help to maintain the posture of the body. In order to fulfil these roles successfully the muscles must possess an adequate amount of strength, a lack of which may reduce the individual's physical capacity to perform specific movements and limit the ability to undertake certain physical tasks.

Muscular strength is a complex aspect of a person's physical capacity which, like all other 'fitness components', is not isolated but is intimately related to other aspects of a person's physical capacity. Muscular strength can be discussed in the form of a continuum. At one extreme muscles have the property of 'maximal strength' which refers to the maximum amount of force a muscle or group of muscles can generate in a single maximal contraction. This may determine whether they are capable of lifting or moving a heavy object. At the other end of the spectrum there is what is often referred to as a muscle's 'strength-endurance' which can also be considered as a person's 'local muscular endurance'. This refers to the individual's capacity to repeat or sustain muscular contractions over a prolonged period of time. If this is put into the context of daily activities it will be a factor in determining a person's capacity to perform household chores such as cleaning, gardening or even carrying shopping. A good level of muscular strength-endurance will enhance a person's capacity to perform these activities without becoming unduly fatigued.

Local muscular endurance is obviously related to the fitness component of endurance, which is linked to people's aerobic capacity and, hence, stamina. However, it is also related to their maximal strength and very often the 'strengthening exercises' which are incorporated into an exercise programme will seek to develop a balance between maximal strength and muscular endurance. This is necessary since both are important to the individual. Although the exercises used to develop both maximal strength and muscular endurance are similar, the precise number of repetitions and the intensity of the exercises will vary quite considerably. In brief, the development of maximal strength will require relatively few repetitions of high-intensity exercises whilst muscular endurance requires a relatively high number of repetitions of low-intensity exercises.

Muscular strength is clearly important in the context of sports activities where the strength requirements will often exceed those required for other everyday activities. When therapists treat injured sportspeople they need to be aware of the specific demands of the individual's sport. If a muscle is weak following an injury, the stresses placed upon it by a particular sport may increase the likelihood of the injury recurring. Therefore, it is important for the therapist to ensure that the muscle is strong enough to cope with a sport before the individual returns to full training or competition.

Another form of muscular strength is 'explosive strength'. This is determined by both the maximal strength of the muscle(s) and the speed with which they contract. This aspect of strength is more often referred to as 'power'. Any dynamic muscular movement requires a certain amount of power, and improvement in the maximal strength of a muscle is likely to increase its power. However, power itself is only usually specifically 'trained' for in the sporting context where it is important in activities such as sprinting, throwing, jumping and acceleration. Therefore, in the context of most exercise programmes (where the therapist is concerned with the development of a person's physical capacity for 'normal' everyday activities) the specific development of power is not a major concern. When therapists are involved with the treatment of injured sportsperformers they are again unlikely to be concerned with the specific development of the 'power' of those people. This is because their primary concern is likely to be the strengthening of the muscles; the subsequent development of muscle power being the concern of each sportsperson's coach after that individual has recovered from his or her injury.

THE PHYSIOLOGICAL DETERMINANTS OF STRENGTH

Muscular strength is determined by a number of factors including;

1. The size of the muscle.
2. The structure of the muscle (whether it is fusiform or pennate, etc.).
3. The proportion of the different types of muscle fibres within the muscle.
4. Biochemical and histochemical properties within the muscle fibres.
5. Neurological factors.
6. Coordination, which should enable efficient movement that optimizes the action of the muscles, producing the desired amount of force for the minimal amount of effort.
7. Whether the individual is suffering from a particular disease or disorder which affects the neuromuscular system.

Muscular size

If all other factors are equal, then the larger the muscle, the more contractile filaments it will contain. The more contractile filaments it contains, the more force it can generate and, therefore, the stronger it will be. An exception to this may be in cases of muscular dystrophy where fatty deposits are laid down in the muscle as the contractile fibres degenerate. This may cause the muscle to maintain or increase its size but lose its strength due to the reduction in contractile fibres.

The structure of the muscle

As stated in Chapter 2, all muscle fibres contract in the same way according to the sliding filament model of muscle contraction. However, the precise alignment of the contractile fibres within muscles can vary considerably and this has a profound effect upon the amount of force they can generate. Muscles which have their fibres running parallel to their main axis (fusiform) are capable of a great degree of shortening. If the fibres are aligned at an angle to the long axis (pennate) then more can be packed into the same volume of muscle: this results in a stronger muscle but one which cannot shorten as much as a fusiform muscle.

The type of muscle fibres within the muscle

Although all muscle fibres have the same basic structure they may vary according to certain physiological, biochemical and histochemical properties. Certain kinds of fibre are stronger than others whilst some have greater endurance properties. Muscle fibres may therefore be classified into two broad categories: type 1 fibres (also called red fibres or slow twitch fibres) and type 2 fibres (also called white fibres or fast twitch). The type 1 fibres are smaller than the type 2 but they possess a better blood supply. They are therefore weaker than the type 2 but have greater endurance properties. Type 1 fibres have a greater capacity to produce their ATP aerobically whilst the type 2 fibres are more biased towards the anaerobic production of ATP.

Therefore, the fibre composition of a muscle will affect its strength and endurance. In general, it is suggested that a greater proportion of type 1 fibres will give the muscle more endurance qualities whilst a greater proportion of type 2 fibres will increase its maximal strength. However, the relative proportions of these fibres are only one aspect in the determination of these properties and appropriate exercises may increase both the maximal strength and endurance capacities of both muscle fibre types.

Biochemical and histochemical properties within the muscle fibres

This factor is obviously related to the previous one. However, whilst muscle fibres may be allocated into broad categories of type 1 or type 2, variations exist within these categories. Type 2 fibres may be subclassified into type 2a, type 2b and type 2c, for example. As another example, type 1 muscle fibres may vary between the aerobic (endurance) and the anaerobic (maximal strength) limits of their category. Indeed, as will be discussed later, through exercise it may be possible to slightly alter the properties of muscle fibres without necessarily altering the category in which they are placed.

Neurological factors

Muscle fibres are stimulated to contract by their motor neurons. The force, and hence the strength, of a muscular contraction is determined by the number of fibres recruited into the contraction. Therefore, if the process of stimulation or recruitment is altered then the strength of contraction may be affected. Exercise may stimulate positive alterations in the recruitment of fibres via various neuromuscular changes which will enhance the strength of muscular contraction. Conversely, the strength of a muscle may be adversely affected by neuromuscular diseases such as motor neuron disease, myasthenia gravis and cerebral palsy, which result in an inhibition of effective motor unit recruitment and hence reduce the strength of contraction.

Coordination

Neuromuscular coordination should result in an efficient movement that optimizes the action of the muscles, producing the desired movement for the minimal amount of effort. Complex movements often need to be learnt but practice may result in their becoming a 'conditioned reflex'. Such movements are usually very efficient, but in situations such as stroke where certain neurological motor areas may have been damaged basic movement patterns may need to be re-learnt. In other disorders there may be an imbalance between the excitatory and inhibitory inputs being sent to the motor neurons of the muscle. If the inhibitory inputs are too weak or the excitatory inputs too strong it can result in hypertonic spasticity. This is when muscles which should relax and lengthen during a movement continue to contract. As a result, the limbs possess a degree of rigidity. This will cause much of the force being generated by the concentrically contracting muscle(s) to be resisted by the antagonist(s), which should have relaxed to permit the movement. The overall effect of this is to impede or prevent the desired movement. So, for efficient and effective movement an appropriate and coordinated balance of neurological inputs is required.

Neuromuscular diseases and disorders

The effects of different muscular disorders are mentioned in brief in the previous sections in relation to their specific effects upon the expression of muscular strength. Their physiological basis and effects are also discussed at the end of Chapter 2 in the section on neuromuscular diseases and disorders.

THE ASSESSMENT AND MONITORING OF MUSCULAR STRENGTH AND MUSCULAR ENDURANCE

When evaluating muscular strength and endurance a number of assessment methods are available. The appropriateness of each method will depend upon the individual, their condition and the aspect of muscular strength that the therapist wishes to evaluate. Assessment methods may be considered under the following headings:

1. Dynamometers for assessing maximal isometric strength
2. Tests for maximal dynamic strength
3. Muscular endurance tests
4. Subjective resistance tests
5. Isokinetic machines

An initial assessment which incorporates one or a combination of the listed methods may be used to assist with the design of a programme where it will provide the therapist with an indication of the participant's capabilities and potential. Repeated assessments may then be used to monitor the participant's progress and the effectiveness of the exercise programme.

Dynamometers for assessing maximal isometric strength

Dynamometers require participants to squeeze, pull or push; the dynamometer registers their maximal isometric strength in a quantitative manner. Common dynamometers include those for grip strength, back strength and leg strength. Owing to the maximal nature of the required contraction care should be taken when using the back and leg dynamometers. Overexertion may cause strained muscles and this risk makes this form of assessment inadvisable for some individuals.

Tests for maximal dynamic strength

Any exercise which uses free weights or a multigym may be used to assess maximal isotonic strength. The assessment requires the participant to complete one lift or movement with a set resistance or weight. If he or she is successful, then the weight or resistance is increased. The new load is then attempted and the process is repeated until the participant is unable to complete the lift or movement successfully. The heaviest weight or resistance coped with is then recorded as the participant's maximum for that particular exercise. The maximal exertion required for these tests makes it unsuitable for many individuals and also conveys a risk of injury.

If the test is being used to determine suitable 'training' loads rather than to produce a value for maximal strength it can be modified. In such tests, rather than attempting to lift a maximum, the assessment may proceed with the participant attempting three repetitions of each weight until it is perceived to be difficult. The perception of a resistance as being difficult should inform the therapist of the participant's capabilities and enable him or her to prescribe suitable resistances in the programme. Since the participant is likely to be required to complete 12 to 15 repetitions within the programme, the prescribed weight is likely to be slightly below that attained in the assessment when only three repetitions were required.

Muscular endurance tests

These tests usually involve the participant attempting to complete as many repetitions of an exercise as possible within a set time limit. Examples of such tests would be the number of sit-ups that could be completed in a minute or the number of press-ups in 30 seconds. The selected duration of the test will depend upon the individual: 20 to 30 seconds being appropriate for many individuals whilst a minute may be used for those who are very fit. A time limit is set on the test in preference to asking the participant to do as many as possible, because the rate of performing the exercise significantly influences the number achieved. Performing sit-ups at a fast rate can be more tiring than performing them at a slow rate where the participant has the opportunity to pause between each one.

With this form of assessment and monitoring the therapist is evaluating a combination of strength and endurance. With such tests it is desirable to use the exercises that are incorporated into the exercise programme as this will indicate to the therapist suitable numbers of repetitions that should be included within the participant's programme.

Subjective resistance tests

In these tests the therapist will ask the participant to perform a movement – such as knee extension or elbow flexion – and will resist the movement using his or her hands, as with accommodating resistance exercises. Whilst this form of assessment will not produce a quantitative measure of strength it can indicate to the therapist the participant's general strength for that movement, and any obvious weaknesses.

Isokinetic machines

Isokinetic machines are a specialist area and they register the strength of a contraction at specified speeds throughout the range of movement. In such tests the participant will be required to repeat a movement a specified number of times at a speed determined by the machine. During the movement the participant will have to exert as much force as possible against the resistance, and this is measured by the machine. Such assessments will produce a large amount of detailed information concerning the strength of the muscles and any weaknesses during particular phases of a movement.

THE EFFECTS OF EXERCISE UPON MUSCLE TONE AND STRENGTH

Appropriate exercises can have beneficial effects upon many of the factors which determine muscular strength. In circumstances in which the muscles are weak and lack tone, exercises may improve the muscle's strength, endurance and tone along with the possibility of developing the individual's coordination and muscular control. However, certain aspects of the muscle cannot be altered by exercise, including:

(a) the overall organization of the muscle fibres within a muscle; and
(b) factors which are constrained by biological limitations to change and growth.

A well-designed exercise programme may develop muscular strength by affecting a number of physiological factors to a greater or lesser extent. These are discussed in detail later in this section.

The precise responses of the muscles to an exercise programme will depend upon the individual, the intensity of the strengthening exercises and the number of repetitions performed. The resulting adaptations made by the muscle will therefore vary from those which are associated with the development of maximal strength to those which are associated with 'strength-endurance'. As a general rule: an exercise session which includes exercises of a high intensity (which therefore permit relatively few repetitions) will stimulate adaptations that are orientated towards the development of maximal strength. Alternatively, exercise sessions which include exercises of a lesser intensity (which therefore permit a greater number of repetitions) stimulate adaptations that are in accordance with the development of muscular endurance. However, whereas an exercise programme may be biased towards the development of maximal strength or muscular endurance or even stamina, these fitness components are not completely isolated from each other since they are related along a continuum. Thus an exercise session may have positive effects upon all aspects of a muscle's strength. The ways in which an exercise programme may be primarily orientated towards the development of maximal strength or muscular endurance is discussed in detail in later sections on the practical aspects of planning exercise programmes.

Exercises which are used to develop muscular strength and/or endurance are also likely to have beneficial effects upon hypotonic muscles by improving the general physical properties and general tone of the muscle fibres. The effects of strengthening exercises can be discussed under the following headings:

1. Muscle size
2. Histochemical and biochemical properties of the fibres
3. Fibre composition
4. Neurological factors and coordination.

Muscle size

The size of an individual muscle is determined by the number of fibres within the muscle and the size of the muscle fibres. As stated in Chapter 2, muscle fibres are made up of smaller units called myofibrils which are in turn composed of the contractile filaments of actin and myosin protein. Appropriate exercises will increase the number of contractile filaments and myofibrils within a muscle. This increase will result in the muscle possessing a greater capacity to develop tension and force, which will make it 'stronger'. An increase in the number of myofibrils within the muscle fibres will cause an increase in the size of the muscle fibres (hypertrophy of the fibres). As a consequence, there will be an overall increase in the size of the muscle. There is therefore a link between muscle size and strength, although it is not the only determining factor.

The increase in muscle size through fibre hypertrophy is generally accepted amongst physiologists. However, there is, in addition, some controversial evidence to suggest that some of the observed increase in muscle size may be attributable to an increase in the number of fibres (fibre hyperplasia). The nature of the investigations into this subject makes the collection of conclusive data difficult and many authorities discount the possibility of an increase in the number of fibres, stating that the number of fibres in a muscle is fixed prior to birth and cannot be altered by exercise. This topic is therefore an area of debate and requires further research.

Histochemical and biochemical properties of the fibres

Whilst there is a clear association between muscle size and strength it is possible for a muscle to increase its strength without a significant alteration to its size. This improvement in strength is caused by changes within the muscle fibres. Maximal strength training exercises appear to increase the strength capabilities of both type 1 and type 2 fibres. There is an overall increase in the amount of contractile protein (actin and myosin) and this is coupled with an overall increase in the size of the fibres and a relative reduction in the size of the capillary network and, hence, the blood supply. (This reduction may be prevented if deemed important by incorporating both strength and endurance activities into an exercise programme.) Also within the muscle fibres biochemical changes occur which enhance the fibres' capabilities of generating ATP anaerobically. This is to be expected since activities which require gross muscular strength tend to be of a high intensity but short duration and therefore are predominantly anaerobic rather than aerobic. There is therefore an associated development of the energy systems that are utilized during the exercise. Such changes are linked with the relative concentrations of the enzymes which mediate the reactions that occur in the energy systems, and the abundance of high-energy molecules such as phosphocreatine.

Exercise programmes that are orientated towards the development of muscular endurance will stimulate a balance of anaerobic and aerobic adaptations within the muscle that are in accordance with the energy demands of the exercise. Similarly, the resultant adaptations to the blood supply are likely to be a compromise between the maximal strength and endurance qualities required by the muscle.

Fibre composition

Strength training exercises can increase the muscle fibre's capacity to develop tension and, hence, produce a stronger force. It has been suggested that the greater the proportion of type 2 fibres in a muscle the stronger and more powerful it will be. Strength training exercises can certainly increase the strength capabilities of all muscle fibres; however, it is further suggested by some authorities that continued maximal strength training may actually convert type 1 fibres into type 2 fibres: a process that is referred to as 'fibre type conversion'. This is again an area of controversy and debate which requires further research if the topic is to be clarified.

Neurological factors and coordination

In earlier chapters it was emphasized that muscle fibres are stimulated to contract by motor neurons. A motor neuron and its associated muscle fibres form what is known as a motor unit. Motor units vary in the strength of stimulus that is required to get the muscle fibres to contract. Some motor units require very little stimulus and are therefore referred to as being low threshold motor units; other motor units require a far stronger stimulus and are therefore referred to as high threshold motor units. The overall strength of a muscle's contraction depends upon the recruitment of these motor units. If more motor units are recruited into a contraction it will be stronger. It is suggested by some authorities that strength training can influence the recruitment of motor units. These adaptations may occur in the central nervous system, and there is some evidence to suggest that it is caused by a reduction in the inhibitory action of the central nervous system. The effects of this would be to increase the ease with which motor units were recruited.

In terms of the ease of movement and the economy of effort, coordination is also an important factor. An uncoordinated movement will be wasteful in terms of the force being generated by the muscles. Appropriate exercises can improve coordination and increase the effective strength of the muscles by making the resultant movements more efficient.

PLANNING EXERCISE PROGRAMMES FOR MUSCULAR STRENGTH

Whenever an exercise programme is planned the following factors must always be remembered. Firstly, that the body takes time to respond and make its adaptations to the exercise and, secondly, that not all parts of the body may adapt at the same rate. In the context of strength training this has specific implications. If the tendons and muscles are overstressed too often they may be damaged. Therefore, strength training should commence at a relatively low intensity and build up gradually over a period of weeks.

The initial stages of a programme may involve exercises that use relatively light resistances but which are repeated a relatively high number of times. For example, a session may consist of 3 sets of 6 to 9 exercises with each set involving 12 to 20 repetitions of each exercise. This would produce a total of 36 to 60 repetitions of each exercise. This type of session should enable the body to become 'familiar' with the exercises and begin to initiate some training adaptations. Over a period of weeks the intensity of the exercise session could be gradually increased, which would normally involve an increase in the amount of resistance or progression onto more demanding versions of the exercises. As part of this progression an increase in intensity is often coupled with a reduction in the number of repetitions. If general muscular tone and a combination of maximal strength and muscular endurance are required, then 3 sets of 12 to 15 repetitions may be advocated for each exercise, making a total of 36 to 45 repetitions for each exercise. If however the development of maximal strength is of primary concern, then the programme needs to incorporate a gradual increase in the intensity of the exercises coupled with a corresponding decrease in the number of repetitions. For example, the programme may progress towards sessions where the participant performs 3 sets of 6 repetitions, with heavy resistances. Conversely, if the development of muscular endurance is of primary concern then the programme may progress towards 3 sets of 30 repetitions. Variations on these guidelines are given later in this chapter.

When making such progressions it is important to gradually increase the number of repetitions or the amount of resistance. This is because it is important not only for the muscles to adapt to the exercises, but also the tendons. The muscles may generate the force, but the force is conveyed to the bones via the tendons. The tendons are often slower to adapt which can mean that even though the muscles may be capable of more work the tendons may not. Increasing the exercise loads when they are in this vulnerable condition makes the tendons prone to being overstressed and susceptible to overuse injuries. Hence, even if the strength of the participant improves quite rapidly, progress must still be gradual if it is to continue unabated without the risk of injury.

It should also be noted that the participant's progress may not be linear and that everyone has a maximum potential. In practice, an individual may find that after some initial improvements they may 'plateau' for a while and appear not to progress before experiencing further improvements. Such plateaux may become longer and more difficult to overcome as the participant's physical potential gets closer. Indeed, the closer people get to their maximum potential the more difficult it will be for them to make further improvements even with substantial increases in the amount of exercise that they do. Such limitations to growth and development are determined by basic biological factors and may also be limited by psychological aspects.

When commencing a strength training programme an initial assessment of strength may help to indicate the type and intensity of exercises that would be suitable for a participant. In practical terms, the therapist should produce a draft of the proposed exercise sessions, which the participant can then attempt. During this initial session the therapist is likely to need to modify the proposed sessions in accordance with the participant's capabilities. This may involve increasing or decreasing the number of repetitions, altering the variation of the exercise included within the session and even adjusting the number of exercises included within a session. When drafting the initial session it is always advisable to underestimate the participant's capabilities. The successful completion of the session, with a subsequent increase in its content, will provide positive feedback to the participant whereas failure to complete the session may be disheartening. Modifications to a session should also take account of the participant's condition one or two days after the exercise, because those who are unfamiliar with exercise may suffer from stiffness in the days immediately following the exercise, even if they did not find it too demanding at the time. Stiffness indicates overexertion and the content of the exercise session may need to be slightly reduced until the necessary physiological adaptations to the exercise have occurred and post-exercise stiffness is no longer experienced. While this method of designing a session may appear to be somewhat random and unspecific, the therapist will soon become experienced at judging a participant's capabilities and the exercises that are suitable for that individual. This experience, coupled with an adherence to the following basic guidelines, should ensure the design of effective and safe exercise sessions:

1. Commence at a level that is well within the participant's capabilities.
2. Progress gradually.
3. Adhere to safety aspects such as warm-up.
4. React appropriately if the participant experiences pain or discomfort with any exercise.

COMPONENTS OF A MUSCULAR STRENGTH-TRAINING SESSION

As with all forms of exercise, a strength-training session should commence with a 'warm-up'. Typically this would include some aerobic exercise, such as cycling on an ergometer for 5 to 10 minutes to warm up the muscles. This should be followed by a series of stretching exercises that incorporate exercises for all the major muscle groups likely to be used during the session. The exact duration and content of the warm-up may also depend upon the relative importance of aerobic fitness and mobility exercises to the individual. For those wishing to develop mobility, a longer duration of time may be spent stretching, while a longer period of time may be spent on the aerobic component for those who need to develop their stamina or cardiovascular fitness. As a final part of the warm-up individuals may then perform some light strength-based exercises using much lower resistances than they use during the main part of the sesssion. For instance, it may include biceps curls with half the normal weight or 'half press-ups'. This final part of the warm-up will specifically prepare the muscles for the more strenuous exercises that follow.

The main part of a strength-training session may be composed of various different forms of exercises, including:

1. 'Body resistance' or circuit-training exercises
2. Free weights
3. Multigyms
4. Exercise machines
5. 'Therapist aided exercises'.

An exercise session could concentrate purely on one form of exercise but more commonly it will include a mixture of the different forms of strength training. The individual exercises within a session are likely to work the muscles concentrically, eccentrically and isometrically. In some cases a single exercise can work many different muscle groups in different ways. The duration of any exercise within the session may be determined by time, repetitions, or, with more advanced participants, by perceived exertion when training to their maximum. The recovery period between exercises or sets may be: (a) determined by a fixed time interval; (b) varied according to the feelings of the participant; or (c) simply determined by convenience, as when working in pairs or sharing pieces of equipment. Examples of such variations are given in a later section. The strength-training aspects of the session may be interspersed with other forms of exercise such as further work on the exercise cycle or additional stretching exercises if desired. This may help to keep the participants warm and provide their muscles with additional 'active' recovery if required.

The main part of the session should be followed by a 'cool-down' period. This will commonly include a few minutes of gentle aerobic exercise and further gentle stretching. The cool-down will help to reduce the risk of stiffness the following day

In the following sections the different types of strength-training exercises that can be incorporated into a strength-training programme will be considered under the following headings:

1. Circuit-training and body resistance exercises
2. The use of multigyms and exercise machines

3. The use of 'free weights'
4. Accommodating resistance work.

The relevant safety aspects and organizational methods used for each type of exercise will be discussed separately under each heading.

CIRCUIT-TRAINING AND BODY RESISTANCE EXERCISES

Circuit-training and body resistance exercises do not require any sophisticated equipment since they either use the person's own body weight as a form of resistance or use simple apparatus such as benches. In general terms, most of the exercises may be broadly categorized into one of three groups, according to which area of the body they work:

1. The legs
2. The trunk
3. The upper body.

However, whilst such categorizations are useful when organizing the exercises into a session they are not always clear cut when considered in detail. For instance, a 'press-up' may be classified as an upper body exercise since it predominantly and obviously uses the arms, but press-ups also require a considerable amount of isometric work from the abdominal muscles which are used to keep the body in a rigid position throughout the exercise.

When incorporated into an exercise session the component exercises are usually performed in a sequence which gives the muscle groups alternate periods of exercise and rest. Therefore, the exercises may be organized into a sequence which works the lower body, trunk, upper body, lower body, trunk, upper body, and so on. For each body part there are a number of possible exercises: these can be graded from easy to hard and it is up to the therapist to determine which versions are appropriate for the participant. The duration aspect within a session may be organized so that the participant completes a predetermined number of repetitions of each exercise before moving on, or the participant may work for a set time interval before progressing around the circuit. Similarly, the amount of recovery may or may not be specified. When specific exercises require various pieces of equipment, such as a mat for sit-ups or a bench for step-ups, they should be situated so that a minimum amount of movement is required between the pieces of apparatus or 'exercise stations'. Not only is this arrangement convenient but it becomes more important if a number of individuals are exercising at the same time. Appropriate spacial organization will minimize the possibility of people colliding as they move around the room. Likewise, apparatus should not be situated where it is possible for a person to fall over it and the safety considerations for each exercise should be adhered to at all times. This section discusses the incorporation of exercises into circuits, though circuit and body resistance exercises need not necessarily be incorporated into a formalized 'circuit' but may be undertaken in a more informal manner along with other exercises and forms of therapy. This section, therefore, aims to present general guidelines for the use of such exercises into exercise sessions rather than setting out fixed, inflexible 'rules'.

In an ideal situation it may be possible to give each participant an individual 'circuit training fitness test' from which the type of exercises and number of repetitions may be determined. This could involve the participant attempting a relatively easy version of the exercise: if 30 repetitions are completed with relative ease, the participant may then be asked to attempt a more difficult version. In this way the appropriate variation of an exercise may be determined. Having established this, it is then necessary to determine the appropriate number of repetitions. This may be found by asking for the exercise to be repeated until the participant begins to struggle to complete the exercise or feels undue local muscular fatigue. It must be realized that in order for any exercise to convey benefits it must 'stress' the body, but it must not 'overstress' it as this may lead to injury. In the early stages of an exercise programme the therapist should always be cautious with the participant's capabilities: minor adjustments to the number of repetitions can then be made during the first few sessions as the participant becomes familiar with the exercises. Increasing the number of repetitions in the early stages also has a positive psychological effect.

By following these general guidelines the appropriate variation of each exercise, and a suitable number of repetitions to be completed, may be determined. This should result in a circuit containing 5 to 12 different exercises that will appropriately stress the participant whilst remaining within his or her capabilities. During an exercise session the participant may complete each circuit one, two or three times depending upon that person's physical capacity in relation to the demands of the circuit. The advantage of this form of exercise programme is that it is very personalized and the therapist can closely monitor the progress of the individual and make appropriate adjustments to the programme. Having performed an initial assessment the results can be used as a means of monitoring the progress of the participant and providing positive feedback.

While the individualized programme may be highly desirable there are occasions when such constant individual attention is not feasible. If the therapist is dealing with a number of individuals but is only able to provide exercise facilities on limited occasions then they are likely to be involved with group sessions. This has the advantage of making the activity more sociable and, as such, does not preclude the use of initial 'fitness assessments' for all individuals. The organization of such sessions may involve a room being made available at particular times with individuals arriving, exercising and leaving when it is convenient for them. In such circumstances, to prevent organizational difficulties, it is desirable for individuals to visit each exercise station in the same sequence even though they may not be doing exactly the same type of exercise. If the amount of space is limited and the participants numerous, it is possible that this will result in queuing for exercise stations especially if, for instance, there is only one mat for sit-ups. To prevent this the therapist may require more specific temporal organization. This may be achieved by allocating to each participant a certain time interval at each station, during which time the participant should complete the predetermined number of repetitions, and then allowing a set time interval for moving to the next station. This may require the therapist to provide instructions in relation to the time and may require participants to start at different stations. However, it will ensure that all participants move between stations and commence each exercise at the same time. It should be noted that with this form of organization there may be an additional slight pause between individuals completing their repetitions and being asked to progress to the next station. Suggested time intervals may be 30 or 40 seconds exercise time with 30 seconds to change stations. In practice, this will depend upon the type of circuit being undertaken and the individuals participating.

With more advanced and 'fitter' individuals a variation on the above theme may be used whereby they do not perform a set number of repetitions but exercise for a given duration. So individuals may exercise for 20 seconds and then be given 40 seconds recovery during which time they change stations. To make it more difficult a ratio of 30 seconds to 30 seconds may be used but this is only likely to apply to the fitter exercisers.

As a final variation there may be circumstances in which the therapist is unable to assess all the participants on an individual basis. As an alternative he or she may set out graded circuits which are often designated by colours such as yellow, red, blue and black. The different levels of circuit may vary in the type of exercises they include or the number of repetitions suggested, or both. For instance, the yellow circuit may represent the easiest circuit which would involve the participants performing relatively few repetitions (say 6 to 12) of the easier versions of the exercises whilst the black circuit may incorporate much higher repetitions (30 to 40) of the more difficult variations. The red and blue circuits could incorporate exercises of intermediate difficulty and/or require the completion of an intermediate number of repetitions.

For such circuits, cards may need to be produced stating the number of repetitions required at each station for each circuit. A problem may be encountered with this form of organization if the participants' capabilities vary considerably over different bodily areas. For instance, if their legs are relatively 'fitter' than their arms, they may be very capable of performing the leg exercises of the black circuit but may only be capable of performing the suggested arm exercise variation and repetitions given in the yellow circuit. This, therefore, emphasizes the value of individualizing such exercise programmes whenever possible.

With all forms of circuit training, diagrams of the exercises may be useful and the participants or therapists should keep record cards which register the number of repetitions they perform for each exercise. In practice, the therapists may like to modify the organizational versions suggested here in accordance with their own experience and resources. For example, it may be appropriate to encourage the participants to gently jog on the spot during the recovery period between each exercise. However, this will depend upon the fitness of the individuals.

EXAMPLES OF BODY RESISTANCE AND CIRCUIT-TRAINING EXERCISES

As with most forms of strength-training exercises these exercises will require a combination of eccentric, concentric and static work involving many different muscle groups. Therefore, where an exercise is classified as 'exercising' a particular muscle group it should be remembered that, although this may be the major site of activity, other muscles will undoubtedly be involved.

Abdominal exercises

1. *Knee raises* (Figure 6.1). This exercise predominantly involves the hip flexors but can be used as a prelude to 'sit-ups' if the participant's abdominal

muscles are weak. The participant sits in a chair and raises one knee by flexing the hip and then slowly lowers the leg to the starting position before repeating the exercise. This may be performed using one leg at a time or with both legs together.

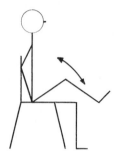

Figure 6.1

2. *Sit-ups* (Figures 6.2–6.5). The degree of difficulty of a sit-up may be altered by varying the position of the hands and arms. With all basic sit-ups the participant should sit on a mat (for comfort and protection of the back) with the hips and knees flexed at about 90 degrees. Flexion of the hips and knees (as opposed to doing sit-ups with 'straight legs', hips and knees extended) should prevent any back problems. All movements should be performed in a slow and controlled manner: this includes both the upward concentric phase and the lowering or eccentric phase. With all variations of the sit-up the feet should be free and not hooked under a support. Use of a support makes the exercise somewhat easier, slightly alters the nature of the exercise by affecting the relative demands placed upon the muscle groups involved and may cause undue strain on the thigh muscles and hip flexors. Similarly, sit-ups on an incline with the feet elevated and hooked under a support are not recommended in these circumstances.

Version 1 (Figure 6.2). The participant lies on the mat with the hips and knees flexed and the hands resting comfortably on the thighs. The body is then raised and the hands are moved so that each hand touches the corresponding lower leg just below each knee cap. During the movement the arms should be kept virtually straight with the elbows being only slightly flexed so as to minimize the amount of trunk movement (flexion). From this point the body

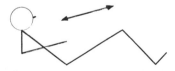

Figure 6.2

is then gently lowered so that the shoulders touch the mat and in doing so the hands slide back up the thighs to their starting position. The movement can then be repeated. With this exercise it is unnecessary to flex the trunk more than specified since the abdominal muscles perform most of the 'work' involved in a sit-up during the early phases of flexion and would perform very little additional work if the trunk was made to flex further.

Version 2 (Figure 6.3). The participant lies on the mat with the hips and knees flexed and the arms crossed over the chest so that the hands touch the opposite shoulder. The trunk is then flexed and raised so that it is almost vertical. The trunk is then slowly lowered so that the shoulders once again touch the mat. The trunk movement is virtually identical to that described in the previous version but the exercise is made more difficult by the positioning of the hands and arms.

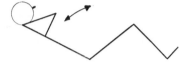

Figure 6.3

Version 3 (Figure 6.4). The participant lies on the mat with the hips and knees flexed and the hands touching the ears. The trunk movement performed in this exercise is identical to that described in versions 1 and 2 of the sit-up but the exercise is made more difficult by the positioning of the hands and arms. With this exercise it is stressed that the hands should be touching the ears and not clasped behind the neck which could cause unwanted strain in this region.

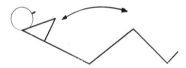

Figure 6.4

Version 4 (Figure 6.5). The participant lies on the mat with the feet elevated and resting free on a chair or bench. While this exercise may not look very spectacular the elevation of the feet makes the movement considerably more demanding on the abdominal muscles. Therefore, when initially performing this exercise the hands should be placed on the thighs and moved to touch just below the knee cap as the trunk is flexed (as in version 1). Further progression may then be achieved by repositioning the arms across

189

the chest as in version 2, or by placing the hands just behind the ears as in version 3.

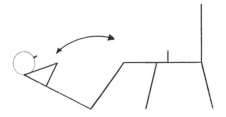

Figure 6.5

3. *Twisted sit-up* (Figures 6.6 and 6.7). The 'twisted sit-up' is a simple variation of the sit-up and involves a small amount of trunk rotation as well as flexion.

Version 1: rotation to alternate sides (Figure 6.6). The participant lies on the mat with the hips and knees flexed and the hands touching the ears. The trunk can then be flexed and rotated so as to bring the right elbow close to the left knee (at this stage there is no necessity to make the elbow touch the knee). The body is then slowly lowered back to the starting position and the movement is repeated, but this time the participant rotates in the opposite direction so that the left elbow is brought close to the right knee. The exercise may then be repeated for the desired number of repetitions.

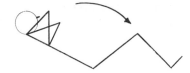

Figure 6.6

Version 2: Rotation to one side (Figure 6.7). The right hand is positioned so that it is touching the right ear whilst the left elbow and lower arm are positioned flat on the mat in line with the trunk. The participant then flexes and rotates the trunk so that the right elbow is brought towards the left knee. In doing this the left elbow will need to be flexed but the lower arm should

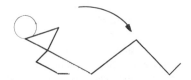

Figure 6.7

remain on the mat. The participant then slowly lowers the body back to the starting position and the movement is repeated. This exercise therefore involves repeated flexion and rotation to the left. To exercise the muscles of the opposite side of the body the positions will need to be reversed such that the left hand is positioned by the left ear whilst the right arm is positioned on the mat. The body can then be flexed and rotated to the right.

4. *Crunches* (Figures 6.8 and 6.9). This is a more advanced form of exercise, requiring good coordination, which exercises the hip flexors as well as the abdominal muscles.

   Version 1 (Figure 6.8). The participant starts by lying flat on the floor in the anatomical position. The hips and knees are then flexed, bringing the knees towards the head. At the same time the trunk is flexed by raising the head and back off the floor. In this position the participant should be able to touch both knee caps with the hands. The hips, knees and back are then extended to return to the starting position.

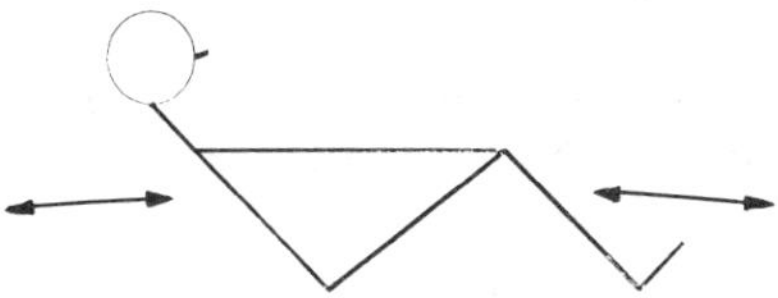

Figure 6.8

Version 2 (Figure 6.9). This version involves the same movements as version 1 but during the second phase of the movement when the knees, hips and back are being extended they are not fully lowered back onto the floor but are kept elevated just a few inches above the floor. This requires constant work from the abdominal muscles and others in order to maintain this body position throughout the set of exercises. This exercise may be performed quite rapidly up to a rate of about one cycle per second and is not suitable for those who have weak abdominal muscles.

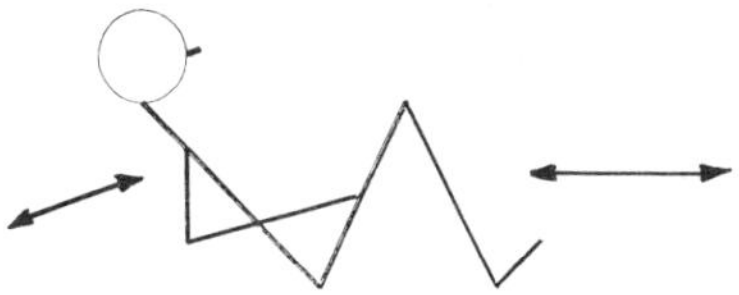

Figure 6.9

Back-strengthening exercises

It is the opinion of many authorities that in most people the constant use of the back muscles prevents them from becoming 'weak'. One of the primary functions of the back muscles is the maintenance of posture, and in this context they are used isometrically. Many exercises such as press-ups and the military press when performed correctly will exercise the back muscles isometrically and thus no further exercises may be required. While many exercise programmes may appear to concentrate upon the abdominal muscles (which are often weak), they are not in fact neglecting the back muscles, as these are usually strengthened by other exercises already included in a programme. However, should the therapist wish to include specific back-strengthening exercises, there are a few to choose from.

1. *Back extensions* (Figure 6.10). Care should be taken with this exercise and it should not be undertaken by those suffering from back complaints. The participant lies face down on a bench with the hips level with the end of the bench, and the upper body extending over the end. In this position the participant will flex at the waist so that the head is close to the ground. In this starting position the lower body will be in a horizontal position on the bench whilst the upper body will be at 90 degrees to it with the head close to the floor. During the exercise the participant's feet will need to be held down by the therapist or a fixed support. The participant then clasps the hands behind the head and raises the upper body so that it becomes parallel with the floor and level with the lower body. Slight hyperextension may be permissible provided that it does not cause any back discomfort. The participant then slowly lowers the upper body so that the head once again almost touches the floor before repeating the movement. The exercise therefore involves both concentric and eccentric contractions of the back muscles. Whilst this exercise may be used for strengthening the back muscles, it should be omitted if it causes discomfort since, as previously stated, it may not be necessary for everyone. Additional back-strengthening exercises are presented in the section referring to free weights.

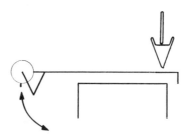

Figure 6.10

Upper body exercises

1. *Press-ups* (Figures 6.11–6.15). Press-ups are primarily aimed at the muscula-ture of the upper body, arms and shoulders. However, the activity also requires postural muscles, such as back and abdominal muscles, to work in order to maintain body position. Therefore, such exercises may statically exercise these

muscle groups as well as dynamically exercising those more obviously involved in the movements.

Version 1: press-ups aginst the wall (Figure 6.11). These exercises provide a basic beginning for the press-up movement. The participant stands with arms outstretched and the palms of the hands flat against the wall at shoulder height, and then moves the feet back approximately 1 foot and lowers the hands about 1 foot down the wall. This will cause the participant to lean in towards the wall slightly and forms the starting position. The participant then flexes the elbows and leans forwards until the face almost touches the wall. Throughout the movement the body should be kept fairly rigid with the lean coming from the flexion of the ankles, not the back. From this position the participant then straightens the elbows by pushing against the wall and returns to the starting position from which the movement may then be repeated.

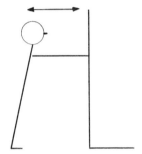

Figure 6.11

Version 2: kneeling or half press-ups (Figure 6.12). The participant kneels on the floor with the knees positioned slightly behind the hips rather then being directly underneath. In this position the participant may elevate the feet slightly and cross them if that is found to be more comfortable. From this position the participant then flexes the elbows and lowers the upper body until the face almost touches the floor. The elbows are then extended, pushing against the floor in order to return to the starting position. Throughout the movement the body should be kept fairly rigid so that it pivots where the knees are touching the ground and the back does not bend.

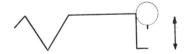

Figure 6.12

Version 3: Press-ups with the upper body elevated (Figure 6.13). This exercise represents an intermediate version between version 1 and the full press-up described in version 4. To perform this version the participant needs the aid of a step or similar fixed object. The higher the step, the easier the exercise. The participant places the hands flat on the step with the body extended out behind in a straight line. This should position the body at an angle of about 45 degrees to the horizontal. The exercise commences with the elbows extended, and the press-up movement is achieved via the flexion of both elbows, which lowers the body, followed by the extension of both elbows, which raises it. Throughout the movements the body should be maintained in a straight line such that it pivots about the ankles and feet without any flexion of the back.

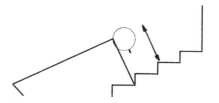

Figure 6.13

Version 4: press-ups flat on floor (Figure 6.14). This exercise may be described as the classic press-up position. Therapists will find that few of their female participants will reach this stage; indeed it is likely to be beyond many of the men. The movement sequence is the same as that described in version 3 but the participant has the hands on the floor rather than being elevated.

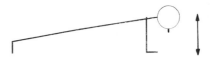

Figure 6.14

Version 5: press-ups with the feet elevated (Figure 6.15). This is an advanced press-up which will only be achieved by those who possess a strong, well-

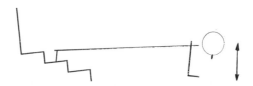

Figure 6.15

developed musculature. In this version the feet are elevated on a bench or chair whilst the hands are positioned on the floor. Elevating the lower body makes the exercise considerably more difficult with the degree of elevation influencing the degree of difficulty. The higher the positioning of the feet, the more difficult the exercise becomes.

2. *Bench dips* (Figures 6.16 and 6.17).

Version 1 (Figure 6.16). The participant places the hands behind them on a bench or fixed object. The feet should extend out in front and the participant should flex at the waist. The feet should be placed flat on the ground and the knees should be slightly flexed. The exercise commences with the elbows extended, the participant then flexes at the elbow and lowers the body down until it almost touches the floor. The elbows are then extended, pushing against the bench to raise the body back up again. Throughout the movement the emphasis should be upon elbow flexion and extension whilst flexion of the trunk is minimized and the back is kept relatively straight.

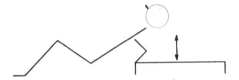

Figure 6.16

Version 2: bench dips with feet elevated (Figure 6.17). In this version the basic movement sequence is identical to version 1 but the participant's feet are elevated on another bench. This permits a greater degree of body lowering and hence elbow flexion which makes the exercise more difficult. In this position it should be possible to lower the body sufficiently for the elbows to be flexed at 90 degrees and hence the upper arms, which extend behind the body, will be parallel to the floor.

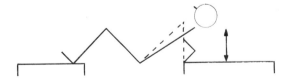

Figure 6.17

3. *Bench raises* (Figure 6.18). This exercise requires some basic apparatus such as a bench and wall bars which are commonly found in exercise areas. One end of the bench is securely hooked over the wall bars at approximately shoulder height. The participant then holds the other end level with the shoulders, and this forms the starting position. From this position the

participant raises the bench above the head, fully extending the elbows. The bench is then lowered back down to the starting position, carefully controlling the movement with eccentric contractions. Throughout the movement the back should be kept straight and the exertion should not cause the participant to hyperextend it. The degree of difficulty of the exercise may be altered by changing the weight of the bench or, with a strong participant, the exercise may be performed using just one arm. Back hyperextension indicates over-exertion and the exercise may need to be modified accordingly. Some individuals may prefer to keep their feet flat on the floor throughout the duration of the exercise whilst others may wish to remain on the balls of their feet with their heels elevated off the ground throughout the entire exercise. Having to push with the legs or rising up and down on the feet indicates that the bench is too heavy.

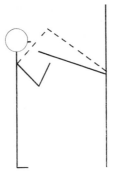

Figure 6.18

4. *Bench curls* (Figure 6.19). This exercise uses the same apparatus as the 'bench raises'. However, it exercises a somewhat different group of muscles through a different range of motion. The participant commences the exercise in almost the same position as the 'bench raises' (with the bench at shoulder height) but with an underhand grip on the end of the bench. During the first phase

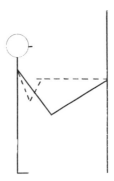

Figure 6.19

of the movement the bench is lowered by extending the elbows and shoulders until the elbows are fully extended. The elbows and shoulders are then flexed to return the bench to shoulder height. This exercise primarily works the elbow and shoulder flexors ('bench raises' primarily worked the elbow extensors).

Leg exercises

Owing to the involvement of the large muscle groups of the legs and the relatively long duration of some of these exercises, such exercises as step-ups, step-overs, ski jumps, astride jumps and bench jumps may convey benefits to the participant's cardiovascular system as well as enhancing leg strength. These benefits will be most pronounced if the exercises are of a suitable intensity to permit a relatively long duration and are repeated a number of times within an exercise session.

1. *Step-ups* (Figure 6.20).
    Version 1. Step-ups may be performed in a number of different ways. Firstly, they may use a low bench or step with the participant stepping up with one foot, and up with the other, then down with one foot and down with the other – thus following the cycle up, up, down, down, up, up, down, down. This may be performed at a set rhythm such as 20 steps per minute, a consistent stepping rhythm may be achieved with the use of a metronome set at 80 beats per minute. Each beat will then correspond to one component of the four-stage cycle (up, up, down, down). When performing this exercise the participant should change the leading leg at intervals. This may be every fifth step, tenth step or fifteenth step depending upon the individual and the duration of the exercise. During the exercise the participant should fully extend both knees when stepping onto the bench. The degree of difficulty of the exercise may be altered by adjusting the height of the step or changing the rate of stepping to make it slower or quicker as desired. A rhythm of 30 steps per minute (120 beats per minute) is fairly brisk.

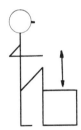

Figure 6.20

Version 2. As an alternative version the exercise may be modified to put a greater emphasis on the use of the quadriceps muscles. This can be achieved by using a relatively high step which is slightly higher than the participant's knee (two benches usually suffice). The bench(es) should be placed next to a wall or support as this will reduce the risk of the participant overbalancing and falling forward. During the exercise the participant places one foot on the bench(es) and then uses that leg to raise the body so that both feet are on the bench. During the movement the participant should try to minimize the amount of assistance given by the foot that was on the floor. The foot that was initially on the bench is then lowered so that the opposing foot is left on the bench. From this position the exercise is repeated. During the exercise the participant always has one foot on the bench, and with each step it alternates between the right and left foot. With this exercise the therapist should again ensure that the participant straightens both legs when standing on the bench. The exercise should be performed slowly and precisely since a rapid rate will cause the lower leg to 'bounce' back up when it hits the floor and remove the emphasis from the hip and knee extensors of the upper leg.

2. *Step overs* (Figure 6.21). This requires the use of a low bench or step. The participant stands with one foot on the bench and one foot positioned on the floor behind the bench. The participant then raises the back foot and steps over the bench so that the foot is now on the floor in front of the bench. Throughout this movement the other foot remains on the bench. The participant then brings the foot on the floor in front of the bench back over the bench and places it on the floor behind the bench whilst again keeping one foot on the bench. Throughout the exercise one foot remains firmly positioned on the bench whilst the participant steps over and back across the bench with the other leg. During the exercise the non-stepping leg should be extended as the other foot is brought across the bench. After the desired number of repetitions the position of the legs should be swapped so that the other leg becomes the 'stepping leg'.

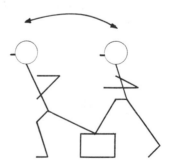

Figure 6.21

3. *Side leg raises* (Figures 6.22 and 6.23).

   Version 1: single leg raises (Figure 6.22). This exercise primarily involves the abductor muscles of the legs. The participant lies on the side in a comfortable position with the legs extended and the upper body 'propped' up by the arms to provide support and stability. From this position the participant then raises and lowers the leg which is uppermost (if lying on the right side this will be the left leg, if lying on the left side it will be the right leg). This

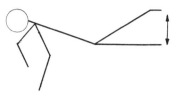

Figure 6.22

movement therefore involves the concentric contraction of the abductor muscles in raising the leg and eccentric contraction of these muscles in controlling its lowering. With this exercise the participant must remember to change sides in order to exercise the abductor muscles of both legs.

Version 2: double side leg raises (Figure 6.23). This exercise is similar to the previous one with the participant starting the exercise in the same position. However, during the exercise the participant attempts to raise and lower both legs at the same time. This exercise therefore works both the abductor and adductor muscles. When lying on the right side, raising and lowering the legs will work the abductor muscles of the left leg and the adductor muscles of the right, with the raising movement requiring concentric contractions and the lowering phase requiring eccentric work. Conversely, lying on the left side will exercise the abductor muscles of the right leg and the adductor muscles of the left.

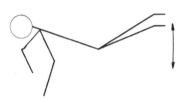

Figure 6.23

4. *Ski jumps* (Figure 6.24). This exercise may be performed over a white line or two white lines positioned approximately 12 to 18 inches apart. The participant stands on one side of the white line(s) with the feet aproximately 12 inches apart and the ankles, knees and hips slightly flexed. The participant then takes off with both feet and jumps sideways (in the frontal plane) across to the other side of the line(s) slightly flexing the ankles, knees and hips on landing. After landing the participant immediately jumps back in the same manner to the starting position. The exercise involves repeated two-footed sideways jumps back and forth across a line or lines. In this exercise there is no need to flex the ankles, knees and hips beyond that which is sufficient to cushion the landing and provide sufficient power for take off. Indeed, assuming a 'deep squatting' position may cause knee problems for some people when performing this exercise.

5. *Astride bench jumps* (Figure 6.25). The participant begins by facing along the length of a bench with the feet positioned on the floor, one on each side of the bench (a). The participant then jumps up, and places both feet

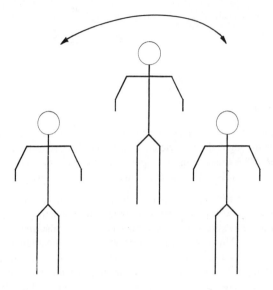

Figure 6.24

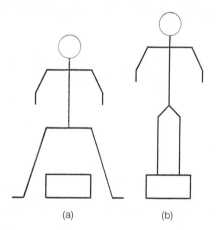

(a)   (b)

Figure 6.25

simultaneously on the bench (b), and immediately jumps back down to the starting position (a). The exercise involves repeated jumps on and off the bench. A reasonably good level of coordination is required for this activity since a lack of coordination, expecially if fatigued, may result in the person tripping over the bench.

6. *Bench jumps single leg* (Figure 6.26). This is a more advanced exercise which, although not significantly more demanding than the previous one, requires a greater degree of coordination. The participant stands facing along the length of a bench with the feet positioned on the floor, one on each side of the bench.

One foot is then placed on the bench whilst the other is kept on the ground. This forms the starting position. In a rapid movement the participant then places the other foot on the bench whilst at the same time, placing the first foot on the ground. The movement is then repeated by moving the foot that was on the ground onto the bench whilst, at the same time moving the other foot from the bench to the floor. So in effect they rapidly hop from one leg to the other with one foot on the floor and the other on the bench.

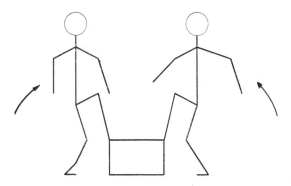

Figure 6.26

7. *Bench clears* (Figure 6.27). This is an advanced exercise which can be very demanding and requires good coordination. It is similar to the astride bench jumps. The participant begins in the same manner with both feet positioned astride of a bench (a). However, when jumping up the feet are brought together to touch in the air (b) and are then moved apart rapidly so as to land astride

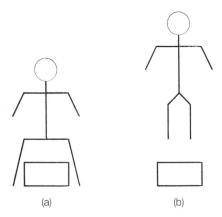

(a)   (b)

Figure 6.27

the bench in the starting position, rather than on the bench. During the exercise the bench is not touched. It is a fast exercise which requires good coordination as well as strength. Alternatives may be used instead of a bench since, clearly, if the person becomes fatigued he or she risks stumbling on the bench.

General exercises

As stated earlier, many of the above exercises will involve muscle groups other than those specifically stated. Some of them, if performed rapidly, will also require a good level of cardiovascular fitness; indeed, if organized in such a way, circuit exercises may be used as a means of developing cardiovascular fitness along with aspects of muscular strength and endurance. The following exercises are more advanced general exercises which may be incorporated into a circuit session for those who are considered to be 'fit' and capable of more demanding activities. The exercises tend to involve a combination of the major muscle groups to a greater or lesser extent.

1. *Sprint starts* (Figure 6.28). This exercise commences in the press-up position (a). From this preliminary position the hip and knee of one leg are flexed to bring the leg under the body with the knee almost touching the chest (b). This forms the starting position: from this position the flexed leg is rapidly extended while at the same time the extended leg is rapidly flexed and brought up to almost touch the chest. This motion is then repeated with the legs flexing and extending in opposition to one another. During this exercise the person's weight tends to be over the hands, which makes it tiring on the arms and shoulders which are working statically, as well as the leg muscles which are working dynamically.

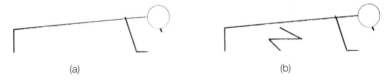

(a)   (b)

Figure 6.28

2. *Burpees* (Figure 6.29). This exercise is similar to the 'sprint start', however it commences in the 'press-up position' (a). From this position both hips and knees are rapidly flexed to bring the knees under the body and close to the chest (b). The legs are then rapidly extended in a thrusting movement which extends the hips and knees to return them to the starting position (a).

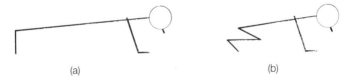

(a)   (b)

Figure 6.29

Throughout the exercise the palms of the hands remain on the floor and, as with the 'sprint starts', much of the person's weight is taken over the hands.

3. *Star jumps* (Figure 6.30). The participant starts in the anatomical position, with the feet slightly apart and the hands by the sides (a). They then jump into the air, opening the legs (abduction) and at the same time bringing the arms over the head, again using an abduction movement (b). The participant then lands in this position, with the feet slightly wider than shoulder width apart and the hands over the head (c), and jumps into the air again, this time adducting both arms and legs (d) to land back in the anatomical position (a). This activity may be performed quite rapidly and hence involves jumping with the simultaneous abduction of the legs and arms followed by a second jump which is accompanied by the simultaneous adduction of the arms and legs.

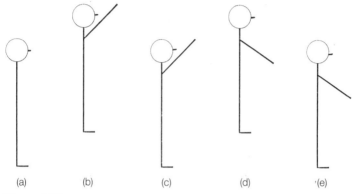

(a)   (b)   (c)   (d)   '(e)

Figure 6.30

4. *Jumping jacks* (Figure 6.31). This exercise is a combination of the 'star jump' and 'burpee'. The 'star jump' is performed as before ((a) – (e)) but as the participant lands back in the anatomical position a crouched position is assumed (f) and the participant places the palms of both hands flat on the floor (g). From this position the weight is then placed on the hands and the hips and knees are extended back in a thrusting movement to assume the 'press-up position' (h). From here the movement is reversed, with the hips and knees flexing rapidly to once again put the participant into a crouched position (i) from which to commence a star jump (j) and the cycle is repeated. These movements should be performed in a smooth, continuous manner producing a fast coordinated action. Overall it is a rapid and demanding exercise which is only suitable for the 'physically fit', and even these individuals are unlikely to achieve many repetitions.

5. *Leg cycling* (Figure 6.32). This exercise may be performed in a number of different ways and in doing so may convey a number of different benefits. The starting position involves the participant lying on their back and then flexing both knees and hips to bring the knees towards the chest. If the exercise is to be performed slowly (conveying benefits to leg muscle strength, muscle control and abdominal muscle strength), participants should raise themselves

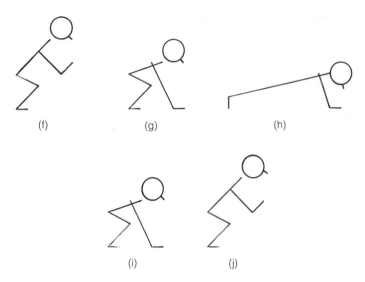

Figure 6.31

up and support their upper body on their elbows, which will help to prevent any unwanted strain being placed on the back. The participant commences the exercise by slowly extending the knee and hip of one leg until it is fully extended. This leg is then slowly flexed whilst the opposite leg is extended. This movement is then repeated and a slow controlled cycling motion is achieved. As a preliminary version of this exercise the extended leg may touch the floor during each cycle; however, as the participant progresses, both legs should remain elevated throughout the exercise.

If, however, more aerobic benefits are sought from the exercise then it should be performed at a faster rate but with a reduced amount of leg extension.

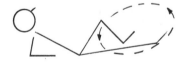

Figure 6.32

6. *Shuttles* (Figure 6.33). This is a simple running exercise which may be incorporated into an exercise session. It simply involves running or jogging from one side of the room to another for a specified number of repetitions or time duration. It is physically demanding and places overload on the cardiovascular system. When doing this exercise care should be taken to ensure that participants do not collide with each other, equipment or the wall. As a variation, the exercise could involve hopping rather than jogging.

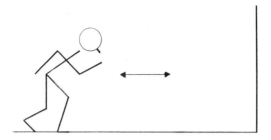

Figure 6.33

THE USE OF MULTIGYMS AND EXERCISE MACHINES

Multigyms and exercise machines provide the opportunity for the muscles to work through a given range of motion against a resistance. These machines often involve the use of levers and pulleys with the resistance being provided by weights. When the use of such equipment is first introduced into the participants' exercise programmes it is important for them to become familiarized with the exercises by beginning with relatively light resistances. Even so, exercises such as the military press may still be too difficult for many. Indeed, if the participants are relatively weak, it is often advisable to start them with alternative forms of exercise prior to commencing this form of training. In the situation where participants are rehabilitating from an injury, it is important for the muscles to be capable of moving the limbs with ease before resistance is applied, since, if the muscles are too weak, they may be overstressed by resistance training. In practice, any exercise session is unlikely to involve the sole use of exercise machines such as multigyms but will incorporate a combination of activities such as circuit-training exercises, dumbells and exercise machines.

Therapists should also remember that exercises using multigyms and related exercise machines may be used in contexts other than the primary development of muscular strength. Since the exercises require a degree of muscular control and coordination and are relatively safe, they may be used to develop an individual's coordination and muscular control. If prescribed in the correct way these exercises may convey great benefits to individuals with neuromuscular disorders such as cerebral palsy or similar disabilities where movement patterns are difficult to perform or need to be 're-learnt'.

The equipment used with these types of strengthening exercises may be in the form of a single exercise station or very often they will be combined in the form of a 'multigym' which will provide a number of exercise stations that may be used concurrently. Other more sophisticated exercise machines that involve the use of hydraulics and accommodating resistances will be discussed later. Exercise machines can convey certain advantages and disadavantages over other means of strength training.

Advantages

1. The amount of resistance may be adjusted by altering the amount of weight used.

2. The muscles may be worked through specified ranges of motion.
3. As with other forms of strength training, the exercises involve a combination of concentric, eccentric and isometric work.
4. Because the movement of the weights themselves is limited there is no necessity for assistants or 'spotters' who are essential for the safe use of free weights.

Disadvantages

1. The machines determine the precise movement during the exercise, which can be a slight disadvantage when compared with free weights. For example, with multigyms, where both sides of the body are being exercised together, it may be possible for one side to perform more of the work.
2. Because of the controlling and guiding influence of the machine the individual's muscles do not have to work as hard to control the movements as they would with free weights.

However for those involved in general strengthening exercises as compared to 'weight training for competition', the advantages of safety and convenience often far outweigh the disadvantages. An exercise session involving the use of exercise machines should always commence with a 'warm-up' that involves some form of aerobic activity and stretching exercises. If the participant is relatively strong, and hence the resistances being used are relatively high, then a few repetitions of the exercises using light resistances may form the final phase of the warm-up prior to the use of heavy resistances. This will ensure that the body is fully warmed up and prepared for the stresses that the exercise will place upon it. The main part of the session is likely to involve a combination of exercises using exercise machines, free weights such as dumbells and traditional body resistance exercises such as sit-ups and press-ups, thereby producing a varied combination of activities. As with almost any exercise session the final phase should involve a gentle aerobic cool-down and further stretching exercises which will gradually return the body to its 'resting state' and help to reduce the likelihood of stiffness the following day.

SAFETY ASPECTS ASSOCIATED WITH MUSCULAR-STRENGTHENING EXERCISE MACHINES

In order to produce the desired resistance given by an exercise machine such as a multigym, it is first necessary to 'select' the desired weight by inserting a 'selector key'. In some situations the selector keys will be attached to the equipment as permanent fixtures: in other situations they may be removable. If the keys are removable it is important that only the manufacturer's recommended and specifically designed key is used. Therefore, for convenience it may be useful to purchase some spares or to provide each user with an individual key for personal use during the session. On no account should substitute keys such as nails or screwdrivers be used as these present a potential hazard to both the user and the machine. Substitute keys can easily become wedged in the machine and may even damage it. In either case this may require some maintenance work or dismantling of the machine to remove the offending 'key'. In addition, substitute keys may not be strong enough to take the stresses placed upon them by the weights and may break. This could cause an unnecessary injury which should have been avoided.

All exercise machines require regular maintenance, which will vary from a weekly lubrication of moving parts to a yearly overhaul and safety check. Both are important for the safety of users, the smooth operating of the machine and the general condition of the equipment. The manufacturer's handbook will usually provide guidance on such matters as the nature and frequency of maintenance.

It is also important that all exercise machines are carefully positioned to allow free access and ease of movement when performing the exercises. Where appropriate they should be securely and expertly fixed to the wall or floor. In all cases the equipment should be situated so as to minimize the possibility of people colliding with it or being too near each other whilst exercising, as this would present a safety hazard as well as an inconvenience.

THE DETERMINATION OF 'TRAINING LOADS'

As mentioned earlier, when commencing any muscular-strengthening exercise programme it is important to start gradually with light resistances. Therefore, in the initial stages the therapist will need to determine appropriate resistances for each exercise. In practical terms this usually involves setting the individual a fairly light resistance and then seeing if the exercise can be performed 15 times with a moderate amount of exertion. If this is found to be very easy then the weight should be increased, or if it is found to be too difficult then the weight should be reduced. This means that a number of minor adjustments are likely to be required during the first few sessions. Therefore, it is important that the therapist keeps comprehensive records which give details of the exercise, weights used and number of repetitions performed.

Once the programme has commenced a record should be kept of each session as this will help to determine when the participant is ready to progress to greater resistances, repetitions or additional exercises. It will probably be necessary for the participant to stay at one initial training load for a least six sessions before gradual progression should be considered. As progress is made, the participant should again remain at the new level of each individual exercise for a number of weeks. To ensure gradual progression it is desirable to increase just one or two exercises at a time in each session, thus each successive session may be made slightly more demanding although each individual exercise may remain constant for six or more sessions before being once again increased. For therapists or advisers the assessment of initial workloads and the determination of appropriate progressions will become easier with experience as they become more familiar with the activity.

EXAMPLES OF MULTIGYM AND EXERCISE MACHINE EXERCISES

These descriptions refer to the exercises that are being performed at a single isolated station or at one of the stations which forms part of a multigym. Owing to the complexity of muscle action it is sometimes inappropriate to specify which muscles are being worked by a particular exercise and therefore it is often more appropriate to refer to the movement and relate it to the many muscle groups which could be involved in the activity, such as arm extension or knee flexion.

Exercises for the lower body

1. *Leg press* (Figure 6.34). The participant adjusts the seat so that when sitting with the feet resting on the footplate, the hips and knees are flexed at approximately 90 degrees (a). Flexing the hips and knees further will make the exercise more difficult (see section on muscular length tension relationships and angles of pull in Chapter 2). Therefore, in the participant's programme it is important to note the seat position as well as the amount of weight being used. Some machines will provide more than one possible foot position, and as this will also affect the degree of difficulty of the exercise it should be noted in the exercise programme. Since this exercise tends to use levers the foot position which provides the longest lever will provide the easiest version of the exercise, while the selection of a foot position which gives a shorter lever will make the exercise more difficult.

   When performing the exercise the participant should ensure that the feet are securely positioned on the correct foot placement. The participant then pushes against the footplate, extending the hips and knees and thereby lifting the weights (b). This action should be smooth and controlled, not jerky or erratic. It is especially important to control the movement near the point of full knee extension since, if the movement is too rapid, the legs will become fully extended but due to the momentum of the movement the weights may continue to rise slightly. The weights will then fall under the influence of gravity and in doing so exert an additional force on the participant's legs, which, with the knees fully extended, are not in a position to absorb this additional force. Therefore, in order to protect the leg joints from this unwanted stress the movement needs to be controlled at all times. Following full extension the weights are then lowered by flexing the hips and knees. This should again be a controlled movement with the leg extensors regulating the movement via eccentric contractions. The weights being lowered should not be allowed to touch the remaining weights of the stack but should be held about an inch

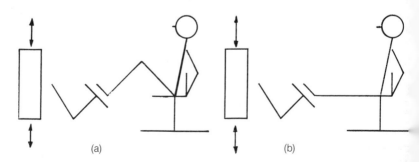

(a)   (b)

Figure 6.34

above them and the movement can then be repeated. This, therefore, requires good eccentric control of a movement which involves muscular coordination as well as strength. As a variation on this exercise it may be performed using one leg at a time rather than with both legs together.

The controlled eccentric phase of the exercise places a considerable amount of overload on the muscles. In those unfamiliar with the exercise this can result in delayed muscle soreness 24 to 48 hours after the exercise. This is due to microtrauma and slight inflammation within the muscle which will fade within a few days. Therefore, as with all forms of exercise,this exercise needs to be gradually introduced into a programme.

2. *Calf press* (Figure 6.35). The calf press may be performed at the same station as the leg press. The starting point for the calf press is at the point of full extension of the leg press. At this point the knees should be fully extended but the ankles will be flexed. From this position the participant then extends and flexes the ankles which will cause a slight rise and fall of the weights.

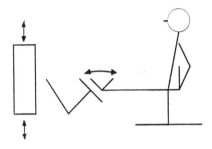

Figure 6.35

3. *Pushbacks* (Figure 6.36). This exercise may be performed at the 'leg press' station of some multigyms. The exercise is performed in a standing position with the participant facing away from the machine. The participant stands on one leg, flexes the knee of the other leg and places the sole of that foot on the footplate of the machine. Then holding onto the machine or another object

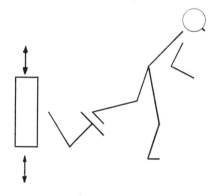

Figure 6.36

for support the participant pushes back with the leg, extending the hip and knee, thereby raising the weights. The weights are then carefully lowered by the controlled flexion of the hip and knee (using eccentric contractions of the extensor muscles). As with the leg press the lowered weights should not touch the remaining ones but should be held just above them, from where the movement can then be repeated. When performing this exercise it is important that the foot of the leg performing the work should be placed firmly on the footplate and is not liable to slip. With some multigyms the angle and positioning of the footplate makes this difficult, which could result in the foot slipping and hence the footplate could hit the back of the participant's legs. With such machines it is advisable not to undertake this exercise.

4. *Hamstring curls* (Figure 6.37). This exercise is performed with the participant lying face down on a bench, legs extended and ankles hooked under a padded bar to which the weights are attached. From this position the participant repeatedly flexes and extends the knee. The flexion movement causes the weights to rise due to the concentric activity of the knee flexors, whilst the lowering action is regulated by the eccentric activity of the knee flexors. The movement should go to full flexion and, as with the previous exercises, should be smooth and controlled. A variation on the exercise could involve the use of one leg at a time. This could be valuable if one leg is weaker than the other, as the strong leg tends to do most of the work when both legs are used. If the appropriate exercise station is not available then an alternative exercise may be performed using a strong elasticated strap. One end of the strap is attached to the participant's ankle whilst the other is connected to a wall or similar fixed object. The participant then lies face down with one knee slightly flexed, and attempts to fully flex this knee whilst working against the resistance provided by the elastic strap.

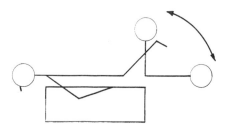

Figure 6.37

5. *Knee extensions* (Figure 6.38). This exercise is usually performed using the same bench as used for hamstring curls. In this exercise the participant sits at the end of the bench with the knees flexed so as to hang vertically over the end of the bench. The ankles are then hooked behind a padded bar to which weights are attached. From this position the participant then extends the knees, working against the resistance of the weights. Upon reaching full extension the weights are lowered by the controlled flexion of the knees and the movement

can be repeated. As with many of these exercises the knee extensions have the option of being performed either with both legs at the same time or each leg, separately, if preferred.

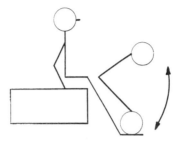

Figure 6.38

6. *Adductor pulls* (Figure 6.39). The station for this exercise is not commonly found either separately of as part of a multigym. The participant performs the exercise in a standing position with one ankle attached to a cord, and commences with the leg abducted and then adducts this leg (which is attached to the machine). Pulling the leg in towards the midline of the body raises the weights and causes the adductors to work against a resistance. In performing this exercise the participant may require some support in order to maintain his or her balance. If an appropriate exercise station is not available this exercise may be performed using a strong elasticated strap. One end of the strap is attached to the participant's ankle whilst the other is attached to the wall or similar immovable object. The adduction movement therefore works against the resistance of the strap.

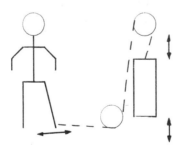

Figure 6.39

7. *Knee raises* (Figure 6.40). Whilst this is really a 'body resistance' exercise, an exercise station for this exercise commonly forms part of many multigyms. To commence the exercise the participant lifts, and holds, the body in position above the ground with the aid of arm rests and handles. The exercise therefore requires a considerable amount of upper body isometric strength and endurance. The exercise starts with the hips and knees extended.

The participant then flexes the hips and knees, raising the knees as high as possible towards the chest. The knees are then lowered by a controlled extension of the hips and knees.

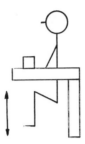

Figure 6.40

Exercises for the upper body

1. *Bench press* (Figure 6.41). The participant lies face up on the bench with the bar positioned so that it is approximately level with the chin. It is important that during this exercise the participant does not arch the back but that it should be kept firmly on the bench at all times. To ensure this and to provide a comfortable position from which to perform the exercise the feet may be placed either with one on each side of the bench with the soles flat on the floor, or together, with the soles of the feet flat on the bench. The latter position may be more comfortable for many people, especially those who are not exceptionally tall and find the foot placement on the floor slightly awkward. To commence the exercise the participant grasps the bar and pushes upwards, extending the elbow in a controlled movement. Once both elbows have been fully extended, the bar is gently lowered using eccentric contractions of the elbow extensors until the weights being used almost touch the remaining weights in the stack. The extension movement is then repeated. The exercise therefore involves aspects of control as well as concentric and eccentric muscular work.

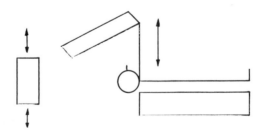

Figure 6.41

2. *Military press* (Figure 6.42). In muscular terms this exercise is similar to the bench press but it is performed from a seated rather than a lying position.

The participant sits on a stool facing in towards the exercise machine or multigym. In this position the bar should be positioned just above shoulder height and slightly to the front. This should ensure that when the exercise is performed the participant pushes upwards and slightly away from the body. This helps to prevent the back from arching during the exercise. For this exercise the taller participants may place their feet flat on the floor whilst others may place them firmly on the rungs of the stool (if present). These positions should provide the individual with a firm stable base from which to push. When performing the exercise the participant grasps the bar firmly and then pushes up and slightly away from the body, extending the elbows in a controlled movement. When the elbows are fully extended the bar is then gradually lowered so that the weights being used almost touch the weights remaining in the stack. From this position the exercise is then repeated.

As with most of the exercises described in this section the military press includes elements of control, as well as concentric and eccentric muscular activity. During the exercise the back should not be arched, but should be kept straight. Arching the back indicates that the exercise is too strenuous and the amount of weight or number of repetitions should be reduced to prevent undue stress being placed on the back. As indicated, therefore, the military press not only exercises the arm and shoulder muscles but also requires the back muscles to work isometrically in order to maintain back posture throughout the movement.

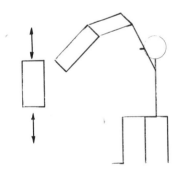

Figure 6.42

3. *Shoulder press* (Figure 6.43). In terms of the muscles used, the shoulder press is very similar to the military press. However, the shoulder press is performed with the participant facing outwards, away from the machine rather than towards it. The individual commences the exercise with the bar level with the shoulders, then pushes directly up, or up and slightly behind, when performing the exercise. This alignment and movement can cause some individuals to arch their backs when performing the movement. It is therefore less preferable than the aforementioned military press for most participants and owing to the overall similarity of the two exercises it may be omitted from most programmes.

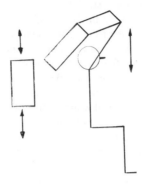

Figure 6.43

4. *Biceps curls* (Figure 6.44). This exercise involves the use of weights and a pulley system. The participant commences the exercise facing the machine, and holding the bar with arms down and elbows extended (almost in the anatomical position). To get into this starting position the weights may need to be lifted slightly if the wire to which they are attached is relatively short. If this is the case, then care should be taken in getting into this position. Firstly, the participant should face the machine and then flex the knees and hips in order to crouch down and reach the bar which will be resting on the floor. From this position the participant will grasp the bar using an underhand grip (Figure 6.45) and straighten the back, looking up directly ahead whilst doing so. The participant then stands up by straightening the hips and knees, not by bending the back (which should be kept straight throughout the movement). This means that the weights are lifted into the starting position by the action of the legs and not the back. Lifting with a curved back or using the back to lift rather than the legs can put too much stress on the back. With some machines it is possible to alter the length of the wire, and if this can be done then it should be adjusted so that the weights being used are lifted a couple

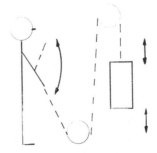

Figure 6.44

of inches above the others when the participant assumes the starting position. Once in the starting position the exercise may commence. The participant flexes the elbows raising the weights whilst keeping the upper arm and elbows close to the body and as still as possible. This ensures that the movement is caused by the elbow flexors rather than the shoulder flexors. Throughout the movement it is important that the back is kept still and not hyperextended to assist the movement. Any undesired back movement may make the exercise easier but puts unwanted stress on the back and should be avoided. During the exercise the shoulder muscles will be used statically to hold the shoulder in position. If, however, the therapist wishes the participant to use the shoulder flexors dynamically then some shoulder flexion may be used in the lifting action, but again the back should remain static throughout. The weights are lowered by extending the elbows. The downward movement is controlled by the eccentric contraction of the elbow flexors.

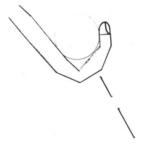

Figure 6.45

5. *Reverse curls* (Figure 6.46). Reverse curls provide a slight variation to the biceps curl. For the reverse curl the movement is performed with an overhand grip (Figure 6.47). In all other respects the movement and safety considerations are identical to those described for the biceps curl.

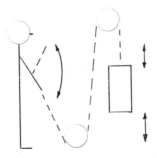

Figure 6.46

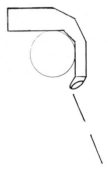

Figure 6.47

6. *Chinning* (Figure 6.48). Chinning is an exercise which may be performed at the same station as the biceps and reverse curls. The exercise commences in the same position as the reverse curl – that is, with an overhand grip, facing the machine with the weights being used already raised slightly above those remaining in the stack. From this position the participant raises the bar directly upwards so that it almost touches the chin. This is achieved by the simultaneous abduction of the upper part of the arms at the shoulder joint and the flexion of the lower arms at the elbow joint in the frontal plane. The bar is then lowered using the reverse movement and the exercise is repeated.

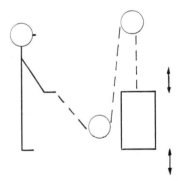

Figure 6.48

7. *Seated rowing* (Figure 6.49). Seated rowing may also be performed at the same station as the biceps curls and chinning exercises. The basic movement is similar to that of chinning. However, this exercise is performed in a seated rather than a standing position. To get into the starting position the participant sits down and places the feet against the foot placements provided. In this position the knees and hips should both be flexed. The participant then takes hold of the bar with an overhand grip and extends the elbows. From this position the participant then straightens the back into a vertical position whilst

continuing to hold the bar to the front with extended arms. At this point the wire or cord attached to the weights should still be slack. The participant then pushes against the foot placements to straighten the hips and knees whilst keeping the back straight and upright. This will push the body away from the machine, causing the wire to tighten, and should result in the weights rising slightly. During this phase it is important to keep the back and arms straight so that the initial lifting of the weights off the stack is caused by the action of the legs. If the wire is too slack then it may need to be adjusted so that the weights are lifted a couple of inches off the stack. This then forms the starting position. From this position the participant then pulls the bar towards the chest using a similar arm action to that described for chinning, however in this case the arm movements will be in an oblique plane with the overall bar movement being upward and outward towards the participant's chest. The weights are then carefully lowered using a reverse movement and held just above those remaining in the stack. Throughout this exercise it is important to ensure that the back is kept vertical and is not used dynamically during the movement. Flexing and extending the back during this exercise may place unnecessary stress on the back. This exercise works the back muscles statically as well as dynamically exercising the arm and shoulder muscles.

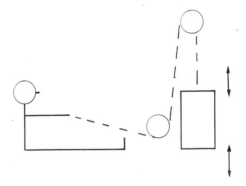

Figure 6.49

8. *Lats pulldowns* (Figure 6.50). This exercise is for the arms and upper back. It derives its name from one of the muscle groups involved, the latissimus dorsi. There are a number of variations of this exercise, which may be performed kneeling on one knee, kneeling on both knees or even seated. Participants should select the one they find most comfortable. The exercise uses the station which is commonly called 'the lats bar'. The 'lats bar' is suspended overhead and is pulled down during the exercise using a combination of shoulder muscles and elbow flexors as well as the forearm muscles which are involved in holding the bar. To get into the starting position for the exercise the participant holds the bar with an overhand grip, with the hands positioned towards the ends of the bar. In this position the hands will be approximately two feet wider than shoulder width apart. From this standing position the participant may then assume a kneeling or seated position whilst

keeping the arms extended above the head and bending the knees to lower the body. Owing to the length of the pulley this will have the effect of raising the weights slightly. This movement into the starting position is preferable to one in which the participants immediately assume a kneeling position with flexed arms, as this makes the weight more difficult to control and may put unwanted strain on the back.

In the starting position the pulley of the machine should be directly above the participant's head. If the participant is positioned too far from the machine the exercise will be awkward to perform. The exercise then commences from this starting position (standing, kneeling or seated) with the arms extended above the head, holding the bar. The participant pulls the bar down behind the head so that it almost touches the back of the neck, thereby raising the weights. The weights are then lowered by slowly extending the arms using eccentric contractions to control the movement. Once the arms are again fully extended the movement may be repeated. Upon completion of the desired number of repetitions the participant extends the arms above the head and then slowly stands (if performing the exercise from a kneeling or seated position), keeping the arms extended until the weights are lowered to the stack. This movement is preferable to the participant standing up with the arms flexed which makes the weight more difficult to control and could place unwanted strain on the back.

As a variation of the lats pulldown exercise the participant may pull the bar down in front of the body until it is level with the chest or until the weights almost reach the top of the machine. As a further variation the participant could pull the bar down alternately behind and in front of the head.

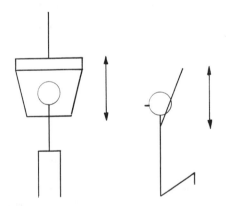

Figure 6.50

9. *Triceps pushdowns* (Figure 6.51). This exercise uses the same station as the lats pulldowns. The triceps pushdowns are performed in a standing position with the participant holding the bar with an overhand grip and the hands approximately one and a half to two feet apart. To get into the starting

position the bar is pulled down so that the elbows are positioned close to the body just above the hips. The elbows are fully flexed, with the bar being held at approximately shoulder height. From this starting position the participant then extends the elbows pushing the bar down whilst keeping the elbows close to the body just above the hip. Once the elbows are fully extended the bar is slowly returned to the starting position by flexing the elbows, controlling the movement with eccentric contractions. Again the elbows should remain close to the body and when full elbow flexion is reached the movement may be repeated.

The exercise involves elbow flexion and extension with the minimum amount of shoulder movement. Shoulder movement (flexion and extension) will make the exercise easier, therefore it may be modified depending upon whether the therapist wishes the particpant to use the shoulders or keep the dynamic aspects of the exercise as primarily elbow extension. Upon completion of the desired number of repetitions the weights are lowered back onto the stack by allowing the bar to rise above the participant's head, again controlling the movement with eccentric contractions.

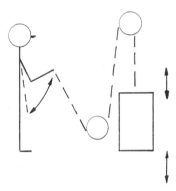

Figure 6.51

10. *Chins* (Figure 6.52). Chins are a body resistance exercise but are included in this section because stations for performing this exercise are commonly included in most multigyms. Chins require good upper body strength and are therefore only likely to be appropriate for individuals who are exceptionally strong. The 'chinning bar' is fixed to the multigym several feet above head height (as an alternative, appropriately fixed bars may be used). To perform the exercise the participant reaches up and holds the bar with both hands. Shorter individuals may need to be lifted into this position, or use a chair. The bar is held with the hands positioned so that they are slightly wider than shoulder width apart. An overhand or underhand grip may be used and indeed may be changed to provide a variation of the exercise. The exercise commences with the arms extended and the participant holding onto the bar with the feet above the ground. For comfort some individuals prefer to cross the feet as they are suspended in mid air. The participant then raises the body using

the shoulder and arm muscles so that the chin is raised slightly above the bar. The body is then slowly lowered until the elbows are again fully extended. The movement can be repeated for the desired number of repetitions.

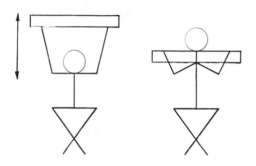

Figure 6.52

11. *Dips* (Figure 6.53). Like the 'chins', dips are a body resistance exercise for which a station is often incorporated into a multigym. The dips described in the earlier section on body resistance involved the participant having the feet on the ground or on another object, thereby supporting some of the participant's weight. The dips described here involve the feet being off the ground and therefore all the participant's weight is being supported by the upper body. This makes it a much more advanced exercise which is only suitable for those with good upper body strength. The participant commences the exercise holding the bars with the elbows extended and feet elevated off the floor. From this position the body is then lowered (via elbow flexion and shoulder hyperextension) using eccentric contractions until the upper arm is parallel to the floor. In this position the elbows should be positioned behind the body, flexed at right angles with the lower arms in a vertical position. The body

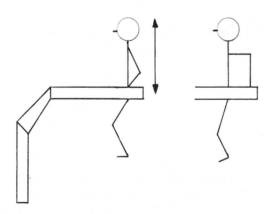

Figure 6.53

is then raised back into the starting position by extending the elbows and flexing the shoulders. For the duration of the exercise some participants may prefer to slightly flex the knees and cross the legs if they find it makes the exercise more comfortable.

THE USE OF DUMBELLS

Dumbells may be used in a large variety of resistance exercises to develop muscular tone, local muscular endurance and muscular strength. Dumbell exercises are usually very simple and safe.

Some dumbells are designed to be a fixed weight whilst others have the facility to adjust the weight by adding or removing weights. Dumbells should be stored in a rack for easy access and should be replaced immediately after use to reduce the risk of someone falling over them. Although dumbells tend to be relatively light (1 to 10 kg each) care should still be taken when lifting them from the stack, especially the heavier ones. When preparing to lift a dumbell from the stack or off the ground always bend the knees, keep the back straight and look up. The dumbells should then be lifted by straightening the legs, assuming the anatomical position. From this position individuals may then walk to the area in which they are going to perform the exercise and carefully, without any hurried movements, assume the starting position for the exercise. Equal care must be taken when returning the dumbells to their storage area.

EXAMPLES OF DUMBELL EXERCISES

1. *Biceps curls* (Figure 6.54). The participant begins the exercise in the anatomical position. From this position the elbow is flexed and the dumbell brought up to shoulder height in a smooth and controlled movement. It is then carefully lowered back to the starting position, controlling the movement with eccentric contractions of the elbow flexors. Throughout the movement the upper arm should be kept close to the body and shoulder movement should be minimal. In addition to this the back should be kept straight and still (the back should not be used dynamically to assist with the movement). Biceps curls may be performed in a variety of ways:

   (a) The arms may be worked separately, with one arm completing its full set of repetitions before the other one is exercised.

   (b) The arms may work alternately, with one arm completing one full cycle of the exercise whilst the other remains in the starting position, the roles then being reversed. This means that each arm completes one repetition and then rests whilst the other arm completes one repetition and so on for the desired number of repetitions.

   (c) Both arms work together in parallel, raising and lowering the dumbells in synchrony.

   (d) Both arms work at the same time but in opposition. One arm raises its dumbell using concentric contractions whilst the other arm is in the process of lowering its dumbell using eccentric contractions.

There is little difference in the effectiveness of each of these variations so the choice of which version to use will depend upon individual preference.

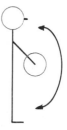

Figure 6.54

2. *Running arms* (Figure 6.55). The arm action used in this exercise is similar to that when a person is walking or running. From the anatomical position the arms are pronated so that the palms are facing the thighs and both elbows are flexed at 90 degrees. This is the starting position. From this position the arms are moved with a running/walking action. The arms are therefore moved in opposition with one moving back as the other moves forwards. On completion of the forward movement the dumbell may reach shoulder height, whilst on completion of the backward movement the upper arm may be flexed at the shoulder so that it is not quite parallel to the ground.

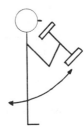

Figure 6.55

3. *Dumbell raises* (Figure 6.56). This exercise requires the use of a bench, and one arm is exercised at a time. When exercising the right arm and shoulder the participant stands on the left leg and places the right knee on the bench so that he or she is looking down the length of the bench with the right arm (which is holding the dumbell) extending over the right side of the bench. The participant then flexes the back to approximately 60 degrees and places the left hand on the bench for balance. This then forms the starting position. From this position the dumbell is raised by flexing the right elbow and extending the right shoulder so that the dumbell is brought up to the height of the right hip. The dumbell is then lowered using the reverse movements and the

exercise repeated for the desired number of repetitions. To exercise the left side the positions are reversed.

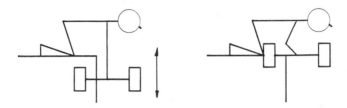

Figure 6.56

4. *Triceps pullovers* (Figure 6.57). During this exercise one arm is worked at at time. In this example the movements are described for the right arm, therefore to exercise the left arm the roles need to be reversed. To get into the starting position the participant stands in the anatomical position. The right arm, which is holding the dumbell, is then pronated so that the palm faces the right thigh. The arm is then fully flexed at the shoulder (keeping the elbow extended) until the dumbell is held vertically overhead. The left arm is then moved to hold the right elbow in position. This forms the starting position. From this position the right elbow is flexed so that the dumbell is lowered behind the head until it is level with the neck. The right elbow is then extended to raise the dumbell back to the starting position.

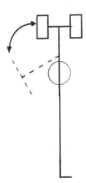

Figure 6.57

5. *Dumbell flies* (Figure 6.58). This exercise is performed with the participant lying face upwards on a bench with the feet firmly positioned flat on the floor or on the bench. The participant holds a dumbell in each hand and abducts both arms so that the arms are at 90 degrees to the body and parallel to the

223

floor or slightly hyperextended in the transverse plane (a). From this position both dumbells are slowly raised so that the arms are held vertically, directly above the chest (b). This movement could be described as shoulder flexion in the transverse plane or as an anticlockwise rotation of the right arm and clockwise rotation of the left arm in the transverse plane. The arms are then lowered back to the starting position using the reverse movements.

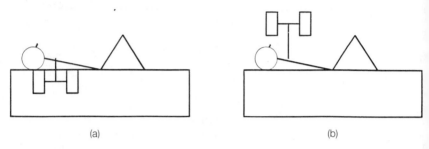

(a)   (b)

Figure 6.58

THE USE OF FREE WEIGHTS AND ANKLE WEIGHTS

Many 'free weights' exercises described in the following section have similar versions that could be performed using an exercise machine. However, exercises that use free weights require the participants to not only work with a resistance (provided by the weight) but to be in complete control of the movement. Conversely, exercise machines provide some degree of control over the movement of the weights (the advantages and disadvantages of this were discussed in an earlier section). In summary, exercise machines provide an extra safety dimension because the weights can only move in a very limited direction (up and down the stack). The participant's control of the movement is therefore limited to the speed of the movement up and down. Exercises which use machines are therefore not likely to cause injury, as losing control of the weights will only cause them to fall onto the stack. However, with free weights the participant not only has to control the speed of movement but also the direction and this makes the exercise more difficult. The additional control needed with free weights may require the fixator muscles to work harder than when performing the equivalent movement on an exercise machine. This may be desirable in some cases; however, if the participant loses control of the weights they are liable to cause an injury as the participant struggles to regain control or drops them. Therefore, free weights have certain advantages over exercise machines but have the potential to cause injury if the participant has a poor technique, becomes fatigued or drops them through carelessness.

Also, when using exercise machines for such exercises as the bench press, leg press and military press it is possible for one side of the body to do more than the other. Free weights require both sides of the body to work equally hard in moving the weights and controlling the movement. Therefore, if one side of the body is stronger than the other it may be desirable to use free weights. Alternatively, each side of the body could be exercised separately.

In practical terms it should also be remembered that exercises using free weights often require the assistance of a helper or 'spotter' especially in exercises such as the bench press. The spotter will assist if the participant becomes too fatigued during the exercise or the weight becomes too heavy, and will also assist with the initial movement of the weight off the stand and its replacement after the desired number of repetitions. A spotter is therefore important to ensure the safe use of free weights. Additional safety considerations associated with the use of free weights include ensuring that all weight 'collars' are firmly secured to prevent the weights from falling off the bar. On a final note of safety, it is very easy for free weights to be left around the exercise area after use. This is not only untidy but presents a serious safety hazard as they can easily cause someone to trip and fall. Free weights must always be returned to their storage area after use, and when in use strong matting is advisable in the exercise area to protect the floor. A mirror is also a standard inclusion in most exercise areas as it can help to ensure that the participant uses the correct technique for each exercise. The factors of safety, control, and potential bias must therefore be considered when setting an exercise programme, and the therapist should then select the desired free weights and/or exercise machine exercises accordingly.

In some cases ankle or wrist weights may be used as an alternative to heavier free weights. Examples of such exercises include the leg extension and hamstring curl which were described earlier. During these exercises the overall movement is the same and the relevant sections should be referred to for details.

EXAMPLES OF EXERCISES USING FREE WEIGHTS

1. *Bench press*. This exercise utilizes the same movements as the multigym bench press described in a previous section (see Figure 6.41). However, as stated earlier, it requires the presence of an assistant or 'spotter' to ensure that the exercise is performed safely. It also requires a set of stands which are positioned on each side of the bench. This supports the weight prior to the exercise and the weight is returned to the stands upon completion of the desired number of repetitions. As the movement of the weights to and from the stand requires good control and coordination, the spotter is therefore likely to assist with this aspect of the exercise, especially if the particpant is fatigued.

2. *Squats* (Figure 6.59). This exercise also requires the use of stands and a 'spotter' to assist with the weights. This is an advanced strength-training exercise and is therefore not likely to be appropriate for those requiring basic exercise therapy. The stands are positioned so that the weights bar is situated just below shoulder height. The participant then stands under the bar with the knees flexed, supporting the bar on the back of the neck. For comfort additional padding should be positioned between the neck and the bar (a folded towel will often suffice). The participant's hands are positioned towards each end of the bar to provide optimum control and balance. From this position the participant extends the knees, lifts the bar off the stands, and then moves forwards a few paces to get clear of the stands. The exercise can then commence. The participant should stand with the feet slightly wider than shoulder width apart, and, from this standing position (a), assume a slight squatting

position (b) (not a deep squat) by flexing the hips, knees and ankles whilst keeping the back straight and looking forward directly ahead. For most individuals the knees should be flexed no more than 90 degrees since additional flexion will place unwanted strain on the knee. With this exercise a mirror is useful. If the participant stands in front of the mirror, this can help to ensure that the head is kept up throughout the exercise. From this semi-squatting position the participant then extends the hips, knees and ankles to return to the starting position. During this exercise the heels of both feet may be elevated by getting the participant to stand with the heels on a block of wood (1 to 1.5 inches high) whilst the balls of the feet remain flat on the floor. This appears to help some individuals keep their back straight and their head up throughout the exercise. The exercise should be performed slowly and in a controlled manner without bouncing (as this puts strain on the knees). When the desired number of repetitions have been completed the participant is guided back to the stands by the spotter and assisted in returning the weights bar to the stands.

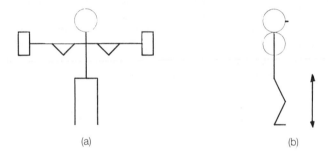

(a) (b)

Figure 6.59

3. *Good morning exercises* (Figure 6.60). As previously stated, many of the exercises described in earlier sections will strengthen the back. However, should the therapist wish to include a specific back exercise into a programme then these exercises may be prescribed for those who already have relatively strong back muscles but wish to develop their strength further. This is therefore not an exercise for beginners, who will probably develop their back strength sufficiently through other exercises such as press-ups and the military press. The starting position (a) for the 'good morning exercises' is the same as for the squats previously described, though much lighter weights are used. From the starting position the back is flexed at between 30 and 45 degrees (b). This should be done slowly and should not go too far such that the participant feels stretch on the hamstrings. From this flexed position the participant then slowly extends the back and straightens up into the starting position before repeating the movement. Throughout the exercise the movement should be slow and controlled, without bouncing. Upon completion of the exercise the participant returns the weights to the stands with the assistance of the spotter.

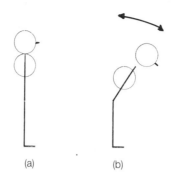

(a)   (b)

Figure 6.60

ACCOMMODATING RESISTANCE WORK

As previously discussed, a feature of most exercises is that during the different phases of the movement the muscles experience a different degree of difficulty. With accommodating resistance work the amount of resistance experienced throughout a movement is altered such that the muscles are worked throughout their entire range of movement. This accommodating resistance may be achieved through the use of specific 'isokinetic' machines or with the aid of a therapist. Exercises such as the knee extension and flexion exercises, as well as various upper body exercises, are commonly provided for with isokinetic machines. More sophisticated versions of such machines also have a diagnostic use and can record the strength of the muscles during different phases of a movement, thereby informing the therapist whether the muscles are significantly weaker at any particular phase of their range of movement. With isokinetic machines the muscles may be exercised at specific speeds. Therefore, if isokinetic machines are included in a programme the speed of movement will need to be considered as well as the number of repetitions. Since such machines are very specialized and any therapist encountering them is likely to receive specific instructions concerning their operation, they will not be discussed further in this text.

Alternative accommodating resistance work can easily be incorporated into a programme if the participant is able to exercise with the therapist who will apply the required resistance instead of the machine. Accommodating resistance can be applied to virtually all dynamic muscular movements and therefore only one specific example will be given in this section to illustrate its application. An advantage of including accommodating resistance exercises in a programme is that movements which normally occur under the influence of gravity (and hence require very little muscular activity) can be made more difficult and the exercises can work certain muscle groups which could be neglected by many other exercises.

1. *Knee extensions* (Figure 6.61). The participant sits on a bench with the knees flexed at 90 degrees so that the lower legs hang vertically over the edge of

the bench. One leg is exercised at a time. The movement for the exercise is the same as that used in the knee extension exercise previously described in the section on exercise machines (see Figure 6.38). The participant simply extends one knee so that the leg is straightened. However, during the exercise the therapist will place a hand on the ventral side of the ankle of the participant and push, thereby resisting the movement. The pressure applied by the therapist should not be so great as to prevent the movement but it should be sufficient to retard its speed considerably. Throughout the exercise the participant should push as hard as possible throughout the full range of movement and, likewise, the therapist should provide resistance throughout, thereby keeping the speed of movement consistent and making the muscles work hard throughout the full range of movement. Accommodating resistance may be simply applied to other movements such as knee flexion, elbow flexion and extension, shoulder movements and indeed virtually any body movement that requires concentric muscular contractions.

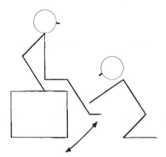

Figure 6.61

7

Aerobic and activity-based exercises

INTRODUCTION

Exercise that is of a relatively low intensity but can be maintained for a prolonged period of time is often referred to as being 'aerobic'. Examples of such exercise include walking, steady cycling, gentle jogging, steady swimming and aerobic dance. The term aerobic is applied to these activities because of the way in which the energy needed to perform them is obtained. During 'aerobic' exercise the muscles are supplied with ATP (required for contraction) via the aerobic pathway. Biochemically this involves the stages of glycolysis or beta-oxidation, the Krebs cycle and the electron transfer chain (see Chapter 3 for details). With this system oxygen is used up during the final stage of the electron transfer chain and therefore the individual's oxygen consumption increases while performing such activities. This is why, during these activities, individuals breathe harder and their heart rates increase.

The aerobic system (unlike the anaerobic lactate system) does not produce waste products that result in the rapid onset of fatigue. Thus, while the aerobic system is being used as the major energy pathway, the activity may be continued for a prolonged period of time. Conversely, if the intensity of the activity is substantially increased, so as to require the use of the anaerobic systems, the muscles will rapidly fatigue. This occurs when a person rapidly climbs stairs, lifts heavy weights, runs fast, cycles fast or swims fast. However, fatigue can eventually occur in aerobic activities as a result of dehydration or when the activity is so prolonged that the body's energy stores become depleted. In practice, fuel depletion and dehydration only usually occur after hours of exercise, as in the case of marathon running. In summary, the term aerobic may be applied to any activity that utilizes the aerobic energy pathway as its prime source of energy.

Like all other components of physical fitness the aerobic aspects cannot be completely isolated. Any activity that may be considered as being 'aerobic' will still require a certain amount of muscular strength, flexibility and coordination. For instance, swimming, cycling and walking all require a certain amount of muscular strength in order to pull the body through the water or push down on the pedals or push against the ground to propel the body along. Activities such as walking, cycling and swimming may be considered as being 'steady-state' activities as the intensity of the activity will remain fairly constant throughout the exercise session.

Other forms of activity, such as badminton, are 'intermittent', as the level of activity may be quite high during a rally but then fall to a relatively low level when the shuttle-cock or ball is not in play. These 'intermittent' activities will also have a major aerobic requirement along with the other aspects of physical fitness. During these activities the aerobic system, and possibly the anaerobic systems, will be used during inten-sive phases. Following these bouts of intensive activity the aerobic system will then continue to be used during the recovery phases of lower intensity activity. During these phases the aerobic system will not only be used to maintain the body's level of basic activity but will also be used to get rid of any metabolic waste products that had accumulated during the intensive play. Hence, it will be used to help the body to recover from the intensive activity. Intermittent activities include certain racquet games and team games such as badminton, tennis, basketball and volleyball. Owing to the aerobic requirement within these activities they may be used to enhance a person's aerobic capacity and, hence, physical fitness. Indeed, such activities may provide a major means of therapy for many individuals as they will involve social as well as physiological aspects.

Exercises and games are often utilized as part of the rehabilitation and recovery process of many individuals, including those who have suffered a heart attack, major illness or amputation. However, as with all forms of physical exercise the intensity of the activity must be appropriate. In this context it should be noted that the intermittent type activities can vary considerably in their intensity, depending upon the skill of the player, the competitiveness and the opposition. Therefore, care must be taken to ensure that such activities are not too demanding for the physical condition of the individual. Other activities which may convey aerobic and social benefits include golf, which requires a considerable amount of walking, and exercise to music, such as low-impact aerobics.

THE IMPORTANCE OF AEROBIC FITNESS

Aerobic fitness is associated with a person's capacity to undertake prolonged forms of activity. These may range from household tasks such as cleaning, gardening and shopping to more obvious forms of physical exercise such as badminton or swimming. The greater a person's aerobic capacity, the more capable will that person be of per-forming such activities without becoming fatigued; and thus aerobic fitness is associated with a person's stamina and endurance. A clear link can therefore be made between the enhancement of people's aerobic capacity and their overall ability to cope with the physical demands of their lifestyle. The participation in aerobic activities may also provide them with a social activity, enhancing the overall quality of their life. In addition to these general benefits, regular participation in aerobic exercise and its resulting good level of aerobic fitness are also associated with a number of positive health benefits. These include a reduction in the risk of certain diseases such as high blood pressure, coronary heart disease, obesity and a number of stress-related disorders. The details of these benefits are discussed in Chapter 8. In summary, an appropriate level of aerobic fitness has implications for all individuals. The role of the therapist may therefore be to enhance this aspect of fitness in accordance with the individual's needs and circumstances.

THE DETERMINANTS OF AEROBIC FITNESS AND THE ADAPTATIONS MADE IN RESPONSE TO AEROBIC EXERCISE

An individual's aerobic fitness or aerobic capacity is determined by a large number of interrelated factors. Primarily it is determined by the individual's capacity to utilize oxygen. A person's maximum capacity to use oxygen is referred to as that person's $\dot{V}O_2$max. It is measured as the maximum volume of oxygen that can be utilized in a minute and is therefore a measure of the individual's maximum rate of oxygen consumption. It is usually measured in litres of oxygen per minute (l/min) or, if it is being related to body weight, as millilitres of oxygen per kilogramme of body weight per minute (ml/kg/min). It should be emphasised that $\dot{V}O_2$max refers to the amount of oxygen that people can utilize, not simply the volume they can get in and out of their lungs. A person's $\dot{V}O_2$max can be assessed using sophisticated laboratory equipment, by measuring the oxygen consumption whilst the individual is working at maximum aerobic capacity on a cycle ergometer, treadmill or similar apparatus. However, because of the maximal nature of the exercise required for such methods they are not suitable for most individuals and therefore a number of submaximal methods of estimating aerobic fitness are often used as an alternative. Details of a number of methods used to evaluate aerobic fitness are presented later in this chapter.

There is a positive relationship between the amounts of oxygen individuals can use ($\dot{V}O_2$max) and their capacity to perform prolonged bouts of physical activity (their aerobic capacity or aerobic fitness). The more oxygen individuals can use the more able they are to perform basic activities with ease and the more capable they are of undertaking and maintaining prolonged forms of activity without becoming fatigued. Therefore the prime physiological objective of aerobic exercises is to increase an individual's capacity to utilize oxygen.

The factors which determine a person's capacity to utilize oxygen include:

1. The condition of the lungs and the muscles associated with breathing.
2. The oxygen-carrying capacity of the blood.
3. The condition of the heart.
4. The condition of the blood vessels.
5. The amount of myoglobin in the fibres.
6. The condition of the mitochondria within the fibres.

1. *The condition of the lungs and the muscles associated with breathing.* The functions of the respiratory system are to get air (containing oxygen) into the body and to remove waste products, such as carbon dioxide. The site of this gaseous exchange which occurs between the air and the blood are the small air sacs of the lungs (the alveoli). For an efficient gaseous exchange the airways of the lungs must be unobstructed, the muscles associated with breathing need to work effectively and the lungs need a good blood supply. Any disorder which restricts these factors will inhibit the entry of oxygen into the body. However, for most people, unless they are suffering from a specific respiratory disorder, this is not the major limiting factor which determines their aerobic capacity. Appropriate forms of aerobic exercise may, however, enhance the respiratory process and enhance an individual's capacity to get oxygen into the body and hence oxygenate the blood.

2. *The oxygen-carrying capacity of the blood.* Oxygen is transported, by the blood, around the body to the various organs which need it, including the working muscles. Virtually all of the oxygen that is carried by the blood is transported in association with the red blood cells (erythrocytes). Specifically the oxygen combines with molecules of haemoglobin which are contained within the red blood cells. This results in the formation of oxyhaemoglobin. The oxygen-carrying capacity of the blood is therefore largely determined by the amount of haemoglobin in the blood. Increases in both blood volume and the number of red blood cells will enhance the delivery of oxygen around the body. Aerobic exercise has been shown to increase all these factors and thereby promote the oxygen-carrying capacity of the blood. This will therefore enhance the delivery of oxygen to the muscles.

3. *The condition of the heart.* The blood is pumped around the body by the action of the heart. Aerobic exercise has been shown to increase the size and strength of the heart. This results in an increase per beat (the stroke volume) in the amount of blood pumped out of each ventricle of the heart. As a consequence, the heart has to beat less often to deliver the same amount of blood to the muscles. The overall effect of this is a more efficient cardiovascular system. It also means that the heart has a greater capacity to deliver more blood, and, hence, more oxygen to the muscles if it needs to. In practical terms this means that when the muscles are working at a relatively high intensity they will have an increased supply of oxygen and are therefore less likely to need to resort to the anaerobic pathways for the production of ATP. The effect of this is to reduce the likelihood of fatigue.

4. *The condition of the blood vessels.* The blood is delivered to the muscles via a series of blood vessels. If these vessels are constricted, as in the case of atheroma (fatty deposits on the walls of the arteries), then the blood supply will be impeded. Aerobic exercise can help to maintain these blood vessels in good condition.

   Within the muscles there is an extensive network of minute blood vessels called capillaries. These capillaries are in close association with the muscle fibres and provide the site of gaseous exchange between the blood and muscle. Aerobic exercise can increase the size of this capillary network by increasing the number of effective blood capillaries in the muscle. The increased number of capillaries will greatly enhance the delivery of blood to the muscle fibres and thus increase the effective delivery of oxygen to the working muscle fibres and the removal of waste products.

5. *The amount of myoglobin in the fibres.* Oxygen moves out of the blood and into the muscle fibres via the process of diffusion. This process is enhanced by the presence of myoglobin within the muscle fibres. Myoglobin molecules have a great affinity for oxygen. They can therefore act as a temporary store for the oxygen within the muscle and enhance the extraction of oxygen from the blood. Aerobic exercise can increase the amount of myoglobin in the muscle fibres. This will therefore enhance the muscle's extraction of oxygen from the blood and effectively increase the muscle's oxygen supply.

6. *The condition of the mitochondria within the fibres.* Once in the muscle fibre the oxygen is ultimately used in the aerobic synthesis of ATP (see Chapter 3). The oxygen is specifically used in the final stages of this process which occur in specialized organelles called mitochondria. Aerobic exercise will increase both the size and number of mitochondria within a muscle fibre. This will therefore increase the muscle's capacity to utilize oxygen in the synthesis of ATP.

It can therefore be seen that a person's capacity to utilize oxygen depends upon a number of factors. Aerobic exercise will bring about certain adaptations within the body which will enhance both the delivery of oxygen to the muscles and the muscles' capacity to use the oxygen. The adaptations will also increase the muscles' capacity to get rid of metabolic waste products such as carbon dioxide and will even enhance the body's ability to oxidize lactic acid during relatively intensive forms of exercise when the anaerobic systems may be used in addition to the aerobic system.

The body's adaptations to aerobic exercise can be considered under two headings: (a) those which are central and (b) those which are peripheral. Central adaptations include changes to the lungs, blood and heart, whilst peripheral changes refer specifically to the muscles. All forms of aerobic exercise will bring about central adaptations and will therefore enhance the body's overall capacity to deliver and utilize oxygen. The peripheral changes are, however, more specific and will only occur in those muscles being exercised. Thus, the specificity of the exercise needs to be considered. For instance, swimming will bring about a number of central adaptations and changes to the muscles used whilst swimming, whereas running may bring about similar central changes but will only bring about peripheral changes in the muscles that are primarily used whilst running. For the therapist this may have slight implications when considering the variety of exercises that should be included in an exercise programme. However, for most people it is of relatively little importance unless they are training for competitive sport. In practical terms this means that when considering which activities to include in an exercise programme, the choice of aerobic exercise is likely to be determined by individual preference, physical capabilities and convenience rather than the relatively slight differences in the physiological adaptations they promote.

FURTHER BENEFITS OF AEROBIC OR ACTIVITY-BASED EXERCISE

The adaptations to aerobic exercise described in the previous section are relevant to virtually all individuals regardless of age or gender. Improvements in aerobic capacity can be observed in all individuals ranging from the very young to the over-70s. Therefore, there are likely to be relatively few individuals for whom the therapist will be unable to devise some form of beneficial aerobic or activity-based exercise programme. In addition to these generalized benefits, it is also worth considering a number of specific benefits which are most relevant to either the elderly or the young.

When considering an exercise programme for the elderly it is important that it should commence at a very low intensity and progress very gradually. Whilst this is a recommendation for all participants, it is especially important with older individuals where there is a possibility of asymptomatic cardiovascular disease and extra care should be taken to ensure that any form of exercise is not too vigorous.

In association with the ageing process there is a steady decline in aerobic capacity, maximum heart rate, flexibility, muscular strength and a demineralization of the bones. However, the regular participation in appropriate forms of exercise would appear to reduce the decline in these bodily functions. Indeed, improvements in cardiovascular function, strength and flexibility have all been observed in the elderly although these adaptations tend to occur more slowly than in younger adults. Activities which require muscular and/or gravitational forces to be exerted upon the bones, which would include almost all forms of physical activity, appear to be effective in reducing the demineralization of the bones (osteoporosis) and thus reduce the risk of the individual developing weak bones that are liable to fracture. It should also be realized that, whilst exercise can be effective in reducing the extent of these aspects of the ageing process in the elderly, it is also appropriate in reducing the decline in physical capacity in adults of all ages. Indeed, research would suggest that adults who exercise regularly throughout life are often physiologically younger than their sedentary colleagues of the same chronological age. There are many examples of individuals who, whilst being over 70, still participate in fairly vigorous forms of activity and even in competitive sport at an appropriate level.

For the elderly, swimming, walking, cycling and flexibility exercises are likely to be the most appropriate forms of activity. Nevertheless, for those who have the capacity and inclination, weight training may also convey considerable benefits in preventing a reduction in lean tissue mass (and hence strength) which tends to accompany the ageing process. For those individuals with specific problems such as arthritis, activities such as swimming may be ideal although this should not be pursued if it causes pain. Swimming is frequently recommended for a number of disorders because of its beneficial effects on joint mobility, muscular strength and cardiovascular fitness. It is often preferable to other forms of activity because of the buoyancy aspect which supports the body and thereby reduces the pressure on the joints. The water also provides a form of resistance against which the muscles have to work.

For the young, exercise conveys numerous benefits as well as a few potential hazards. On the negative side, children undertaking too much exercise may be prone to a range of overuse injuries (as are adults). The young are particularly prone to some of these injuries because of their immature bodies. Of particular concern are areas such as the growth plates (epiphyseal plates) of the growing long bones. These are made of cartilage rather than bone in the immature skeleton and this makes them more prone to damage from excessive or repeated stress. Epiphyseal injuries only occur when the exercise loads placed upon the child are too great. These injuries are therefore only likely to occur in children who undertake too much exercise or training in the pursuit of excellence in competitive sport, and even within sport they are relatively uncommon. The causes of such overuse injuries include: running too many miles every day on hard surfaces; or repeated over-hyperextension of the back in gymnastic type movements. These problems are unlikely to be caused by the type of exercise programmes prescribed by the therapist or any other form of regular participation in physical activity, including the training for competitive sport, if appropriately coached.

In contrast, the vast majority of children are more at risk from the effects of underactivity rather than overactivity. It may therefore be the role of the therapist to prescribe suitable exercise programmes which will increase children's participation in physical activity. Research would indicate that exercise can help to promote the overall physical development of children. This includes the skeletal, muscular, neuromuscular and cardiovascular aspects of their physical capacity. In addition, exercise may help to develop a child's coordination, reduce the risk of obesity and help with the social development of the growing individual. Various reports would suggest that exercise is beneficial to children of all ages but that the greatest physical responses to exercise occur during or after the growth spurt. The increased responses in these age groups are therefore believed to be associated with various hormonal changes which occur at this time. Such social, physiological and psychological benefits are therefore pertinent to all growing children whether they are suffering from a specific disease or disorder, rehabilitating from an accident or illness or just as part of the 'normal' developmental process. A general lack of physical activity may result in an impaired development of the individual; therefore, the exercise programmes which the therapist devises should primarily aim to enhance the physical and social development of the growing child.

For children as well as adults it is important to ensure that an exercise programme is varied and, for children, an element of fun should be included if possible. Variety will help to ensure a more comprehensive physical experience and development and will also reduce the chances of boredom. Similarly, the exercises or activities should be enjoyable if the child is to persist with them and get the most out of the sessions. Appropriately designed forms of 'play' may be orientated towards the development of the child's strength, cardiovascular system, coordination and muscular control. In reality, a combination of these effects is likely to be sought.

Therefore, in summary, when considering exercise programmes which are aerobic or activity-based, therapists must always use their experience in making the required adjustments to ensure that the forms of exercise are appropriate for the participants. All individuals are unique and therefore all exercise programmes need to be considered as being unique if they are to fulfil the needs of the individual.

THE IMMEDIATE RESPONSES OF THE BODY TO AEROBIC EXERCISE

To ensure that the body functions effectively a large number of factors have to be maintained within fairly closely defined limits. If these limits are exceeded then aspects of the body's metabolism and physiology may start to deteriorate. The maintenance of the body in an acceptable and relatively steady state is referred to as homeostasis. Factors which need to be regulated in order to maintain homeostasis include temperature, oxygen levels, blood sugar levels, blood pressure and the acidity of body tissues. A bout of exercise has the potential to temporarily disturb this state of homeostasis, since it causes an increase in heat production, utilization of oxygen, and utilization of energy stores, and also the production of metabolites which can cause an increase in the osmolarity and acidity of body tissues and fluids. The body, therefore, needs to respond to the state of exercise by bringing about a number of physiological changes which will help to maintain its homeostasis. These responses include an increase in the cardiac output of the heart, an increase in the rate and depth of breathing, circulatory changes and an increase in the secretion of a number of hormones (such as adrenalin) which help in the regulation of a number of factors within the body. These observed changes tend to be temporary responses to the exercise and are in proportion to the intensity of the exercise. Repeated bouts of exercise will continue to bring about these temporary responses but will, over a period of time, also induce a number of more permanent adaptations or 'training effects' which are discussed separately.

Quite often the body will make slight adjustments to its physiological processes even before a bout of exercise has commenced, i.e. anticipating a bout of exercise will bring about a number of preliminary responses. For example, the thought of exercise will cause a rise in sympathetic nervous activity and the secretion of sympathetic hormones such as adrenalin and noradrenalin. This will result in a rise in the heart rate, breathing rate and the mobilization of certain energy fuels such as liver glycogen and free fatty acids. It may also initiate changes in the circulation of the blood. This will include the vasodilation of blood vessels leading to the working muscles and the vasoconstriction of blood vessels which supply other organs such as the kidneys and gut. This prepares the body for the exercise as it mobilizes its energy stores and increases the blood supply to the muscles which will need it. For this reason adrenalin is sometimes termed as the fright, fight or flight hormone. Physiologically it would appear that the initial responses to the anticipation of exercise result from an increased activity of the cerebral cortex; however, once the activity has commenced the major area for controlling the respiratory and cardiovascular responses is the brain stem, of which the medulla oblongata would appear to be the most important.

Once the exercise has commenced it will cause changes in the levels of certain factors within the body. These include an increase in the temperature of the muscles and blood, a fall in the level of oxygen in the blood and an increase in the level of carbon dioxide in the blood, the latter of which will also affect the acidity of both the blood and the cerebrospinal fluid. In addition to these changes there will also be a rise in the concentration of other metabolites that are associated with exercise, such as potassium and lactic acid. Other factors which may stimulate or influence the homeostatic responses of the body during exercise include limb movement, muscle contractions and an increased activity of the motor cortex which, in addition to sending impulses to the working muscles, also sends impulses to the cardiorespiratory control centre of the brain (the medulla). When exercising, a whole range of factors serve to stimulate the required homeostatic responses. The integrated nature of these stimuli, which tend to occur together, make it inappropriate to discuss them in isolation or even to suggest which are the most significant.

As the body exercises, the immediate changes which occur act as stimuli, and are detected by various receptors or sensors situated in the muscles, cardiovascular system and nervous system. Information from these sensors may then cause intrinsic reflex responses within the muscles, or the information may be sent via sensory neurons to the cardiorespiratory control centres of the brain. Here the information is processed and a number of responses may result. These will include changes in hormonal secretions, and cardiac and muscular activity. The overall effects of these changes include:

1. An increase in heart rate (HR).
2. An increase in the stroke volume (SV) of the heart.
3. An increase in cardiac output (CO).
4. An increase in the rate and depth of breathing, which will increase minute ventilation.
5. Circulatory changes.
6. Changes in blood pressure.

In the following discussion, the values given to illustrate each of the responses are generalized averages: the specific values for an individual will depend upon size, age, gender and level of physical fitness.

1. *An increase in heart rate (HR).* At rest, average heart rates are approximately 72 beats per minute (or bpm). However, during exercise they may rise to 170 bpm. This increase will be as a result of:
   (a) an increased stimulation from the sympathetic neurons which increase the rate of discharge of the pacemaker (sino atrial node) of the heart;
   (b) the activity of the sympathetic hormones adrenalin and noradrenalin which also effect an increase in heart rate.

2. *An increase in the stroke volume (SV) of the heart.* The stroke volume is the amount of blood which is ejected by each ventricle of the heart with each beat. At rest the stroke volume of the heart may be in the region of 70 ml/beat. However, during exercise this may rise to over 120 ml/beat. This increase is believed to be caused by the sympathetic activity of various neurons and hormones, which results in a more forceful contraction of the ventricles. The observed increase in stroke volume during exercise is also suggested to be caused by an increase in the amount of blood returning to the heart. This is the Frank–Starling phenomenon which suggests that the additional amount of blood returning to the heart causes an increase in the filling of the ventricles; this results in an additional stretch on the walls of the ventricles which, in turn, causes a more forceful contraction. However, this mechanism for increasing stroke volume is now under question from some authorities.

3. *An increase in cardiac output (CO).* Cardiac output is the amount of blood ejected by each ventricle each minute. The increases in heart rate and stroke volume will therefore result in an increase in cardiac output (CO). Cardiac output is calculated by multiplying the heart rate by the stroke volume:

CO	=	HR	x	SV
(litres per minute)		(beats per minute)		(millilitres per beat)

At rest the cardiac output of an adult may be in the region of 5 l/min. However, during exercise this can rise, to be in excess of 25 l/min due to the combination of an increased heart rate and stroke volume. This increase in the cardiac output of the heart will increase the supply of oxygen and nutrients to the working muscles and will also aid with the removal of waste products. In addition, it will enhance the removal of heat from these areas and thus assist with the process of thermoregulation.

4. *An increase in the rate and depth of breathing which will increase minute ventilation.* Minute ventilation refers to the amount of air breathed in and out of the lungs in a minute. At rest, this may be in the region of 8 l/min, whilst during exercise it may rise to over 150 l/min as a result of the combined increases in the depth and rate of breathing. These increases will be under the influence of sympathetic neural activity which rises as a result of an increase in the levels of carbon dioxide and, hence, the acidity of the blood and cerebrospinal fluid.

Additional factors which have been shown to increase minute ventilation include joint movements which are detected by sensors around the joints. It is believed to be these sensors which bring about the immediate increases in minute ventilation which occur as soon as the exercise commences. The overall effect of an increased minute ventilation will be an enhanced oxygenation of the blood and a more effective removal of waste products such as carbon dioxide from the body, thereby helping to maintain the state of homeostasis.

5. *Circulatory changes*. Prior to and during exercise a number of circulatory changes are observed. These include the vasodilation of blood vessels leading to the exercising muscles and the vasoconstriction of blood vessels leading to other organs such as the gut. This will have the effect of diverting blood towards the exercising muscles which may be considered as a 'priority area' during exercise. Some of this redistribution of blood flow may be attributable to extrinsic factors which are influenced by the cardiorespiratory system. However, the redistribution of blood through the muscle may also be increased by intrinsic changes such as a fall in the level of oxygen within the muscle or a rise in acidity. This will cause an additional localized response that involves the dilation of appropriate blood vessels leading to the exercising muscle fibres. It is suggested that during exercise the muscles may receive over 80% of the cardiac output as compared with only 20% when the body is at rest. This redistribution of blood flow coupled with an increased cardiac output can effectively increase the blood supply to the muscles by a factor of over 20, from just over 1 l/min at rest to over 20 l/min during strenuous exercise.

6. *Blood pressure changes*. Blood pressure is determined by the force with which blood is pumped around the body and the resistance it encounters in the blood vessels of the circulatory system. During exercise there is a slight increase in systolic blood pressure but relatively little change in diastolic blood pressure. These observed effects are the result of the combined influences of an increase in cardiac output, which would tend to increase blood pressure, coupled with a general vasodilation of the arterioles leading to the exercising muscles, which would cause a reduction in blood pressure. Hence, the overall effect is an increase in cardiac output and circulatory vasodilation, which enhances the delivery of oxygen and nutrients to the working muscles without a substantial rise in blood pressure (which could damage the blood vessels and other organs).

Therefore, it can be seen that during a bout of exercise the body makes appropriate responses which enable it to maintain its condition of homeostasis and permit the continued participation in the exercise despite the significant increases in metabolism. This permits prolonged exercise. However, this may only be continued until the body is no longer able to maintain its homeostasis. At this point fatigue will result, causing a reduction in the intensity of the exercise or its complete cessation. Examples of this loss of homeostasis causing fatigue include:

1. The accumulation of lactic acid causes an increase in the acidity of the body fluids during strenuous forms of exercise. This rise in acidity (fall in pH) is detected by sensors and is registered by the body as pain or discomfort in the exercising muscles. The rise in acidity also prevents the further production of lactic acid by inhibiting a number of the enzymes in the glycolytic pathway. The overall

effect causes discomfort in the muscles and inhibits the further production of potentially toxic metabolic waste products: this is what is generally felt as muscular fatigue. Thus, the homeostatic process ensures that the pH of the body fluids does not fall to a level at which it could result in damage to the cells of the body.
2. A reduction in blood glucose levels and the depletion of muscle glycogen reduces the muscles' supply of energy. This will result in a general feeling of fatigue and a reduced capacity to exercise.
3. The loss of a substantial amount of sweat, without the replacement of body fluids, causing a general feeling of fatigue and a reduced physical capacity.
4. The elevation of body temperature above the homeostatically permitted level causes fatigue and reduces the capacity to exercise.

Therefore, in general, an exercise-induced homeostatic imbalance will result in feelings of fatigue and discomfort which will prevent the body from being exerted beyond its limitations. This imbalance is temporary since cessation of the exercise and, where necessary, the appropriate ingestion of food and/or fluid will permit the homeostatic balance to be restored.

Upon the cessation of exercise the heart rate and minute ventilation will gradually return to their resting levels as the various factors within the body return to their pre-exercise values. The rate of the return to these pre-exercise levels will depend upon the intensity of the exercise and the fitness of the individual. In general, the more intensive the exercise the longer it may take the individual to recover, while fitter individuals are likely to recover faster than the less fit.

DESIGNING AN AEROBIC OR ACTIVITY-BASED EXERCISE PROGRAMME

As with all exercise programmes, a number of factors need to be considered when prescribing aerobic or activity-based exercise programmes. These factors include:

1. The overall objectives of the programme
2. The kinds of activities that could be included
3. How the activities may be integrated into a more holistic programme
4. The frequency of the activities
5. The intensity of the activities.

When devising an exercise programme it is first necessary to define the basic objectives of the programme and to consider the reasons for incorporating exercise into the weekly routine of the individual. The reasons for the inclusion of exercise may have a physiological, social or psychological basis, although in reality it is most likely that a combination of benefits will be sought.

Different types of activity can convey different benefits in different settings and therefore the therapist must seek to obtain a balance of activities that will fulfil the desired objectives. When considering the overall content of the programme careful consideration also needs to be given to the need for variety. A range of different activities will help to ensure that the participant receives a wider physical experience which may be valuable socially, psychologically and physiologically as well as helping to achieve a more comprehensive state of physical fitness. Variety will also help to prevent staleness or boredom, which could prevent the participants from getting the most out of the programme and may even cause them to stop. Therefore a weekly programme may include: a number of formal exercise sessions in the gym where the emphasis may be on muscular strength or mobility: and a number of social sessions such as swimming or bowls, which, whilst having some physiological benefits, will also have psychological and social implications for the participants. In this way the precise content of the programme may be determined to produce an optimal balance of physiological, social and psychological aspects, in accordance with the physical and mental needs of the participants.

The frequency of exercise sessions within a programme are also likely to be determined by a number of factors. These include not only the physiological aspects of the participants' capability to exercise repeatedly and their need to recover, but also the accessibility of facilities or the amount of time the therapist can spend with the individuals. Access to a swimming pool may be fairly easy; however, if the therapist needs to be present at all sessions then this may severely restrict the number of sessions that the participants can undertake in a week. Group-orientated activities will also depend upon the availability of fellow participants.

The intensity of any activity is also a major consideration when devising a programme. If the participants are to gain optimal benefits from the programme and/or the correct balance between sessions the session must provide overload without being overtaxing. This particular aspect of an activity is discussed later in this chapter as a separate issue with each form of activity and type of exercise.

What often tends to be forgotten with activity-based exercise is the importance of 'warm-up' and 'cool-down'. Whilst a warm-up may easily be included as part of the routine of a gym-based session it is often forgotten in other surroundings. It is important to remember the principles of warm-up even when participating in activities such as badminton, tennis or swimming. In such surroundings the principles of warm-up may be included by performing a number of basic stretches prior to commencing the activity, and ensuring that the initial few minutes of activity are relatively gentle and not too vigorous. A swimming session may commence with a few minutes of easy swimming, whilst a land-based activity could commence with a number of loosening exercises followed by a few minutes of aerobic activity such as walking or gentle jogging. This will gradually prepare the heart and the rest of the body for the forthcoming activity, which could be quite strenuous. Similarly, a gentle cool-down phase should be included at the end of a session. This is important as there is often a tendency to end an activity session at the peak of exertion, especially if the activity has a competitive element, such as a game of badminton. Therefore, the final phase of any session should involve a gradual reduction rather than an abrupt cessation of the intensity of the activity. If working within a strict limited timetable, the therapist will need to ensure that sufficient time is allocated at the end of the session for a cool-down.

THE PRINCIPLES OF EXERCISE APPLIED TO AEROBIC OR ACTIVITY-BASED EXERCISE PROGRAMMES

When devising an aerobically based exercise programme the basic factors which need to be considered are:

1. The type of exercise
2. The intensity of the exercise
3. The duration of the exercise
4. The frequency of the exercise

General information concerning these factors was presented in Chapter 4, and a number of specific issues relating to aerobic and activity-based exercise are covered in this section. Support for the inclusion of aerobic type exercises into a person's general lifestyle or specific rehabilitation/recovery programme comes from various sources including the Health Education Authority (UK), the American College of Sports Medicine and the American Heart Association.

The type of exercise

To increase the aerobic capacity of individuals the exercise needs to put their cardio-vascular system under an appropriate amount of stress by applying the principles of overload and specificity. Aerobic exercise has the characteristics of:

(a) primarily using the aerobic system to produce the required ATP;
(b) involving large muscle groups such as the legs;
(c) elevating the heart and breathing rates;
(d) being of an intensity which can be maintained for a prolonged period of time.

Examples of aerobic exercises include: walking, jogging, swimming, cycling, rowing, skipping, aerobic dance, skating and cross-country skiing. These forms of aerobic exercise are also reported to be the most effective in reducing the risk of CHD, reducing high blood pressure, reducing body fat and improving blood lipid profiles. However, for a more complete overall physical fitness an exercise programme should also include activities that are designed to enhance or maintain muscular strength and flexibility (which have been discussed in earlier chapters). Therefore, for a comprehensive exercise programme additional exercises may need to be undertaken to supplement the aerobic aspects.

The choice of aerobic exercise to be included within an exercise programme is important, since, not only does it need to fulfil various physiological objectives, but it may also need to fulfil a number of sociological and psychological functions. Ideally the exercise should be of a type that the participant enjoys. This enjoyment factor is an important consideration for the social and mental well-being of the participant and is also important if the participant is to adhere to the exercise programme. If participants do not enjoy the exercises they are unlikely to stay with them and adherence to an exercise programme is vital if it is to be effective. This is especially so if it is hoped that the inclusion of exercise into a weekly routine represents a permanent positive change in the lifestyles of the individuals. This can be made easier by choosing activities which fit in well with the lifestyles of the individuals, i.e. by considering time factors and the accessibility of facilities.

Whilst the general effects of the different types of aerobic exercise are similar, some forms of exercise may be less suitable than others for particular individuals. For example, obese individuals may be advised to avoid jogging since their additional weight can put excessive strain on their joints, causing overuse injuries. For these individuals alternatives such as swimming or cycling may be preferable.

In addition to the previously mentioned aerobic activities, a number of team and racquet games can provide a good form of exercise. However, the effects of these activities can vary considerably. They may be sociable and very enjoyable, thereby conveying some benefits. However, the level of activity is often unsuitable for the individual's physical condition. In some cases the game may be too leisurely to convey the desired physiological benefits. This can occur in a social game of tennis where, due to the skill aspect, the players actually spend most of their time walking slowly or jogging short distances whilst their cardiovascular system receives very little benefit. The game may be tiring on the muscles but it may not be as aerobically beneficial as a brisk 20 minute walk or swim. Conversely, in some cases the intensity of a racquet game may be far too intensive for the individuals, over-stressing their cardiovascular system. This can occur in the game of squash: as is often said, 'many people play squash to get fit but in reality they should get fit before they play squash'. The demanding nature of the game makes it highly unsuitable for some individuals who would be better advised to adopt an alternative form of recreative exercise.

It can therefore be seen that factors such as age, skill, the opponent and the individual's own perception of exercise intensity will affect the nature of the exercise and hence its suitability for inclusion into an exercise programme. However, a combination of activities is likely to convey diverse benefits and the actual composition of the programme will depend upon the physiological, social and psychological needs of the participant.

When the various factors associated with each activity and its diverse benefits are taken into consideration, it is still possible to broadly categorize types of exercise into groups that relate to their physiological and health-promoting effects.

Category 1: Very good, provided that the intensity and duration are appropriate.

- Brisk walking
- Brisk swimming
- Brisk cycling
- Jogging
- Hill walking
- Good exercise classes (aerobics)
- Skipping.

Category 2: Good, but the aerobic benefits vary considerably depending upon the level of skill of the participants and how vigorously they participate.

- Team games
- Racquet games
- Circuit training
- Dancing
- Martial arts
- Gardening
- Golf.

Category 3: These activities are acceptable and tend to produce relatively small aerobic benefits but may be considered as suitable because of the additional benefits they convey.

- Bowls
- Yoga (primary benefit on suppleness)
- Weight-lifting (primary benefit on muscular strength).

The intensity of the exercise

For aerobic exercise to be of benefit to the participant's cardiovascular system it needs to be of an intensity which provides an appropriate amount of overload. This will then stimulate the desired beneficial adaptations to the exercise. As a general guideline, exercise which makes the participant slightly breathless is likely to improve his or her aerobic capacity. Alternatively, the determination of appropriate exercise intensities can be achieved using either (a) exercise heart rates or (b) the participant's perceived exertion.

As a person's fitness level improves and their heart rate becomes lower at specific exercise intensities, the level of perceived exertion should also fall by a corresponding amount. This means that as a person gets fitter, a certain exercise level will be found to be easier. When embarking upon a programme for the sedentary and/or relatively unfit it is advisable to begin with exercise intensities at the lower end of the training zone, or even just below it. Indeed, some studies have reported significant improvements in the fitness of such individuals when using relatively low exercise intensities. Therefore, as with all forms of exercise it is advisable to begin at a relatively easy level and gradually progress as the participant's level of fitness improves.

Determining exercise intensity by heart rate

To be of aerobic benefit to the individual, the exercise needs to be of an intensity that will elevate their heart rate into what is known as their training zone. As previously indicated, this intensity of exercise is also likely to make them slightly breathless. Exercising within the training zone will stimulate the desired benefits to the cardiovascular system and is also reported to reduce the risk of certain ailments such as coronary heart disease.

An individual's heart rate training zone may be calculated as follows. A person's maximum heart rate is estimated to be (with some variation) approximately 220 minus their age. The maximum heart rate is therefore considered to fall by approximately 1 bpm/year. As an example, an average 45 year old will have an estimated maximum heart rate of approximately 175 bpm (220 – 45). However, there is some evidence to suggest that continued physical activity throughout life can minimize this reduction in maximum heart rate. As a consequence of this, the overall physical capacity of individuals is less likely to decline as they get older.

Having estimated an individual's maximum heart rate it should be stressed that when undertaking aerobic exercise for health the individual should work well below this maximum rate. Indeed, the upper end of the heart rate training zone is often put at approximately 85% of the maximum heart rate, whilst the lower end of the training zone is considered to be approximately 65% of the maximum heart rate. Therefore, for a 20 year old with a maximum heart rate of approximately 200 bpm (220 – 20), the heart rate training zone will fall between 130 and 170 bpm (65% and 85% of 200).

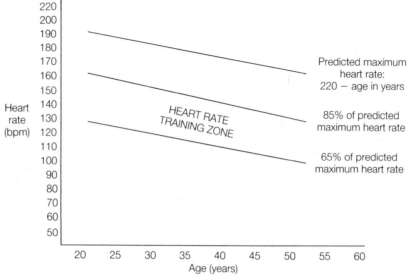

Figure 7.1 Illustrating the heart rate training zone.

That is to say, for the exercise to be effective the heart rate should reach at least 130 bpm but should not exceed 170 bpm. For a 50 year old the estimated training zone will be between 110 and 145 bpm (65% and 85% of 170). The exact values for the heart rate training zone will vary slightly between different authorities but will be similar to those given here. A diagram of the heart rate training zone is presented in Figure 7.1. Whilst such guidelines may be applicable for most individuals certain cardiovascular disorders may require modifications to the suggested training zones, and in some cases may make them inappropriate.

If exercise is to be effective in increasing a person's aerobic capacity the heart rate should be maintained in the training zone for a prolonged period of time. Here again the exact value for the duration of the exercise may vary but most authorities recommend between 20 and 60 minutes per session. A minimum of 20 minutes is recommended for health benefits, with the longer sessions having the potential to promote greater adaptations in those who are relatively fit. It should be noted that the suggested exercise intensities and durations outlined here are for exercise programmes designed to promote a general increase in cardiovascular fitness and health; they are not specifically applicable to those who are 'training' for competitive sport. The objectives of those people may be somewhat different as they strive for a fitness peak and in doing so may push themselves extremely hard. Those individuals may therefore elevate their heart rate in excess of the values recommended here. However, whilst such efforts may be necessary in the pursuit of sporting excellence they are not necessary for those wishing to attain a level of fitness that is associated with good health.

It should also be noted that during the early stages of a training programme individuals may be advised to keep their heart rates at the lower end of the training zone. In addition, if they are unable to get their heart rate into the suggested training zone it should not cause undue concern and may well be due to their muscles not being as fit (relatively speaking) as their cardiovascular system. This can cause 'local muscle fatigue' at relatively low heart rates and prevent the continuation of the exercise. Improvements will occur with continued training and the participants may then be able to walk faster or cycle faster and elevate their heart rates into the recommended zones. As the fitness of individuals improves, they will find that their heart rates will be slightly lower at any given speed of swimming, cycling or walking/jogging. Therefore, to continue the improvement they must jog, swim or cycle a little faster, or perhaps a little longer, thus applying the principle of progressive overload.

Determining exercise intensity by perceived exertion

As an alternative, or in addition, to the heart rate training zone a further indication of the suitability of the exercise intensity can be obtained by using a scale of perceived exertion (Borg, 1974). With participants who are on medication such as beta-blockers (which will suppress the heart rate during exercise) this becomes the major means of assessing exercise intensity since the exercise heart rate is no longer applicable. A table of perceived exertion may also prove to be of greater value when dealing with older participants (60+) since in this age group there is a great diversity in physical capacities. For example, this age group will include those who have a very good level of physical fitness, especially if they have always been active. Conversely, this age group will also include individuals whose physical capacity is relatively poor. This may be due to illness, disability or a sedentary lifestyle. Therefore, although individuals may be of the same chronological age they will vary considerably in their physical capacity.

As previously mentioned, there are occasions when a subject's level of perceived exertion can provide a useful indication as to whether the intensity of the exercise is suitable. A scale of perceived exertion commonly used to assess exercise intensity is that devised by Borg, and is illustrated in Figure 7.2. It can be used very effectively in conjunction with heart rates, especially during the early stages of a programme, to familiarize participants with feelings of perceived exertion, thereby enabling them to correspond their feelings with heart rates within their training zone. In this way they should quickly become familiar with how hard a particular form of exercise should feel if it is to be of benefit to them. In cases where heart rate training zones become inappropriate, the participants could be advised to exercise at a perceived exertion of between 12 and 14.

A less quantitative means of assessing appropriate exercise intensities using perceived exertion is based upon the idea that, whilst exercising, individuals should become slightly breathless, but still be capable of holding a conversation. This can easily be applied by the therapist who can simply ask the subjects how they are feeling whilst they are exercising. If any of the subjects has difficulty in answering then he or she is working too hard.

The duration of the exercise

Many authorities suggest that for optimal health benefits aerobic exercises should

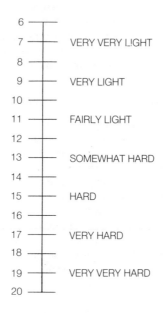

Figure 7.2 Illustrating the Borg scale of perceived exertion.

be undertaken for between 20 and 60 minutes per session, although the exact duration of each session will, of course, depend upon the type and intensity of the exercise and the fitness of the participant, as well as the amount of time available. It is generally agreed that for those unfamiliar with exercise a lower intensity session of relatively long duration is preferable to one that is shorter but more intense. On a practical note, these suggested durations are exclusive of the time spent warming up and cooling down. In the early stages of a programme the participant may be unable to maintain 20 minutes' continuous exercise comfortably. A shorter duration may therefore be used as a starting point, or the session may be split up into several bouts of exercise interspersed with rest or periods of lower intensity exercise. For instance, a 20 minute swim could be split up into four 5 minute periods of brisk swimming, each being separated by 5 minutes of gentle swimming or rest.

The frequency of the exercise

It is generally considered that a frequency of three to five times a week provides optimal aerobic benefits for the amount of time spent exercising, although for the very unfit a frequency of twice a week will still be beneficial, and is certainly preferable to no exercise at all. Exercising more than five times a week may convey further aerobic benefits but physiologically there is a point of diminishing returns and the relatively small additional aerobic benefits gained from the other sessions may not be worth the extra commitment. Exercising with a greater frequency may also increase the risk of staleness or overuse injuries in the participant. Varying the type of exercises included within a weekly programme is likely to reduce the risk of such occurrences. When considering the frequency of exercise sessions within a programme other factors, such as the intensity and duration of the exercise, will also need to be considered. For instance, if an individual is exercising at a relatively low level and for relatively short durations, then an additional exercise session may indeed be deemed to be worth-while. Here again it needs to be emphasized that these suggested frequences are for individuals desiring basic aerobic and health benefits from their exercise participation and not for those individuals who are seeking fractional improvements in performance, as in the case of the competitive sportsperson.

A health-based exercise programme should also include rest days or days where the exercise is of a much lower intensity and duration. These will enable the body to recover from the exercise and make appropriate physiological adaptations to the training stimuli. Therefore, individuals exercising three times a week should be advised to split up their three exercise sessions with a rest or 'easy' day between each. This helps the body to recover and helps prevent staleness and/or overuse injuries, which can even occur in beginners using relatively low exercise loads if their bodies are not physically capable of coping with them. If, however, the exercise sessions are of a relatively low intensity and are being undertaken for reasons other than the primary development of aerobic fitness, then the therapist may advocate exercise every day or even more than once a day on some occasions.

In summary, the information given in this chapter should provide the basis for designing activity and aerobically based exercise programmes which will enhance the individual's physical capacity as well as conveying other social, psychological and health-orientated benefits. Participants who are taking medication (such as beta-blockers), or have CHD, or are recovering from an operation, or have other forms of illness, will often require modifications to the basic programmes outlined here and, where appropriate, such modifications are discussed in a separate section.

EXERCISE FOR THE PROMOTION OF AEROBIC CAPACITY AND GENERAL HEALTH

There is much evidence to link the regular participation in aerobic forms of exercise with the promotion of good health and a reduction in the risk of certain cardiovascular diseases. Some of the evidence in support of this is reviewed in Chapter 8. However, in summary, there would appear to be a link between an individual's level of aerobic fitness and a reduction in the probability of that individual suffering from any of a number of diseases that are common in many western societies: coronary heart disease, obesity, hypertension, stress disorders, etc. When discussing exercises which will promote an individual's aerobic capacity it is important to remember that exercises of this type, duration and intensity are precisely those which are recommended in the context of the promotion of general health. Therefore, they have implications for everyone, not just those individuals who are under the specific guidance of a therapist. When considering an exercise programme that is designed to increase aerobic capacity it is also possible to regard the same programme as a means of promoting the general health of the individual. Since the two topics are so intimately related they may be considered together, with the promotion of aerobic fitness being a major component in the more holistic topic of 'health'.

As a general guideline many authorities advocate that for the development of aerobic fitness, and hence the promotion of health, an exercise programme should include at least 20 minutes of vigorous exercise three times a week. In this context the term 'vigorous' is important as it implies a level of exercise which is sufficient to cause slight breathlessness but is not exhaustive. However, whereas this prescription provides some general guidelines and indications as to the nature and intensity of the exercises which should be included, it should be noted that an exercise programme is more likely to produce optimal benefits if it is personalized. Thus, as previously stated, an exercise programme needs to be specifically designed for the individual according to goals and current physical condition. Individualizing a programme requires personal contact with the participant and a degree of experience. However, basic guidelines can assist the adviser in designing such programmes, enabling the appropriate adjustments and manipulations to be made to suit the condition of the individual.

The aims of a programme may vary considerably, depending upon the age and circumstances of the individual. An exercise programme is likely to have a number of objectives, but should also be dynamic and subject to change as the circumstances and condition of the participant change. Hence, the aims as well as the content of the programme may alter with time. Various goals may be set in the initial stages of the programme but may then be altered accordingly, especially if the programme extends over a period of years. Firstly, the age of the participant may have a significant influence upon its objectives and hence its content. In the young, up to about 16 to 20 years of age, exercise programmes may be orientated towards optimal growth and development, minimizing the risk of disease later in life and initiating healthy lifestyle habits. These kinds of objectives can be observed with the introduction of 'health-related fitness' into aspects of the school Curriculum. Within the programme these basic objectives may then be modified if the individual is suffering from certain physical or mental conditions. These may be temporary, as in the case of rehabilitating from a fracture, or more permanent in the case of genetic disorders.

For young adults who have reached physical maturity the programme may concentrate on developing or maintaining their physical capacity as well as on reducing the risk of hypokinetic diseases such as obesity, atherosclerosis and diabetes. These basic objectives will again need to be individualized because of the diversity of conditions which the therapist is likely to encounter, ranging from a temporary loss of physical fitness due to the participant being bed-ridden following a fracture, to more debilitating and permanent conditions such as multiple sclerosis.

In older age groups the emphasis of the programme may again be modified. In addition to the previously stated objectives it should also be orientated towards preventing individuals from assuming too sedentary a lifestyle. The programme should help them to maintain their physical capacity as they get older, and thus their independence, as well as reducing the risk of diseases such as osteoporosis. Therefore, in summary, similar basic objectives may be set for all exercise programmes but their specific nature and emphasis will vary according to the precise condition and age of the participant.

MEDICAL CLEARANCE PRIOR TO THE COMMENCEMENT OF AN AEROBIC EXERCISE PROGRAMME

Many authorities recommend a complete medical check-up prior to the commencement of an exercise programme. This is particularly prudent if the individual has not exercised for some considerable time. A check up may include a basic questionnaire, assessment of blood pressure, analysis of body composition, resting ECG, analysis of blood cholesterol and even an exercise stress test where the activity of the heart is monitored during strenuous exercise. Such medical evaluations may be performed at various venues and may be conducted in several stages, with only those deemed to be of a high risk going on for the more extensive form of evaluation. In practice, these evaluations tend to be a precautionary measure, with most individuals being cleared for exercise. For the therapist such extensive measures will rarely be necessary and it is more likely that individuals will be sent to the therapist by their medical consultant for a programme of exercises or, when this is not the case, clearance may be gained by simply conferring with the medical consultant about whether any specific factors need to be considered when devising an exercise programme for any individual. However, in some cases extensive forms of physiological assessment do serve a useful function, and if the therapist considers a person to have several risk factors then the therapist may well be advised to seek further medical advice before proceeding with the programme.

THE PHYSIOLOGICAL ASSESSMENT AND MONITORING OF AEROBIC FITNESS

Introduction

The rationale behind physiological testing and monitoring was discussed in Chapter 4. Therefore, this section will concentrate its discussion on the practical aspects of assessing aerobic fitness. This will be followed by examples of aerobic fitness tests along with comments on their suitability for different individuals.

The aerobic capacity of individuals is largely determined by their ability to utilize oxygen. This capacity to use oxygen ($\dot{V}O_2max$) can be measured using sophisticated laboratory apparatus and may be used as a specific measurement of aerobic fitness. However, such methods of assessing aerobic fitness are complex and require maximal exertion on the part of the participant. They are therefore not likely to be suitable for the vast majority of individuals that the therapist will encounter. Maximal tests are only usually employed in the contexts of 'sport science' when evaluating the fitness of competitive sports performers or in specific exercise-related areas of research. The protocols for such tests will therefore not be discussed in detail since any therapists working in these fields are likely to be specialists who already have expertise in these testing procedures. For those therapists with a general interest in the area a brief outline of ($\dot{V}O_2$ max) and the onset of blood lactate accumulation (OBLA) tests were presented in Chapter 4. For additional details see the list of recommended further reading.

As an alternative to these tests there are a variety of less complex and more appropriate assessments which, if utilized correctly, can provide valuable information for both the therapist and the participant. These tests may be classified as maximal tests or submaximal tests.

Maximal tests, as the name implies, require the participant to exercise at maximum capacity. These tests are therefore only suitable for the relatively fit and highly motivated. Any form of physical disability or disorder which is likely to be adversely affected by exercise of such high intensity will make this form of testing unsuitable for certain individuals. Submaximal tests require the participant to exercise at much lower exercise intensities. These tests are primarily based upon the findings that the 'fitter' an individual is the lower will be that individual's heart rate during a specified bout of exercise. The observed lower heart rates of the 'aerobically' fit are related to the increased stroke volume and the improved efficiency of the cardiovascular system that is associated with regular exercise.

When considering whether to evaluate an individual's fitness, and if so what tests to use, it is important to consider the reasons for doing the assessment and the ways in which the results may be used. To assist the therapist with this process a general outline of the potential uses of physiological assessments is presented. Further reference should also be made to the general rationale behind physiological assessments, which was discussed in Chapter 4.

Considerations for the application of physiological assessment

1. A basic physiological assessment may be used to determine appropriate training loads in subsequent exercise sessions.
2. If applicable, the quantitative results obtained from an assessment may be used to compare the participant's fitness with standardized norms.
3. The results of repeated assessments will provide objective data which may be used to monitor the participant's fitness over a period of time.
4. The data obtained from a series of repeated tests may be used to give positive feedback to the participant since they will provide objective as well as subjective information on the state of the participant's fitness and the effectiveness of the exercise programme.
5. A fitness assessment may be used to evaluate the individual's strengths and weaknesses and may also provide a focus on the components of fitness.

The relevance and applicability of each type of test will depend upon the participant being assessed and the reasons for assessing them. Simple non-quantitative assessments may involve a basic evaluation of an individual's capacity to perform prolonged forms of exercise such as walking. A more quantitative assessment could attempt to evaluate how far a person could walk in 10 minutes or how long it takes that person to walk a mile. These examples would require quite a reasonable level of fitness and therefore the therapist will need to devise variations that use times or distances that are appropriate for the individual being assessed. Substantially shorter tests should be devised for the less fit with whom it may also be important to ensure that there is no element of competition in order to prevent overexertion. Conversely, for active individuals who are already physically fit more strenuous variations of these tests are available. Examples of these include a number of 'shuttle running' tests, or simply recording how quickly a person can run 1.5 miles. These latter tests are obviously maximal and will only be appropriate for those who are already physically fit and have the motivation to perform such tests.

Assessment tests which utilize submaximal protocols tend to rely upon the measurement of the heart rate during exercise and/or the measurement of post exercise recovery heart rates. The relevance of these heart rates relates to the fact that if the body is given a specified and standardized amount of exercise to do then those individuals with a 'fitter' cardiovascular system will be able to perform the exercise with a lower heart rate and, as a consequence, will have lower heart rates immediately after the exercise. For example, when monitoring an individual, he or she may initially perform a standardized test with an exercise heart rate of 150 bpm. Following the completion of a six-week exercise programme designed to improve aerobic fitness, that same individual should be able to perform the same test with a lower heart rate.

The simplest and most commonly utilized forms of submaximal testing are the 'step tests'. Submaximal cycle ergometer tests are based upon similar lines but permit a variation in the intensity of the exercise. However it should be noted that if the participant is taking any form of medication, such as beta-blockers which influence the heart rate, then the exercise heart rate no longer becomes an appropriate measurement of aerobic fitness and alternatives will need to be considered.

With most assessment procedures a key aspect of the evaluation is likely to be the comparison between the individual's current scores and previous ones, thereby monitoring any progress. Relating scores to standardized norms is often inappropriate because of the highly individual nature and circumstances of the participant with whom the therapist is working. However, if working in a specialized area, the therapist may accumulate a quantity of data which could enable specialized norms or standards to be produced for use in his or her own setting.

Step tests

There are a large number of variations on the basic step test. However, they are all based upon the same physiological principles. The stepping cycle usually involves starting with both feet on the floor facing the bench or step. The participant then places one foot on the step, then the other, then lowers one foot to the ground, then the other, and this is repeated in a continuous manner. Thus, it involves a repeated four-stage cycle of 'up, up, down, down'. This cycle is performed at a predetermined speed on a bench or step of a specified height. A speed of 30 cycles per minute is fairly brisk and will be appropriate for most individuals in the general population; however, with individuals whose levels of aerobic fitness may be 'below average', a slower stepping rate of 20 cycles per minute may be more suitable. During the assessment a metronome may be used in order to set the pace, and it is usual to set it to coincide with each phase of the cycle. Thus, for a stepping speed of 20 cycles a minute the metronome should be set to 80, while for a stepping speed of 30 steps per minute the metronome should be set to 120.

The height of the bench may also vary in accordance with the physical condition of the individuals being assessed. Step heights of 12 to 18 inches are fairly standard and will be appropriate in most situations. In reality the therapist is likely to use whatever is accessible, but if monitoring fitness over a period of time it is important to maintain the same step height and stepping rate if the results are to be comparable. When performing the activity it is also important that the participant maintains a consistent stepping technique; this will include extending the knees when on the bench. Alternating the 'leading leg' a number of times during the test may be desirable as it tends to fatigue more rapidly than the other.

The duration of step tests vary from 3 to 5 minutes, although in some variations it is not necessary to complete the full duration of the test as long as the duration for which the individual exercised is recorded. In practical terms, the participant will stop exercising either upon the completion of the specified duration, or when the participant feels that he or she has had enough, or when the therapist perceives that the exercise should stop. Following the cessation of the exercise a number of post-exercise heart rates may be recorded. Ideally, the participant's heart rates should be recorded immediately the exercise has ceased; however, for practical reasons of locating the pulse, etc., a post-exercise heart rate taken 30 seconds after the cessation of the exercise is more realistic, unless apparatus for the continuous monitoring of the participant's heart rate is available. When measuring the heart rate the pulse should be monitored for between 15 and 30 seconds. This figure is then used to calculate the heart rate in beats per minute (bpm). Additional post-exercise heart rates may then be taken at minute intervals as a means of recording the rate of recovery. The fitter the individual, the lower the heart rate will be during exercise, the lower it will be after exercise and the sooner it will return to its pre-exercise level.

In practical terms the therapist may therefore devise a 3 minute step test using a gymnasium bench and a stepping rate of 25 steps per minute. Prior to the test the subject's pre-exercise heart rate may be measured for later comparison. Upon completion of the 3 minutes the participant's heart rate may be measured 30 seconds after the exercise and then at 1 minute intervals. This will give four post-exercise heart rates. Repeating the test a number of weeks later will produce a comparable set of results which may be used to evaluate any substantial changes in the fitness of the participant, with lower heart rates indicating an improvement in aerobic fitness.

If the facilities are available it may be possible to monitor the participant's heart rate during the exercise, which will give a 'working heart rate'. The working heart rate will increase during the exercise and then level off at a peak some minutes into the test. This working heart rate can then be used in addition to the post-exercise heart rates as a means of evaluating the participant's fitness. The working heart rate is often more informative than the recovery heart rate as it indicates the amount of 'physical stress' the body is experiencing during the exercise. A lower working heart rate during the exercise indicates a greater capacity to cope with the exercise. Significantly lower heart rates should also be associated with a general feeling that the exercise is easier and this provides a further subjective indication of an improvement in aerobic fitness.

If the participant does not complete the specified duration of the exercise the therapist may record the length of time for which the exercise was sustained, and this may then be used as an initial evaluation of their fitness. Alternatively, the duration of exercise and the recovery heart rates may be incorporated into a mathematical equation to produce a 'fitness index' which will increase as the participant is able to exercise for longer and/or their recovery heart rates are reduced. An example of such an equation is given below and, as with other aspects of the testing procedures, therapists may like to devise norms for participants in accordance with their own circumstances and the individuals with whom they work.

$$\text{Fitness index} = \frac{\text{Duration of exercise in seconds} \times 100}{\text{Sum of the three recovery pulse rates}}.$$

So, if the participant exercised for the specified 5 minutes (300 seconds) and then recorded the following post-exercise heart rates of 152 bpm 30 seconds after the exercise, 140 bpm 1 minute 30 seconds after the exercise, and 123 bpm 2 minutes 30 seconds after the exercise, their fitness index would be calculated as follows:

$$\text{Fitness index} = \frac{300 \times 100}{(152 + 140 + 123)} = \frac{30\,000}{415} = 72.3.$$

In subsequent tests any decrease in the post-exercise heart rates would be manifested in an increased fitness index which would indicate an increase in aerobic fitness. Similarly, if the participant was unable to exercise for the full 5 minutes on the first test and only managed 2 minutes 16 seconds, then the duration of exercise would be 136 seconds. If on a subsequent test the participant was able to continue the exercise for a longer period, this would result in a larger value on the top line of the equation and therefore a higher fitness index. The example presented above is intended to provide some form of general guidance of how an individual's aerobic fitness may be quantified. It is not intended to represent a rigid testing procedure that is applicable for all individuals. Indeed, therapists are likely to wish to produce modifications of this assessment procedure and adopt their own form of assessment and calculation of a fitness index that is appropriate for the individuals with whom they are working.

Submaximal cycle ergometer tests

When compared with step tests, a major advantage of the cycle ergometer tests is the variability of the workloads. Within the duration of a cycle ergometer assessment it is possible to increase the intensity of the exercise gradually by altering the resistance of the ergometer. This means that a test can commence at a very easy level and gradually increase in intensity until it reaches a level that is appropriate for the individual. This has a distinct advantage over the step tests, which have a fixed exercise intensity that may be too strenuous to assess some individuals effectively and yet not be sufficiently strenuous for others. The data collected during cycle ergometer tests can be used to produce an objective evaluation of an individual's fitness and, where appropriate, to calculate suitable exercise loads which can be used in the subsequent exercise programme.

When using a cycle ergometer the recommended speed of pedalling is approximately 50 to 60 pedal revolutions per minute (rpm). Specifying a pedalling rate is more practical than suggesting specific speeds since different exercise cycles will possess differently sized wheels. This means that for some ergometers a pedalling rate of 50 rpm will correspond to a speed of approximately 18 km/h whilst in other ergometers it may only correspond to 12 km/h. In exercise terms it is the speed with which the legs are moving that is important rather than the fictitious speed shown by the ergometer. Pedal rates faster than 60 rpm tend to be too rapid and require an anaerobic contribution to the exercise, thereby causing the rapid onset of fatigue. Conversely, pedalling rates of less than 50 rpm are often considered to be somewhat too leisurely. Therefore rates between 50 and 60 rpm are generally considered to be optimal for comfort, convenience and for producing a suitable intensity of exercise. However, the therapist may wish to modify the rate slightly in accordance with the participants and ergometers he or she is working with.

During a cycle ergometer fitness assessment and/or during an exercise programme it is usual to maintain a constant pedal speed throughout the exercise. The intensity of the exercise is altered by adjusting the amount of resistance applied to the pedals of the cycle whilst keeping the rate of pedalling constant. With most ergometers an increase in the resistance is produced by increasing the tightness of a 'resistance belt' which is positioned around the rim of the 'flywheel'. Alternatively, some ergometers are 'electronically braked' whilst others use 'wind resistance'. The intensity of the exercise performed by the participant therefore depends upon the speed of pedalling and the amount of resistance offered by the ergometer. Different exercise cycles display their scale of resistance in different ways. In the simplest examples it may be in the form of an arbitrary scale from 1 to 10 where the units of resistance are not specified. In other ergometers the resistance or power output is displayed in kilograms or watts. If it is possible for the therapist to describe the power output in terms of watts, then this is preferable since watts are internationally recognized units in this field of exercise physiology. This will then make any dialogue on the topic easier and more meaningful.

The following example protocol for a submaximal cycle ergometer test is presented to illustrate the general design of such tests. The therapist may then modify this protocol in accordance with requirements.

1. Check the medical history of the participant and ask if any medication is being taken. This may be important if beta-blockers are being taken, as they will keep the heart rate low (making it an inappropriate measure of exercise intensity).
2. Take the pre-exercise pulse to check its regularity.
3. If appropriate, take a blood pressure reading to ensure that the participant is not suffering from hypertension. These preliminary procedures may have been performed by nursing or medical staff prior to the individual embarking upon the exercise programme.

4. Ensure that the participant is seated comfortably on the ergometer. When seated the knees should be slightly flexed at the bottom of the down stroke. This is the optimum position for ease of pedalling. It will also ensure that the participant will be working the knee joint extensively, but will not be overstretching.

5. Describe the test procedure. The assessor should inform the participant of the exercise protocol and emphasize that the test is not maximal.

6. The therapist should make it clear that the participant can stop the test at any time. The test should stop if the participant feels dizzy, uncomfortable or distressed. The aim is to get the participant to work moderately hard but not to exhaustion. The test is likely to make the participant slightly warm and breathless but should not cause any distress or discomfort.

7. The test should commence with the participant pedalling at the desired speed against a light resistance. A power output of approximately 25 watts (or ½ kg resistance) is recommended. Even if the participant is fairly fit the initial workload should still be light as it will serve as a warm-up. Commencing at a substantially higher resistance is liable to result in premature fatigue as the body is unprepared for the exercise.

8. The participant should pedal for 2 minutes at the initial workload whilst the therapist monitors the heart rate. This may be performed using a cardiometer or pulse meter throughout the tests. Alternatively, the pulse could be taken at the end of the 2 minutes at the exercise intensity. Whilst the pulse is being recorded the participant should not stop pedalling.

9. If at the end of 2 minutes the heart rate is still relatively low and the participant is feeling comfortable and is able to continue, the workload may be increased. It is usual to increase the workload by small increments to enable the body to adjust gradually to the increased exercise intensity. Increases of between 25 and 50 watts (½ and 1 kg) are recommended. The precise increase will depend upon the fitness of the subject and how easy the exercise is found to be. Whilst the resistance is being increased the participant should continue to pedal, and thus will pedal continuously throughout the assessment without a break.

10. Stage 9 is then repeated until either the participant feels that enough effort is being made, or until the heart rate reaches the top end of the training zone, or until the therapist perceives that the assessment should be concluded. During the assessment the participant may get slightly breathless but should still be able to hold a conversation and should not experience any discomfort or pain. The subject is also likely to become warm, so any excess clothing should be removed prior to or during the assessment to prevent overheating.

11. Following the completion of the final workload the subject should cool down by pedalling steadily for at least a minute against a very easy resistance. This will allow the heart rate to gradually lower until it returns to just above the pre-exercise level.

12. Upon completion of the test the assessor should have a number of heart rate measurements which were taken whilst the participant pedalled against a known resistance. These data can then be used in the evaluation of fitness and may also be used to determine future exercise loads on the ergometer if that is to be included as part of an exercise programme.

13. The heart rate data collected during the assessment may be tabulated and/or compared to previous results. Lower heart rates at the specified workloads indicate an improvement in aerobic fitness. Alternatively, the data can be plotted onto a graph and used to calculate a measure of aerobic fitness called the physical working capacity (PWC) value. The resultant graph can also be used to determine appropriate exercise loads.

The PWC value and exercise loads are calculated by plotting a graph of heart rate (bpm) against the workload (which may be in watts or other units). A 'line of best fit' may then be drawn through the points on the graph (Figure 7.3). This graph may be used to predict the workload that would be needed to elevate the participant's heart rate to a specified rate. A PWC 170 value refers to the exercise intensity required to elevate a person's heart rate up to 170 bpm. The specific PWC value selected for an individual will depend upon his or her age and condition. As a general guideline, the PWC value should be towards the upper end of the training zone (see page 243 and Figure 7.1). This means that for a 20 year old a PWC 170 value may be appropriate, whereas for a 50 year old a PWC 140 value may be more applicable. The PWC value is calculated by drawing the line of 'best fit' through the points on the graph (Figure 7.3). At the point where this line crosses the horizontal line corresponding to the desired heart rate a vertical line is drawn down to the x axis. The point where this line crosses the x axis will represent the workload required to elevate that person's heart rate to the specified level.

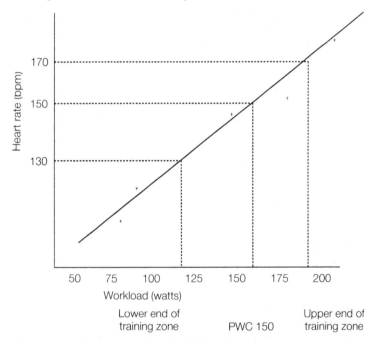

Figure 7.3. Illustrating how the data obtained from a PWC test may be used to determine appropriate training loads and a PWC value.

In terms of monitoring fitness these graphs and PWC values may be used in the following way. An improvement in aerobic capacity will result in a correspondingly lower heart rate at each of the exercise intensities. This will result in a 'line of best fit' that is below the previous one and is also likely to have a shallower gradient. This will therefore produce a higher PWC value since a greater workload will be required to elevate the individual's heart rate up to the same level. In basic terms this means that the fitter the individual, the higher the PWC value will be.

Suitable training loads can also be determined using the graph obtained from a PWC test. Firstly, the participant's heart rate training zone is calculated in accordance with age (see page 243 and Figure 7.1). Horizontal lines are then drawn from the points on the y axis which correspond to the lower and upper ends of the training zone. Where these lines cross the 'line of best fit' through the points on the graph, vertical lines are drawn down to the x axis. The points where these lines cross the x axis represent the suggested minimum and maximum exercise loads that should be used in the participant's programme. Any exercise intensity between these values will therefore elevate the heart rate into the training zone. For example, if the lower end of the participant's training zone was 130 bpm, a horizontal line should be drawn from 130 until it crosses the 'line of best fit' and then directly down until it crosses the workload axis. The point that it crosses should then correspond to the minimum exercise intensity that the participant should work at if aerobic benefits are to be gained from the exercise. This could be 105 watts. Similarly, the maximum exercise intensity can be calculated by using the heart rate at the upper end of the training zone. In this example, the maximum workload could be 155 watts, therefore any exercise intensity between these two extremes (105 and 155 watts) is likely to be suitable for the development of the individual's aerobic fitness.

Where repeated assessments indicate an improvement in fitness the appropriate training exercise loads are likely to increase as the participant's capacity to cope with the exercise increases.

The example described in this section is for a basic cycle ergometer. However, it is possible to devise similar tests that use arm ergometers, rowing machines or even motorized treadmills if desired. Therefore, by using the same basic principles, therapists can devise appropriate methods for assessing and monitoring the fitness of the individuals with whom they are working.

EXAMPLES OF AEROBIC AND ACTIVITY-BASED EXERCISE PROGRAMMES

The programmes that are set out in this section illustrate what may be included within an aerobically orientated exercise programme. Each programme suggests a number of starting points and the way in which the principle of progression can be applied. The programmes are illustrative and therefore the therapist may decide to make appropriate modifications to them or use a combination of different programmes. The central feature of the example programmes is the aerobic component, although for some individuals the activities such as swimming and cycling will also convey benefits to their muscle strength and mobility, especially if these components of their fitness are relatively poor. If, however, mobility and muscular strength are the primary areas of concern then the therapist should include additional specific exercises for suppleness and strength within the overall programme. The inclusion of these additional exercises will also ensure a more comprehensive level of fitness in all participants.

The programmes presented include many levels. It is therefore up to the therapist or adviser and the participant to decide the level at which it is most appropriate to start. In the initial stages of a programme it may be desirable to start at a very easy level. This will give the participant's body time to adapt to the physical demands it experiences. It will also provide motivation and positive feedback as the participant should be able to progress rapidly. If the participant attempts to start at a level that is too demanding, then this may reduce his or her confidence as well as placing inappropriate physical stresses upon the body.

Having commenced the programme it is then up to the therapist and participant to decide how quickly to progress onto a higher level. Progress should be gradual if the body is to be given time to adapt to the increased exercise loads it is given. If progression is too rapid then these adaptations will not occur fully and the body will start to be overstressed. This may result in slight unwanted aches and pains which, if unheeded, could develop into overuse injuries. The final level that the participant eventually attains will vary considerably and will depend upon a large number of physiological factors, as well as motivation. The most physically demanding levels illustrated here are not appropriate for most individuals. These levels of intensity, frequency and duration will be unnecessary and in many cases undesirable for the vast majority of participants. However, they may be appropriate for some and are included to illustrate how such levels may be gradually attained.

Getting started

Knowing how and where to begin an exercise programme can be the most difficult stage for the therapist. Therefore, some basic guidelines and suggestions are presented here. It should be remembered that exercise and physical fitness is very specific. Even if the participant is fairly fit it does not necessarily mean that they will find all forms of exercise easy. If an individual wishes to try something new, they should begin at a relatively easy level and progress gradually. For example, cycling puts slightly different stresses on the body when compared to jogging and, as a consequence, someone who cycles regularly may not be completely fit for jogging. It is therefore important to remember this aspect of specificity and not to place too many unfamiliar stresses upon the bones, joints and muscles. Even the relatively fit may overexert themselves and experience a few unwanted aches and strains the following day. Therefore, if the exercise is unfamiliar even to these individuals, it is better that they start at a level they find relatively easy than attempt to do too much too soon. The therapist should also be aware that if participants are overweight, then activities such as jogging may put too much stress on the joints. For these individuals alternative non-weight-bearing activities such as swimming and cycling are likely to be preferable.

Points that the therapist may consider when designing an exercise programme are:

1. Try to choose exercises that the participant will enjoy and will stick with.
2. Choose exercises that will easily fit in with the participant's daily routine.

3. Gradually increase the amount of exercise.
4. Do not exceed the participant's limits.
5. Vary the exercise routine to prevent boredom.
6. Try to ensure that the exercises are done frequently and regularly.
7. Make exercise part of a daily or weekly routine.
8. If necessary include strength and suppleness exercises as well as aerobic exercises in the programme.
9. Remember that if the participant is serious about his or her physical condition and health, then the commitment to exercise should be for life and not just a few weeks.

A cycling or cycle ergometer programme

The following section gives guidelines for a cycling or cycle ergometer programme. Both the stationary cycle ergometer and the traditional bicycle provide useful forms of aerobic exercise. Each has its advantages and disadvantages and therefore it is up to the therapist to decide which is the most appropriate. As the cycle ergometer will be used in a consistent environment, climatic factors will not affect the exercise. It is also isolated from other factors such as traffic and therefore the exercise will be performed in relatively safe surroundings. The consistency of the environment also makes the precise content of an exercise session easier to control and may be more easily kept under the close scrutiny of the therapist.

For many individuals the exercise ergometer presents a number of distinct and specific advantages. Indeed, for some participants the cycle ergometer will in reality be the only practical option, especially if they are unable to balance or cope with traffic, such as those with a poor level of motor coordination. For example, those suffering from disorders such as cerebral palsy may gain great benefits from the use of a cycle ergometer as this may help them to develop their motor control as they endeavour to pedal at a constant speed and maintain a constant pressure on the pedals.

The determination of exercise intensities for a cycle ergometer programme is discussed in the sections dealing with training zones and physiological assessments for the cycle ergometer. The duration of exercise on a cycle ergometer is more appropriately specified by time rather than a distance, although either may be used.

The major advantages of the traditional bicycle over the stationary ergometer are mobility and variation. When using a bicycle the participant is exposed to a changing and variable environment. The variety may make the exercise more enjoyable and will also present a variety of physiological challenges such as hills. The independence offered by the bicycle may also provide appropriate social and psychological benefits to the participant. When using a bicycle all the various safety aspects concerning the machine, lights, bright clothing and road safety must be considered. Whilst it is not within the realms of this text to discuss these specific details, it will be up to the therapist and/or participant to be aware of such matters.

The therapist must therefore consider the needs of the participant carefully before deciding the form of exercise that is most appropriate and how the exercise loads should be determined. If using the traditional bicycle, the therapist and/or participant should work out the routes carefully. This may help to ensure that the exercise is structured and appropriate rather than random; however, there are occasions when a 'random' cycle ride with no fixed route has its uses. If possible the initial routes should be fairly short and flat. As the participant improves, the routes can gradually be made longer and a number of 'deliberate' hills could be included to increase the intensity of the exercise and, hence, the amount of overload. However, especially during the initial stages or early in a session, participants should not force themselves up hills and if they are tired they should dismount and walk. The required exercise intensity is that which makes them 'slightly breathless', not exhausted.

The cycling programme presented in this section is set out with various stages which may be used as starting points. Precisely at which stage the participant starts will depend upon his or her level of fitness and a few experimental sessions may be needed before an appropriate stage can be determined. Throughout the programme progression should be gradual and steady: if a stage is too difficult then the participant should go back one stage until an appropriate level is found. The times and distances given in the programme may be applied to either the cycle ergometer or the traditional bicycle. However, as with all programmes the therapist will need to make appropriate modifications, especially in the bicycle programme where traffic may be a major consideration. The suggested times and distances which are presented at each stage are therefore given as alternative forms of duration, they are not target times for a specified distance.

Cycling programme with specified time durations

In addition to the examples given here, where the duration and frequency of the exercise are increased, progression should also be applied by increasing the intensity of the exercise. On the cycle ergometer this will involve increasing the resistance of the ergometer, while on a bicycle it may involve cycling faster and/or including hills. In the more demanding sessions the therapist may also wish to include phases of more intensive exercise (against a relatively high resistance for a couple of minutes) separated by phases of lower intensity exercise where the participant pedals against a relatively easy resistance. However, this form of 'interval' training is only for those who are considered to be aerobically very fit.

Stage 1.   10 minutes, 2–3 times a week
Stage 2.   15 minutes, 2–3 times a week
Stage 3.   15 minutes, 3–4 times a week
Stage 4.   15–20 minutes, 3–5 times a week
Stage 5.   20 minutes, 3–5 times a week
Stage 6.   20–30 minutes, 3–5 times a week
Stage 7.   30 minutes, 3–5 times a week
Stage 8.   35 minutes, 3–5 times a week
Stage 9.   40 minutes, 3–5 times a week
Stage 10. 45 minutes, 3–5 times a week
Stage 11. 50 minutes, 3–5 times a week.

Cycling programme where distance is used to determine the duration

Stage 1.   2 miles, 2–3 times a week
Stage 2.   2.5 miles, 2–3 times a week

Stage 3. 2.5 miles, 3–4 times a week
Stage 4. 2.5 miles, 3–5 times a week
Stage 5. 3 miles, 3–5 times a week
Stage 6. 3.5 miles, 3–5 times a week
Stage 7. 4 miles, 3–5 times a week
Stage 8. 5 miles, 3–5 times a week
Stage 9. 6 miles, 3–5 times a week
Stage 10. 7 miles, 3–5 times a week
Stage 11. 8 miles, 3–5 times a week.

Walking/jogging programme

The following section presents guidelines for a walking/jogging programme. It should be stressed that it is not essential for the participants to progress up to the jogging stages for them to gain the desired aerobic benefits from the exercise. Substantial improvements in aerobic fitness and the associated health benefits may be gained from brisk walking. Indeed, for the vast majority of individuals that the therapist will work with, walking will be the preferred activity with jogging only being appropriate for the relatively fit individuals, most of whom will be in the younger age group.

For those individuals who do wish to jog it can be made into a social activity if people exercise in pairs or small groups and, without making the activity competitive, events such as 'fun runs' may be used as goals at various intervals in a programme. Competitive running is a specialist area of exercise and for those wishing to become involved in the sport, local running clubs may be able to supply the required advice and support. In this context the therapist should also be aware of the growing number of 'disabled' runners who run, not just for the exercise, but also to participate in competitive sport. Even relatively severe disabilities such as blindness and amputation will not preclude some individuals from these competitive activities. Blind athletes run with the assistance of a 'guide' and are able to compete in all events from the 100 m to the marathon, while those lacking limbs may run with the aid of specially designed artificial limbs. Whilst jogging or running may not be suitable for all of the people with whom they work, therapists should not automatically preclude any disabled person from such activities. For further advice on such activities, therapists should contact the relevant sporting associations for the disabled.

In the context of the walking/jogging programme presented in this section the same principles as those already discussed apply: participants should commence at a relatively easy stage and progress gradually until they reach the desired level. Attempting to do too much will overstress the body causing minor aches and pains which, if not heeded, may result in overuse injuries. Specific conditions may cause the therapist to begin the prescribed programme at an easier level than that presented here, and throughout the programme appropriate modifications may be needed. If progressing from an initial walking programme it may be desirable to move onto a jogging programme without going through all the walking stages. This is perfectly acceptable, provided that the progression remains gradual and is well within the participant's capabilities. In the following list, stage 20 illustrates a form of intensive training called 'interval training'. This is an advanced form of training and is only likely to be appropriate for those wishing to run competitively.

Stage 1. Walk 0.5 mile, 2–3 times a week
Stage 2. Walk 1 mile, 2–3 times a week
Stage 3. Briskly walk 1 mile, 2–3 times a week
Stage 4. Briskly walk 1.5 miles, 2–3 times a week
Stage 5. Briskly walk 2 miles, 3 times a week
Stage 6. Walk 2 miles, varying the pace between brisk and fast walking, 3 times a week
Stage 7. Walk 2 miles, gradually increasing the amount of 'fast' walking, 3–4 times a week
Stage 8. Walk 2.5 miles, varying the pace between brisk and fast walking, 3–4 times a week
Stage 9. Gradually increase the distance walked and/or the frequency of walking sessions each week.

Those with a good basic level of fitness, and who are familiar with exercise, may wish to start a basic jogging programme.

Stage 10. Try a mixture of brisk walking and jogging. For instance, walk 100 m then jog 100 m, walk 100 m and so on for 2 miles. Repeat 3–4 times a week
Stage 11. As for stage 9 but gradually increase the amount of jogging, 3–4 times a week
Stage 12. Walk for half a mile then jog continuously for 1 mile, then walk for a half a mile
Stage 13. Walk for half a mile then jog continuously for 1.5 miles, 3–4 times a week
Stage 14. Jog for 2 miles, 3–4 times a week
Stage 15. Jog for 2.5 miles, 3–4 times a week
Stage 16. Jog for 3 miles, 3–4 times a week
Stage 17. Jog for 3.5 miles, 3–4 times a week
Stage 18. Jog between 3 and 4 miles, 3–4 times a week
Stage 19. Gradually increase the distance and frequency of the runs, perhaps by half a mile per run each week
Stage 20. On some of the runs try a mixture of fast and slow running, i.e. 200 m fast, 200 m slow, 200 m fast and so on. The fast runs should only be done when the participant is properly warmed up.

Swimming programme

Swimming is an excellent form of exercise and can be used to improve strength and suppleness as well as aerobic fitness. It is especially good for those who are overweight or have certain injuries as the water will help to support the body. Since pools vary in size and the participant's techniques will largely influence how fast they can swim it is not possible to prescribe a detailed swimming programme with suggested distances. However, outlined here are a set of guidelines and suggested progressions.

The times given are for the total amount of time spent on brisk swimming; for instance, if 6 minutes brisk swimming is the target, the participant could split this into six 1-minute swims with several minutes rest or easy swimming between each. The brisk swimming should be preceded by several minutes easy swimming as a warm-up. Therefore, although the target time may be only, say, 3 minutes this refers to 3 minutes of brisk swimming and in reality the session could also include about 15 minutes of easy swimming. The participants should progress up the stages at their own rate and only when they feel ready for it. As with the running programme, the final stages represent fairly demanding exercise sessions which will only be appropriate for fit competent swimmers and should not be considered as a 'goal' for the vast majority of individuals who will gain the desired benefits at the lower stages.

Stage 1.   3 minutes, 2–3 times a week
Stage 2.   5 minutes, 3–4 times a week
Stage 3.   7 minutes, 3–4 times a week
Stage 4.   9 minutes, 3–4 times a week
Stage 5.   11 minutes, 3–5 times a week
Stage 6.   13 minutes, 3–5 times a week
Stage 7.   15 minutes, 3–5 times a week
Stage 8.   17 minutes, 3–5 times a week.

Those with a good level of fitness, and who are familiar with regular exercise, may wish to start at stage 9. At all stages it is possible for the participant to determine the exercise intensity by deciding how fast to swim.

Stage 9.   20 minutes, 3–5 times a week
Stage 10. As for stage 9 but gradually decrease the amount of rest until the participant can swim for 20 minutes continuously
Stage 11. 20 minutes, swim 2 slow lengths then 1 fast, 2 slow, 1 fast and so on, 3–5 times a week
Stage 12. 20 minutes, swim alternate fast and slow lengths, 3–5 times a week
Stage 13. It is now up to the participant to increase gradually the amount of time spent swimming and the number of fast lengths undertaken.

Activity-based exercise

The previous examples of cycling, walking/jogging and swimming programmes provide illustrations of types of exercise for which the physical requirements of the session can be fairly closely defined. Thus the intensity and duration, as well as the type of exercise, may be determined prior to and during the session. Alternative activities, such as team games or racquet games, can be more variable in their intensity and duration for reasons that were discussed at the start of this chapter. So although the type of exercise in these activities may be fairly predictable its intensity may vary depending upon the skill of the player, the opponent(s) and the competitiveness of the game. Similarly, golf courses vary in length and in how hilly they are. Carrying the golf clubs rather than using a trolley would also make a significant difference to the intensity of the exercise. Similarly, the exact type, intensity and duration of exercises which constitute aerobics (a term generally used to describe a form of exercise to music) vary considerably. Some forms will be of a relatively low intensity whilst others will be high intensity. Some will include types of exercises which may be unsuitable for the individual whilst others may provide an ideal exercise session. In summary, these alternative activities can provide a valuable form of exercise provided that they adhere to the desired principles of exercise and are appropriate for the individual. Participating in these activities has social and psychological as well as physiological implications (these were discussed more fully earlier in this chapter).

When deciding upon the inclusion of such exercises the therapist must consider the needs of the participant. Physiologically this includes the type of exercise and the demands it places upon the individual's strength, flexibility and cardiovascular system. The therapist must then consider the amount of overload that a particular activity places upon the individual and consider whether it is appropriate and likely to bring about the desired improvements in physical fitness. Tennis is clearly more strenuous than bowls, but that does not necessarily mean that it is better for everyone; indeed, squash, for example, tends to be even more strenuous and can be too strenuous for some individuals whilst being appropriate for others. Specifically, the intensity and duration of the exercise needs to be considered to ensure that it is sufficiently strenuous without overstressing the individual and to ensure that the duration of the activity is appropriate. For example, to derive aerobic benefits from a game of badminton it should be fairly continuous, make the participants slightly breathless and, if applicable, elevate their heart rates into the training zone for much of the session, which should last a minimum of 20 minutes.

The therapist also needs to ensure that the activity being considered is not likely to cause any injury to the individuals through overstretching or excessive pressure on their joints. Here again the suitability of different activities will depend upon the individuals and their physical capabilities. When participating in such activities it is also important to ensure that the principles of warm-up and cool-down are observed.

In summary, whilst the local resources and clubs may provide a useful setting for these activities it is the therapist who must judge their suitability and apply any restrictions or modifications that they feel are necessary. Appropriate modifications to the rules may be devised in accordance with individual capabilities and the setting within which they are performed. In the context of such activities or training those confined to wheel chairs provide no exception and suitable modifications to most activities can produce a viable alternative which may be enjoyed by all, as well as conveying the desired physiological benefits.

8

The role of exercise in the promotion of good health

INTRODUCTION

The regular participation in physical activity is reported to have implications for the general health and 'well-being' of all members of the population, regardless of age, gender or whether they suffer from a recognized medical disorder or not. In summary, its effects include:

1. The promotion of good health
2. The prevention of 'ill health'
3. The improvement of health and physical capacity following ill health or an accident
4. Reducing the severity of a disorder.

Exercise is therefore advocated as a means of maintaining good health even for those who are apparently free from disease. Indeed, for the vast majority of the population exercise should be considered as a means of preventing ill health, especially since hypokinetic diseases (diseases associated with inactivity) such as coronary heart disease are insidious, only becoming apparent at a fairly advanced stage.

For some individuals the assumption of a relatively sedentary lifestyle is enforced by a disability or condition which makes physical activity more difficult. For others a lack of physical activity may be attributed to: the increased availability of transport; a reduction in the physical demands of many jobs; and also the popularity of leisure pastimes which involve a minimum amount of physical activity. A sedentary lifestyle and a general lack of physical fitness can result in a 'vicious circle' or 'downward spiral', whereby the overall lack of physical activity causes a deterioration of physical capacity, which then makes physical activity more difficult and the individual less inclined to exercise: hence their condition continues to deteriorate.

The consequences of a trend towards inactivity, coupled with dietary factors and the demands of modern society, are believed to be related to large increases in the incidence of certain diseases and disorders. This link has resulted in these diseases being referred to as 'hypokinetic diseases'. Examples include: obesity, coronary heart disease (CHD), hypertension, diabetes, some respiratory disorders, some digestive disorders and even some forms of cancer.

There is much research to support the belief that appropriate forms of physical activity can reduce the risk or severity of many of these disorders and, in addition, exercise is also reported to help control other related problems such as stress. Therefore, inactivity itself is considered to be a health risk by many authorities, which causes them to recommend the participation in appropriate forms of exercise as a means of promoting or maintaining health. For additional information a number of key texts, review and research articles are listed as recommended further reading at the end of this book, including Astrand and Grimby (1986), Bouchard (1989) and Fentem *et al.* (1988, 1990).

In general, research into the topic of health and exercise aims to determine whether there is a definite relationship between the regular participation in physical activity and the development and maintenance of good health. However, as is often the case with research into human epidemiology, the complexities of disease and the human lifestyle make the reported benefits of exercises difficult to prove. Therefore, whilst there is an undoubted relationship between exercise and health, the proof of the cause and effect is often open to debate. Critics of exercise suggest that, rather than regular exercise promoting good health it is only those who are predisposed to good health that exercise. In addition, many of the critics of exercise dispel its benefits by pointing to the incidence of exercise-induced injury (Solomon, 1985). In reality such occurrences are relatively infrequent and, when they do occur, are often due to the individual either undertaking forms of exercise that are inappropriate for their physical condition, or failing to adhere to certain safety aspects associated with the exercise. Thus the advocates of exercise would still suggest that most people are more at risk of underactivity than of overactivity.

The reported physiological benefits of exercise upon health can be considered under the following headings:

1. The growth and development of children
2. The maintenance of health in adults
3. The reduction in the risk of various diseases throughout life
4. Minimizing the effects of the ageing process.

When considering the potential benefits of exercise upon the health of individuals it should be remembered that reducing the risk of disease is only one of the proposed benefits. Exercise can also enable people to get more out of life by:

(a) improving their capacity to cope with the physical demands of life at whatever age;
(b) enhancing the social aspects of their lifestyle; and
(c) improving their mental state.

Thus the diverse benefits of exercise should not be forgotten in any holistic approach to health and, whilst research into its effects upon longevity remain inconclusive, there is no doubt that it can improve the quality of a person's lifestyle, regardless of age.

However, whilst exercise may be advocated as a means of promoting good health, it should also be remembered that inactivity is only one of the risk factors associated with diseases, ill health and incapacity. The regular participation in vigorous physical exercise may indeed reduce a person's risk of suffering from disease or disability, but it cannot guarantee that person against it. Thus, the beneficial effects of exercise must be considered in the context of other factors such as a poor diet, a stressful lifestyle and smoking. Research findings also indicate that it is the current participation in exercise which conveys the benefits and a degree of 'protection' against disease. This means that adults who were active ten years ago but have since then assumed a sedentary lifestyle will have lost much of their physical capacity and appear to be just as much at risk from hypokinetic diseases as those who have never participated in any form of regular physical activity. Conversely, it is also apparent that it is almost never too late to start exercising and, as previously stated, benefits may be gained by individuals of all ages.

Unfortunately, despite the evidence to support the benefits of exercise upon health, many people still participate in relatively little physical exercise. Butler (1987), in his investigations, presented figures which suggested that over 75% of adults in Britain exercised less than twice a week, despite the fact that about half of those interviewed believed that they did not take enough exercise. Similar conclusions have been drawn from numerous studies conducted world wide, and show that, while there is a general belief in the population that 'exercise is good for you', people do not exercise because of a lack of time or incentive. Therefore, despite an apparent awareness of the health-promoting benefits of exercise, relatively few people are willing to make a commitment to exercise on a regular basis. In this context it may therefore be the role of the therapist to provide the opportunity, advice and expertise in encouraging a person to undertake appropriate forms of health-promoting exercise.

EXERCISE AND THE HEALTH OF THE GROWING CHILD

The topic of exercise and the growing child is extremely broad. This is partly due to vast differences in the physical and mental capabilities of children of different ages and also to the variation between children of the same age. Therefore, this section, rather than attempting to provide a detailed series of programmes that are specific for children of different ages and capabilities, will briefly outline a few aspects related to exercise and the health of the child, mentioning a number of issues and guidelines which the therapist may apply. For specific details of the benefits of exercise to children, and exercise programmes for children, see the recommended further reading.

There is no doubt that appropriate exercise can be of great benefit in the development and health of a child (Binkhorst et al., 1985; Rutenfranz et al., 1987). These benefits can extend beyond the basic physical implications to include other social and psychological aspects and may have specific significance if the child is handicapped. In addition to the specific problems associated with certain disorders, inactivity can result in a general underdevelopment of the child's physique and physiology, making the child relatively weak, prone to rapid fatigue and susceptible to certain disorders throughout childhood and adult life. For example, inactivity during childhood may:

(a) limit a person's physical capacity during childhood and later in adult life; and
(b) increase susceptibility to obesity, cardiovascular disorders and even osteoporosis.

Whilst diseases such as CHD are generally associated with mature adults, they do occur in children (Gilliam et al., 1977; Linder and DuRant, 1982; Wilmore and

McNamara, 1974). Of additional concern are reports of the initial stages of these diseases being present in a significant percentage of children. Therefore, it is also suggested that good health and activity in childhood can diminish the risk of these diseases in childhood and in later life.

In this context, concern has been expressed by various authorities about the general lack of activity observed in many children, including those who follow a normal school curriculum; hence the introduction of 'health-related fitness' into many schools. The aims of such innovations are to make children aware of the importance of exercise and to attempt to elevate their participation in physical activity up to a level which is considered to be beneficial for health. For a child with a specific physical or mental disability these concerns are magnified, especially if they are restricted from participating in the regular forms of physical activity that are available to most children.

For children the primary roles of exercise may include the development of:

(a) their cardiovascular system;
(b) their muscular strength;
(c) joint function;
(d) motor skills; and
(e) social and mental attributes.

The exercises used to develop these factors will vary but may include specific exercise sessions in a gym, exercise sessions with the therapist, games and activity sessions. The effects of these forms of exercise were discussed in earlier chapters along with guidelines for the provision of overload. For the child an exercise programme may need specific modifications and, in general, the exercises are likely to be easier, less intensive and of shorter duration than those prescribed for most adults.

When prescribing exercises for children the basic principles of specificity, duration and intensity need to be applied. However, a number of additional factors also need to be considered, for example: children do not possess the same aerobic or anaerobic capacities as adults; they tend to tire more rapidly; and their bodies are not fully developed. Furthermore, it is important to try to make physical activity fun if at all possible, since a child will not be interested in pursuing an activity just because 'it is good for them'. To achieve this, certain physical activities can be incorporated into games in order to maintain the child's interest. These may be group activities or just between the child and therapist. Children with specific disorders will require specific exercise programmes to develop their cardiovascular system, muscular strength, joint mobility and coordination.

If attempting to put physical activity into the format of a game the therapist needs to carefully consider:

(a) the physical requirements of the game;
(b) the muscle groups that are being used;
(c) how the muscles are being used;
(d) the range of motion through which the joints are being moved;
(e) the demands that are being placed on the cardiovascular system; and
(f) how additional overload could be applied to the activity.

When dealing with any child it is important to remember that the skeleton is not fully developed. This means that the therapist should avoid putting excessive stress on the bones. Appropriate activities include swimming or cycling, which will have the desired strengthening effects on the musculature as well as improving cardio-vascular function without unwarranted stress. If specific strengthening exercises are needed, then body resistance or accommodating resistance exercises are likely to be most suitable, with light weights being used in certain circumstances.

Excessive forms of exercise can result in damage to the immature skeleton, including growth plate injuries. In practice these kinds of injury only tend to occur in children who are involved in extremely intensive training regimens that require them to train for many hours a week and, in general, tend to be associated with competitive sport. This is not to say that sport is necessarily bad for children; it does, however, suggest that if 'training' is taken to an extreme in terms of intensity, duration or frequency, or if it is of an inappropriate type, then the child may be vulnerable to injury. Examples of inappropriate training would include running too many miles on hard roads, lifting very heavy weights or over-hyperextending the back too often in gymnastics. In contrast to these, the basic exercises and exercise programmes that are performed under the guidance of the therapist who is seeking to optimize the child's physical development and health, rather than push them to the limits of their capabilities, are unlikely to cause problems of overuse or injury. Similarly, well-qualified sports coaches and physical education teachers should have the knowledge and experience to devise training programmes that will enhance the physical development and sporting capabilities of the child in relative safety (Gleeson, 1987). It is only when exercise is inappropriate for the child that the child is likely to be in danger of an exercise-induced injury. Indeed, as previously implied, most children are more likely to be at risk of underactivity than overactivity.

EXERCISE AND THE HEALTH OF THE ADULT

For the adult, the reported health-related benefits of exercise are diverse and often interrelated. However, for convenience they may be considered under the following broad headings:

1. The promotion of physical capacity, to enhance a person's capacity to cope with the physical demands of his or her lifestyle
2. The provision of a social environment
3. A reduction in the risk of certain hypokinetic diseases
4. The enhancement of recovery from, or minimizing the effects of, an accident, illness or trauma.

A number of these aspects have been discussed in earlier sections and therefore will not be repeated in this chapter in detail. However, they should not be forgotten in a holistic approach to health. The remainder of this chapter will therefore centre upon a number of specific health topics for which exercise has implications. The extensive amount of research into these areas often suggests an important role for exercise at all ages, from childhood to old age. Where appropriate, these findings are discussed within each section.

EXERCISE AND THE ELDERLY, AGEING AND LONGEVITY

The variety and complexity of human lifestyles, along with the natural genetic variation between individuals, makes the study of the relationship between exercise, ageing and longevity extremely difficult. A person's maximum physical capacity is generally considered to increase during childhood, reach a peak during the late teens to early 30s and then decline as the person gets older. There is no doubt that in the population as a whole there is a gradual decline in general physical capacity from middle age onwards. This decline involves all aspects of fitness, including aerobic capacity, strength and flexibility. The basis of this decline relates to many physiological parameters, including: maximum heart rate, stroke volume, cardiac output, the ratio of blood capillaries to muscle fibre area, the speed of nerve impulse transmission and pulmonary factors. However, what still remains to be answered is: 'How much of the decline is due to an inevitable ageing process and how much is due to a change in lifestyle with age?'

It is suggested that in many cases the observed ageing process can be attributed to a combination of: the inevitable ageing phenomena, the presence of disease, and a regression of physical capacity through inactivity. As people get older there is a tendency for them to become less physically active and more sedentary. This reduction in physical activity may be related to their job, which often tends to become less physically demanding, and other pressures such as family commitments, which can greatly reduce the amount of time a person spends in physically active leisure pursuits. In addition, society has certain expectations about how physically active someone should be at different ages. Therefore, a factor for consideration is whether the 'inevitable' reduction in physical capacity can be minimized through the continuous participation in vigorous physical activity throughout life, and if so, to what extent can the decline be retarded. Whilst there may be much individual variation in the ageing process, the findings of Bruce (1984) indicated that as people aged, the decline in aerobic capacity of sedentary individuals was twice as fast as those who exercised regularly. This would suggest that much of the observed reduction in physical capacity is often premature.

In western society it is becoming more acceptable for 'older' people to be seen to be physically active and for them to pursue physically demanding hobbies. With these trends, the physically active older person is becoming more common, as are some middle-aged individuals who through the continued participation in exercise programmes find themselves still as physically fit as they were ten years ago. Unfortunately, such individuals are still in the minority and for the population as a whole there is still an overall trend towards inactivity. Strauzenberg (1981), in a review of the literature, concluded that the ageing process was slowed down by the regular participation in exercise and that older people who had regularly participated in vigorous physical activity since their youth were biologically younger than their sedentary counterparts. Such research into the topic is always open to criticism, since in long-term studies the participants are almost inevitably volunteers and therefore self-selected. Therefore, it can always be argued that it is only those who are biologically younger that are capable or willing to participate in vigorous exercise. Hence, whilst there may be a link between exercise paticipation and biological age the exact cause and effect is still not proved conclusively (Holloszy, 1983; Kasch, 1976; Thornton, 1984).

When compared to younger adults the 'elderly' exhibit similar beneficial adaptations to exercise although they tend to occur more slowly. Therefore, when devising a programme the starting point may need to be at a very easy level and subsequent progression should be applied very gradually. Furthermore, since the maximum physical potential of the participant is likely to be lower owing to the effects of ageing, the goals of the programme will also need to be set accordingly. However, the general content and type of exercises included within a programme can be very similar to those for younger adults, with the inclusion of activities such as walking, swimming, cycling, flexibility and strengthening exercises. (MacHeath, 1984; Rikkers, 1986).

Research into the effects of exercise upon life expectancy are complex. There is a wealth of evidence supporting the notion that exercise reduces the risk of CHD and thus will increase life expectancy in that respect. However, its effects upon the incidence of other diseases requires further research. Many of the animal studies which have been conducted under laboratory conditions indicate that animals which exercise regularly have an increased life expectancy. However, how relevant these findings are for human beings remains to be seen. Human studies on the topic, including that of Karvonen *et al.* (1974) who studied endurance skiers, tend to indicate an increased life expectancy of two or three years. Since such increases in longevity are relatively small, most of the advocates of exercise emphasize the benefits of exercise in increasing physical capacity during life, and hence the quality and vitality of life, rather than the quantity of years.

EXERCISE AND CORONARY HEART DISEASE

The heart is made up of specialized muscular tissue called cardiac muscle which, like other muscles in the body, requires a constant supply of blood to provide it with the oxygen it needs to contract. However, whereas skeletal muscle can resort to anaerobic metabolism for short periods during intensive exercise, cardiac muscle cannot work anaerobically. The heart therefore possesses a very extensive network of arteries and blood vessels (coronary arteries) which supply the cardiac muscle with all the blood and oxygen it needs, even during intensive forms of exercise. These blood vessels form an extensive network in and around the heart muscle itself (Figure 8.1).

In the case of what is usually referred to as coronary heart disease (CHD) the coronary arteries become constricted by a build-up of fatty deposits (atheroma) on the inside of the artery wall (Figure 8.2). This is the condition referred to as atherosclerosis. The exact details of the processes leading to atherosclerosis are not clearly understood. However, factors such as high total blood cholesterol levels, hypertension, damage to the walls of the arteries, high carbon monoxide levels in the blood, cigarette smoking and a relatively low ratio of high-density to low-density lipoproteins in the blood are all thought to increase the risk of atherosclerosis. The overall effect of atheroma is to reduce the diameter of the blood vessels, thereby restricting the flow of blood to the area of cardiac muscle that they supply. A further restriction to the flow of blood through the arteries may be caused by a hardening of the elasticated walls of the arteries (arteriosclerosis). Although this may occur to some extent as an inevitable consequence of ageing it is believed to be worsened by the presence of the fatty deposits. In such cases the walls of the hardened arteries fail

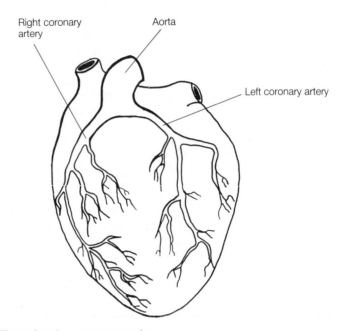

Figure 8.1 Illustrating the coronary arteries.

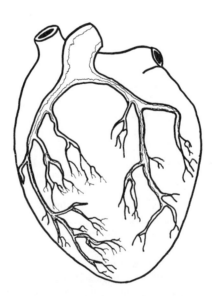

Figure 8.2 Illustrating the build-up of atheroma.

to stretch fully when blood is pumped through them, which further restricts the supply of blood to the cardiac muscle.

At rest the flow of blood, and hence oxygen, reaching the cardiac muscle is usually adequate even if the arteries are partially constricted. However, if the heart has to work harder, for instance when walking upstairs, then the restricted flow of blood may be insufficient to supply the oxygen needed by the cardiac muscle. When an area of cardiac muscle receives an inadequate supply of blood the condition is known as ischemia. An inadequate supply of oxygen to a region of the heart may result in chest pains and the conditions known as angina pectoris or angina decubitus.

Angina symptoms tend to appear when the process of atherosclerosis is already somewhat advanced, with the diameter of the coronary artery (or arteries) having been reduced by about 75%. Angina is a serious condition which often requires medication; it also predisposes the sufferer to a greater risk of the coronary arteries becoming completely blocked. If this occurs, the flow of blood to the corresponding region of cardiac muscle will be stopped, and hence that part of the heart will be severely deprived of oxygen. If the lack of oxygen persists then an area of cardiac muscle in that region will die (Figure 8.3). This is what is typically referred to as a myocardial infarction (MI) or heart attack. (The death of the cardiac muscle cells may also be referred to as necrosis.) On some occasions, if the area of damage to the heart muscle is relatively small, this occurrence may go almost unnoticed by the victim (a silent infarction). On other occasions it can cause severe chest pains, and if the area of damage is sufficiently large, it can of course be fatal.

According to figures published by the British Heart Foundation (1986), heart and circulatory diseases account for 44% of all premature deaths in the United Kingdom.

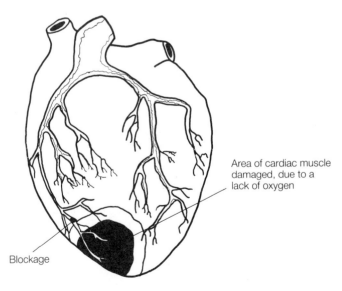

Area of cardiac muscle damaged, due to a lack of oxygen

Blockage

Figure 8.3 Illustrating a myocardial infarction.

While in the United States the American Heart Association (1984) estimated that more than 51% of all American deaths were caused by cardiovascular disease. Similar figures are reported by Hutchinson (1985) and Kannel (1985), who also report that in addition to the premature fatalities, over 8 million people in the USA suffer from some form of disability as a result of CHD. Additional reports on the scale of the problem and the effects of CHD were presented by the British Cardiac Society (1987) who stated that by the age of 40–44 one in six men in Britain will have clinical evidence of CHD and by the age of 55–59 the figures will have increased to one in three. Thus the scale of the problem is apparent.

It is widely known that cardiovascular disease is far more common in men than in women. The reason for this observed inequality is believed to be due to hormonal differences between the sexes. The key difference seems to be the significantly higher levels of oestrogens in women. These hormones appear to convey a form of protection to women prior to the menopause. After the menopause, when the hormonal differences are greatly reduced, women appear to be as much at risk from CHD as their male counterparts. Further support for the suggestion that oestrogens convey protection against CHD comes from clinical investigations in which oestrogens were administered to male patients recovering from myocardial infarction. In these trials oestrogens were shown to be effective in reducing the risk of a further attack.

A major and increasing concern over the incidence of coronary heart disease is its frequency in the relatively young. Autopsies conducted upon United States soldiers killed in the Korean War indicated that over 77% of them had signs of coronary artery disease despite the fact that their average age was only 22 (Enos *et al.*, 1953). Similar findings have also been found in more recent studies conducted on American soldiers killed in Vietnam (McNamara *et al.*, 1971). Indeed, CHD is not just a disease associated with old age, it is a major killer of men in the 35–44 age group and there is also an apparent increase in CHD in women of this age group. To further this concern, some investigations have shown that the early stages of cardiovascular disease can be observed in young children, including some under 5 years of age (Kannel and Dawber, 1972).

Therefore, it is clear that CHD represents a major health problem for a large proportion of the population. It is not a disease which just affects the elderly and any preventive measures that can be taken to reduce the magnitude of the problem are of great importance. One of the major difficulties in trying to persuade people to take preventive measures such as exercises, is that though CHD is a gradual process which may begin in childhood or even infancy, the symptoms and debilitating effects of the disease do not become apparent until it is fairly advanced.

It is evident that some individuals are inherently more likely to suffer from CHD than others. This may be due to factors such as age, sex, race and other inherited (genetic) traits over which the individual has no control. However, research has also shown that there are a number of other 'risk factors' which can also increase the chances of a person suffering from CHD. These include:

1. Hypertension
2. Smoking
3. Obesity

4. High total blood cholesterol levels
5. A relatively low ratio of high-density lipoproteins to low-density lipoproteins
6. A stressed emotional state
7. A lack of physical exercise.

These factors can be influenced by individuals and thus in this respect individuals are able to exert some influence over their chances of suffering from CHD. Whilst these 'optional' risk factors are listed separately they are often interrelated, and altering one factor, such as taking up exercise, can have beneficial effects upon the others. For example, exercise may reduce body fat levels, lower blood pressure, reduce blood cholesterol levels and alleviate stress. These changes will all contribute towards decreasing an individual's chances of suffering from CHD. Evidence in support of exercise as a means of reducing these risk factors comes from a large number of investigations which are reviewed by Astrand and Grimby (1986), Bouchard (1989), the Coronary Prevention Group (1987), Fentem *et al.* (1988, 1990), and Morris *et al.* (1987). Overall the research suggests that death due to ischemic heart disease is twice as frequent in the physically inactive as in the physically active. There is also general agreement within the published literature that before exercise can reduce the risk of CHD effectively it needs to be 'aerobic', undertaken regularly and be of sufficient duration. Thus, these findings lead many authorities to recommend activities such as swimming, cycling, jogging and brisk walking as possible health-promoting forms of exercise. Most authorities would recommend a frequency of about three times a week, with each session lasting a minimum of 20 to 30 minutes (see Chapter 7 for details). However, whilst there is an association between physical activity and a reduced risk of CHD, it is also apparent from the available literature that the exact physiological process(es) which reduce the risk still remain somewhat unclear. In general, it is widely accepted that exercise produces its effects by improving the overall condition of the cardiovascular system and by exerting numerous effects upon the various risk factors associated with CHD. The suggested effects of exercise include:

1. Improving blood lipid profiles
2. Reducing arterial blood pressure
3. Improving overall body composition by reducing the percentage of body fat
4. Reducing sympatho-adrenal activity
5. Reducing or inhibiting atheroma
6. Improving the efficiency of the heart
7. Providing a means for controlling stress.

Other proposed effects include promoting the growth of collateral blood vessels and inhibiting the formation of unwanted blood clots. Thus, there is much evidence to support the role of exercise in beneficially affecting a number of CHD risk factors, which even without the implications of CHD are considered in themselves to be detrimental to the overall health and well-being of the individual.

Support for the effects of exercise in promoting the growth of additional coronary blood vessels comes from the work of Eckstein (1957), Schaible *et al.* (1981) and Wyatt and Mitchell (1978) who suggested that if CHD is present then exercise may promote alternative coronary arteries to perform the function of blocked ones and hence reduce the impact of atherosclerosis or even a myocardial infarction.

In summary, it is suggested that exercise can induce the development of additional blood vessels within the cardiac muscle. This growth of additional blood vessels is referred to as 'vascularization' and has been extensively observed in skeletal muscle following a programme of aerobic exercise. Similar effects are believed to occur in cardiac muscle; however, research into the subject is difficult and most studies supporting the idea have involved the use of other animals or are based on indirect evidence (Barnard, 1975; Blumgart et al., 1940; Connor et al., 1976; Ferguson et al., 1974; and Stevenson et al., 1964). Therefore, whilst this suggested benefit promotes much interest it is still subject to speculation and debate.

The results of such research are complicated by indications that the deprivation of oxygen to part of the heart muscle, caused by a blockage within a coronary artery, also appears to be a stimulus for initiating the development of collateral arteries within the myocardium. These by-pass the blockage, forming what is known as a collateral circulation, and hence the heart muscle in this area can be supplied with the blood it requires via an alternative set of blood vessels (Ferguson et al., 1974; Schlesinger, 1938; and Zoll et al., 1951). Therefore, in studies where exercise has been used and coronary collateralization has been observed, the extent to which the exercise itself was responsible for the changes is not entirely clear.

In addition, aerobic exercise has been shown to increase the size of blood vessels in skeletal muscle, thus enhancing blood flow to the muscles. Studies on rats would indicate that a similar process may also occur in cardiac muscle (Bloor and Leon, 1970; Stevenson et al., 1964; Tharp and Wagner, 1982; and Tepperman and Pearlman, 1961). This would again enhance the delivery of blood to the myocardium and have further implications since the larger diameter of the coronary arteries would reduce the risk of a complete blockage and, hence, a myocardial infarction. Once again studies into this aspect in humans are complicated by possible genetic and other lifestyle factors, but some indirect evidence does support these suggestions (Currens and White, 1961; Qu Xia, 1990).

Further support for the role of exercise comes from the work of Tharp and Wagner (1982) who suggest that one of the major benefits of exercise upon cardiac function, and hence reducing the risk of ischemic heart disease, is the training effect, which causes a reduction in the heart rate at a given submaximal exercise intensity. The slower exercise heart rate will result in a longer diastolic period in the cardiac cycle. This will enable a greater perfusion of blood into the heart muscle itself and thereby enhance the supply of oxygen to the cardiac muscle.

In summary, these research findings suggest that exercise has an important role to play in reducing the risk of CHD and may therefore be prescribed as a form of preventative medicine. Furthermore, in addition to its reported preventative effects, exercise is also used very extensively in the rehabilitation programmes of many heart attack victims. Here it is used to both help restore their physical capacity and to try and reduce the risk of a further attack. (For details see Exercise and coronary rehabilitation, page 290.)

If evidence from research studies does support the notion that exercise can reduce the risk of CHD, the question may then be asked: 'Can the participation in very large amounts of exercise provide complete immunity against CHD?' This question was investigated by Noakes et al. (1984) who studied the incidence of CHD in marathon runners. From their findings they concluded that, while exercise did indeed reduce the incidence of CHD, very large doses of exercise did not provide complete immunity, especially when other risk factors such as smoking and poor blood fat profiles were involved. Thus, most authorities recommend a basic level of exercise participation with appropriate levels of intensity, duration and frequency and few would advocate excessive amounts of exercise as a means of substantially reducing the risks still further. Therefore, in summary, there is much evidence to support the belief that exercise can reduce the risk of CHD but any health-promotion programme must also consider the other risk factors associated with CHD and advise the participants accordingly.

EXERCISE, BLOOD PRESSURE, HYPERTENSION AND CHD

Blood pressure is a measure of the pressure exerted by the blood on the walls of the arteries. Owing to the pumping action of the heart the blood travels through the arteries in surges rather than in a steady flow. This causes the pressure exerted on the walls of the arteries to vary. The greatest pressure occurs as the heart contracts causing the blood to surge through the arteries in a wave. This surge of blood can be felt as the pulse in certain arteries, such as the radial and carotid arteries which are close to the surface of the body. The pressure occurring during the surges is known as the systolic pressure. Between the surges, whilst the heart is refilling with blood, the pressure in the arteries is at its lowest and is known as the diastolic pressure.

Blood pressure is usually measured at the left brachial artery whilst the subject is seated, or occasionally lying down. It is measured using a sphygmomanometer which is strapped to the upper arm over the artery. When measuring 'blood pressure' both the systolic and diastolic pressures are taken. The blood pressure is then expressed as the systolic pressure over the diastolic pressure.

Although they appear to be expressed as a fraction they are always expressed as two figures, with the difference between the two being the 'pulse pressure'. There are a range of accepted values for both systolic and diastolic pressures. For adults, typical systolic values range between 120 and 145. Typical diastolic pressures range between 60 and 85. However, owing to the stiffening of the arteries there is a slight rise in blood pressure with age, and some authorities suggest a much wider range of acceptable values.

If a pressure exceeds the 'normal range' it is said to be high; if it is below, it is said to be low. Blood pressure is expressed in units of millimetres of mercury: mmHg (Hg being the chemical symbol for mercury). This is because mmHg is the standard unit of pressure and indeed most traditional sphygmomanometers measure blood pressure using a column of mercury. Digital sphygmomanometers, whilst not using mercury, still express blood pressure in the same units. Therefore a blood pressure reading may be written as:

Systolic   125 mmHg

Diastolic   75 mmHg

An individual's blood pressure is influenced by a number of factors, including their emotional state, posture, recent exercise, smoking and recently ingested food or drink. However, a persistently high resting blood pressure is known as 'hypertension';

for example, a reading of 175/100. High blood pressure is due to the occurrence of a greater than normal amount of pressure within the arteries. This may be caused by the arteries being constricted, possibly as the result of tension or fatty deposits. It may also be caused by the arteries losing their elasticity and, hence, capacity to stretch as the blood passes through them.

High blood pressure is not only undesirable in terms of overall health, it is also a major risk factor in many diseases including CHD. Contributing factors include stress, diet, smoking and an inherited tendency towards high blood pressure. Therefore, changes in diet, medication and exercise are various methods which may be employed to reduce hypertension.

Studies and reviews investigating the value of exercise in reducing resting blood pressure include those of Boyer and Kasch (1970), Duncan *et al.* (1985), Kiyonaga *et al.* (1984), Kukkonen *et al.* (1982), Roman *et al.* (1984), Seals and Haberg (1984) and Tipton (1984). In other investigations (Goldberg *et al.*, 1980) it has also been shown to be effective in reducing the amount of medication required to control hypertension, and thus exercise has gained much support in the control of hypertension, especially in patients where the condition is considered to be relatively slight.

As previously mentioned, the arteries have a tendency to lose their elasticity as part of the ageing process and, as a result, there is a slight increase in blood pressure with age. However, the investigations of Blair *et al.* (1984) and Kasch and Wallace (1976) indicate that this loss of elasticity, and hence rise in blood pressure, may be largely prevented by the continued participation in forms of endurance exercise throughout life.

During exercise itself the increased cardiac output of the heart causes blood pressure to rise; however, much of the potential rise is offset by the dilation of blood vessels thereby reducing the peripheral resistance and thus resulting in measured blood pressures rising to only slightly above their resting values. Studies, such as that of Choquette and Ferguson (1973), have shown that appropriate exercise programmes are effective in reducing blood pressure, not only at rest but also during exercise. In summary, research would suggest that exercise can be used to reduce the risk of hypertension, reduce hypertension itself and reduce the amount of medication needed to control it. It should also be remembered that high blood pressure can also occur in children (Blumenthal *et al.*, (1977) and therefore appropriate forms of exercise may be recommended for this age group as well as for adults as a means of controlling blood pressure and hence promoting good health.

However, it should also be mentioned that isometric exercises should not be recommended for those with high blood pressure. Therefore any exercise programme devised for those with hypertension should include exercises that are of a dynamic nature such as walking, swimming or cycling. The reason for avoiding isometric exercises is that a muscle which is held in a strong static contraction may restrict the blood flow through that muscle, thus causing a build-up of metabolic waste products which can then stimulate an unwanted rise in blood pressure as the cardiovascular system attempts to send more blood to the muscle. Dynamic exercises tend to avoid this problem owing to the cyclic contractions and relaxations of the muscles which facilitate the venous flow of the blood out of the muscle and back towards the heart.

EXERCISE, STRESS AND CHD

Various pieces of research have also indicated that a person's emotional state, or the amount of 'stress' experienced, is another significant risk factor for CHD, as well as contributing to a number of other stress-related disorders (Friedman and Rosenman, 1959, 1974; Friedman, 1969). A major problem encountered when trying to assess the significance of stress on a person's health is that it is difficult to measure quantitatively. Therefore, it is difficult to separate its potential effects from other factors and its precise relationship with certain disorders, and its significance as a risk factor for CHD remain largely unknown. However, some authorities consider it as a major determinant both directly and indirectly because of its influence upon other factors such as blood pressure.

The individuals most at risk from stress are those exhibiting 'type A behaviour' – that is to say, those with a strong competitive drive at work and/or in their leisure time. They also tend to work in a tense state with some degree of urgency. Studies have indicated that exercise can be effective in reducing the amount of stress a person experiences and may therefore be an effective means of controlling it, thereby reducing the risk of CHD and other disorders (Blumenthal et al., 1980; Folkins and Amsterdam, 1977; Ledwidge, 1980; Seals and Hagberg, 1984). In addition, work by Long (1983) suggests that the psychological aspects of exercise programmes are an important factor in reducing stress and may indeed be more significant than the more easily measured physiological effects. Thus, exercise may be used to control this increasing problem in modern society which affects both children and adults. However, therapists will need to ensure that any exercise programme does not become too competitive as this could increase the amount of stress experienced by the individual rather than reduce it.

EXERCISE, BLOOD LIPIDS AND CHD

According to various authorities, including Grundy (1986) and Martin et al. (1986), there is a link between high levels of serum cholesterol and an increased risk of CHD. Evidence would suggest that high levels of fat in the blood (hyperlipedemia) above 150 mg/dl represent a significant CHD risk factor, with a considerable increase in risk if the level exceeds 200 mg/dl. It is therefore clearly desirable to have blood cholesterol well below these levels in order to reduce the risk of CHD. The value of exercise in reducing blood cholesterol levels has been demonstrated in various studies, including those of Hartung (1984) and Haskell (1984a), thus by implication this research provides support for the notion that physical activity can reduce the risk of CHD.

The most common types of fat found in the blood are triglycerides and cholesterol, which circulate in the blood in association with protein carriers and form what are known as lipoproteins. There are several types of lipoproteins found in the blood and, according to their structure, they are designated as high-density lipoproteins (HDL), low-density lipoproteins (LDL) and very low density lipoproteins (VLDL). The relative abundance of these different types of lipoproteins has been shown to have a significant effect upon the probability of the formation of atheroma in the blood vessels and, hence, the incidence of coronary heart disease. Thus, not only is the absolute concentration of fat within the blood a CHD risk factor but the relative abundance of these lipoproteins can influence CHD risk.

High-density lipoproteins appear to reduce the incidence of atheroma formation by transporting cholesterol to the liver, where it is metabolized and removed from the body via the bile secretions. Conversely, relatively high levels of the low-density lipoproteins appear to cause the formation of atheroma on the walls of the arteries. Numerous studies have shown that exercise increases the ratio of high-density lipoproteins to low-density lipoproteins in the blood (Castelli et al., 1986; Cowan, 1983; Goldberg and Elliot, 1985; Gordon et al., 1983; Huttunen et al., 1979; Roberts, 1984; Rotkis et al., 1980; Thorland and Gilliam, 1981; Wood and Haskell, 1979). Exercise is therefore considered to be beneficial in reducing the risk of CHD through improving the ratio of HDLs to LDLs, thereby reducing the rate of deposition of atheroma on the walls of the arteries and increasing the rate of removal of cholesterol from the blood (Haskell, 1984a, b).

Further interest in the effects of exercise upon blood lipid profiles comes from studies on children (Gilliam and Burke, 1978; Nizankowska-Blaz and Abramowicz, 1983; Widhalm et al., 1978) who found higher levels of HDL in children who were more physically active compared with those who were relatively sedentary. Other studies which investigated the relationship between physical activity levels and blood lipid profiles in children have been less conclusive (Linder and DuRant, 1982; Valimaki et al., 1980) but this may be due to the fact that the children tended to have 'normal' blood lipid profiles even before the exercise programme commenced and, hence, little or no change would be expected. Other factors such as the type, intensity and duration of the exercises undertaken in the different programmes may also go some way to explain the inconsistencies of the findings.

EXERCISE, BLOOD CLOTS AND CHD

A further factor which needs to be considered when discussing the effects of exercise upon the incidence of CHD is the formation of blood clots which can cause blockages in arteries that are already partially closed owing to atherosclerosis. Unwanted blood clots can result in a blockage in a coronary artery and cause a myocardial infarction. A blood clot is called a thrombus if it blocks the artery in which it was formed or an embolus if it is formed in one artery but is then transported in the blood and causes a blockage in another.

The formation of blood clots is a complex process requiring a series of reactions which activate clotting factors within the blood. The initiation of the clotting process is triggered by factors released by damaged tissues and cells. In the case of a small cut or graze on the skin the clotting process will result in the blood coagulating in the vicinity of the damaged tissue and the ultimate closure of the wound. The reverse process, whereby blood clots are dissolved and removed, is called fibrinolysis. It has been suggested that atherosclerotic arteries have similar properties to other forms of damaged tissue and hence stimulate the clotting process thereby increasing the number of blood clots in the circulation. Such an increase in the number of blood clots would increase the chances of one of them causing a blockage in an artery and, hence, the probability of a myocardial infarction and/or stroke.

It has been proposed by some authorities that if exercise were to promote fibrinolysis it could reduce the incidence of blood clots and hence the risk of heart attack (Fentem and Turnbull, 1987). However, research studies to date appear to indicate that exercise increases the rates of both clot formation and fibrinolysis. Thus, if the effects on both processes are of equal magnitude they would offset each other. Therefore, there is currently no conclusive evidence to support the suggestion that exercise directly reduces the risk of blood clot formation (Andrew *et al.*, 1986; Astrup, 1973; Davis *et al.*, 1976; Hyers *et al.*, 1980; Joye *et al.*, 1978; Meade *et al.*, 1979; Vogt and Straub, 1979). However, it must of course be remembered that if exercise has a beneficial effect upon the condition of the atherosclerotic arteries themselves it could indirectly reduce the formation of blood clots. This would be in addition to the reduction in the amount of atheroma and, hence, constriction within the arteries, thereby reducing the chances of a blood clot becoming stuck in a constricted artery and the risk of a complete blockage. Therefore, this is clearly an area of interest and further research into the topic may yield valuable information on its importance in preventing myocardial infarctions.

EXERCISE, OBESITY, HEALTH AND CHD

Obesity refers to the physical condition where an individual has an excessively high amount of fat stored in the body. It is essential for the body to contain a certain amount of fat as it fulfils certain vital functions within the body: it forms a major component in the structure of cell membranes, provides insulation, provides physical protection, acts as an energy store, is essential for the manufacture of certain body chemicals such as steroid hormones, and is also required in the numerous metabolic processes which occur.

It is generally considered that, for health, a man's body weight should be made up of approximately 15% fat whilst the fat in a woman should be approximately 23%, although some authorities recommend values slightly below this. Fat stores in excess of these values are generally considered to be detrimental to health and if excessive amounts of fat are stored in the body it results in the condition of obesity. Although the figures vary, it is generally considered that values in excess of 25% for males and 35% for females represent obesity. At the other end of the spectrum, exceptionally lean individuals such as male and female endurance runners may have body fat values as low as 6% and 12% respectively. These low values are not generally considered to be 'unhealthy' but below this there may be health implications, especially for women, who may become more prone to osteoporosis if they lose too much fat.

In addition to its social implications, obesity also reduces a person's physical capacity and is considered to be a major risk factor associated with a number of diseases and disorders, including:

(a) CHD, possibly through the association between obesity and other CHD risk factors such as hypertension, inactivity and blood cholesterol profiles
(b) impairment of cardiac function
(c) hypertension
(d) diabetes (about 80% of adult onset diabetics are overweight)

  (e) renal disorders
  (f) pulmonary disease and impairment of lung function
  (g) osteoarthritis
  (h) cancer
  (i) gallbladder disorders
  (j) abnormal plasma lipid and lipoprotein profiles.

Obesity is a complex phenomenon which may be caused by a number of factors, including inactivity, overeating, hormonal disturbances, and genetic and socioeconomic factors. The amount of fat stored in the body is dependent upon the number of fat cells a person has and the size of those fat cells, which in turn depends upon the amount of fat that is stored within them. Studies have suggested that there are two basic types of obesity: in one type the individual has an increased number of fat cells (hyperplasia obesity), whilst in the other the individual has a normal number of fat cells but they are larger and contain more fat (hypertrophy obesity).

Problems of excessive fatness in some individuals may originate prior to birth. Research by Udall (1978) showed that mothers who put on too much fat during pregnancy produced fatter babies who appeared to possess a greater number of fat cells (adipocytes) when compared with less fat babies whose mothers had not put on an excessive amount of fat during pregnancy. This hyperplasia is believed to make the overfat babies more prone to obesity throughout their lives (Charney, 1976). A second period of vulnerability to obesity may occur during infancy. According to Brook (1972), if infants are overfed in their first year they may become overfat, with a resulting increase in the number of fat cells. This hyperplasia again has implications for obesity throughout life. A third period of potential hyperplasia may then occur between the ages of 9 and 13, just prior to the adolescent growth spurt (Hirsch, 1972; Salans et al., 1973). It may therefore be suggested that overfatness in childhood can make the individual more prone to obesity in adulthood, although some authorities would dispute these reported changes in the number of fat cells.

Studies on obese adults suggest that if they were not overfat as children then their obesity is likely to be of the hypertrophy-obesity type rather than being due to hyperplasia. Such conclusions are reached because these individuals appear to have a normal number of fat cells, but the fat cells are larger than in non-obese individuals (Bonnet et al., 1970; Hirsch and Batchelor, 1976; Sims, 1974). It is also interesting to note that when the amount of fat stored within the body is reduced the fat cells shrink in size, but there appears to be no reduction in the actual number of fat cells. To support this, studies by Rognum et al. (1982) and Vinten and Galbo (1983) showed that whilst exercise was effective in reducing the fat stores of the body, the effects were on the size of the fat cells and the amount of fat stored within them rather than on the actual number of fat cells. Such findings may indicate why many obese individuals find that having lost fat they are very prone to 'putting it back on again'. In addition, Bjorntorp (1974) suggested that individuals suffering from hyperplasia-obesity have more difficulty in reducing their body fat levels and physiologically do not respond as well as hypertrophy-obesity patients to normal diet and exercise regimens. Therefore, in the case of obesity, as with any disorder, 'prevention is better than cure' and such preventive measures should be initiated early on in the life of the individual.

While obesity is linked with CHD, the exact relationship between the two is unclear due to its association with other risk factors. For example, many obese individuals have high blood pressure, consume too much fat in their diet and take very little vigorous exercise. It is also apparent that obesity limits an individual's physical capacity and puts more strain upon the cardiovascular system, muscles and joints even during relatively low-intensity activities such as climbing stairs. Therefore, an individual's body composition is an important consideration in terms of both physical capacity and general health.

The amount of fat stored in a person's body basically depends upon their calorific balance; that is to say, the relationship between the number of calories that are taken in compared to the number of calories that are used up. If the number of calories taken in greatly exceeds the number used up then substantial amounts of fat may accumulate in the body, with much of this fat being stored in fat cells under the skin (subcutaneous fat). If, however, more calories are consistently used up than are taken in, then their fat stores of the body are reduced. If an individual wishes to maintain his or her body composition, then it is necessary to ensure that the calorific intake and expenditure are balanced. If, however, the individual wishes to reduce their fat stores, then more calories must be used up than are eaten.

Calories are used by the body in the processes of general metabolism and during exercise. This calorific balance, and the tendency to store fat, therefore depends upon a number of factors including diet, the level of physical activity, general metabolism, and certain inherited characteristics of the individual. Of these factors, the amount of exercise undertaken by a person is one which can be altered. Thus, by increasing the calorific expenditure of the body – by undertaking more exercise – it is possible for an individual to reduce the fat stores.

Aerobic exercise programmes have long been advocated as a means of 'losing weight' and have been demonstrated to produce significant reductions in body fat levels in both obese and non-obese individuals, even without being undertaken in conjunction with a calorie-restricted diet (Bjorntorp, 1978; Boileau et al., 1971; Leon et al., 1979; Wilmore, 1983). In support of the role of exercise in maintaining a good body composition, various authors (Chirico and Stunfard, 1976; Mayer, 1980; Mayer and Thomas, 1967) present evidence to suggest that obesity is very often due to inactivity rather than overeating, even in children (Corbin and Pletcher, 1968). These suggestions are supported by various pieces of research which indicate that many obese individuals do not have a higher than average calorific intake (Fry, 1953; Johnson et al., 1956; Peckos, 1953). From such findings it is therefore not surprising that many investigators recommend a combination of exercise and a calorie-controlled diet as the optimal means of controlling and/or reducing body fat, with numerous research papers on the subject of exercise and obesity being reviewed by Bjorntorp (1983), Pace et al. (1986) and Segal and Pi-Sunyer (1989).

As a general basis for reducing body fat levels many authorities recommend a calorific deficiency of about 500 kcal per day. This amounts to a deficiency of 3500 kcal per week, which is equivalent to approximately 1lb of fat. Such a deficit may be achieved through either exercise or dietary modifications or both. Whilst a fat loss of 1lb per week may not appear to be spectacular it should be remembered that people do not become obese overnight and that the more rapid weight losses which are observed under certain regimens may have drawbacks: these are discussed more fully later in this section. As a means of burning up excess calories aerobic forms of exercise appear to the most effective and will, of course, convey other health benefits upon the participant. However, to be effective in burning up excess fat the exercise undertaken needs to be of a sufficient duration, intensity and frequency (see Chapter 7 for details). Authorities such as the American College of Sports Medicine and the Health Education Authority (UK) recommend participating in some form of exercise at least three times a week if the exercise is to be effective in reducing fat levels. It is also recommended that the exercise sessions should be of at least 20–30 minutes' duration; thus during each session the participant should use up approximately 300 kcal.

To lose 1lb of fat it is necessary to burn up about 3500 kcal. This calorific expenditure would be approximately equivalent to about twelve 30 minute exercise sessions, or 35 miles of jogging or walking, or 20 hours golf or 12 hours cycling. Such figures are often quoted by sceptics to illustrate, as they would put it, the 'futility' of exercise in a weight control programme. However, to put these values into perspective: if someone was to walk 3 miles five times a week, this would represent a calorific expenditure of 75 000 kcal per year or the equivalent of 20 lb of fat. In addition to this significant contribution to weight control, the participants would also gain numerous other health benefits from the exercise.

In terms of the duration of exercise it should be noted that in activities such as jogging there is very little difference in the calorific expenditure of jogging 3 miles in 24 minutes and doing the same 3 miles in 33 minutes: that is to say, in terms of calorific cost it is the duration of the exercise in miles that counts, not the speed at which the miles are run.

A major problem encountered by the therapist or health adviser is that many people wish to lose quite considerable amounts of fat very quickly without much effort, despite the fact that they probably put on the fat over a period of many months and years through an inappropriate lifestyle. Those wishing to lose weight are also subjected to much commercial advertising which leads them to believe it can be done without effort or the changes in lifestyle discussed above. However, many of these advertised methods cause a weight loss due to a fluid imbalance and/or a loss of important energy stores such as muscle glycogen, whilst being relatively ineffective in losing fat: they can also convey other health implications for some individuals.

Another factor to note is that in weight reduction programmes that do not include exercise there is a tendency for the subject's resting metabolic rate to fall as the programme progresses. This means that the individual actually needs fewer calories each day and, hence, further fat reduction becomes more difficult. The inclusion of exercise into a fat reduction programme helps to prevent this unwanted fall in resting metabolic rate (Donahoe et al., 1984; Mole et al., 1989) and also helps to prevent the undesirable loss of important lean tissue, which may occur if dieting is the sole means of reducing body fat (Zuti and Golding, 1976). Research has also suggested that the regular participation in exercise can result in an elevated metabolic rate for some time after the exercise session has finished, thereby further enhancing a reduction in fat stores.

It is also important to note that exercise will only be really effective in reducing the fat stores if the calorific content of the diet does not exceed the overall calorific expenditure of the individual. Therefore, in the case of trying to control or reduce an individual's obesity, the level of physical activity and the diet both need to b considered. Depending upon the individual's circumstances, current dietary habits and the amount of fat which needs to be lost, a calorie-restrictive diet may not be essential to produce the desired reduction in fat (Leon et al., 1979). However, it is often argued that exercise alone is ineffective in reducing body fat levels, since it stimulates an increase in appetite which more than compensates for the calorific expenditure of the exercise. This appears to be an area of some controversy, with a number of investigations indicating that there is little or no increase in calorific intake as a result of exercise (Katch, 1969) whilst others would suggest that there is (Woo et al., 1982a, b; Woo and Pi-Sunyer, 1985). A further consideration on this matter is that in some investigations it has been shown that whilst the non-obese individuals may tend to increase their calorific intake to compensate for the additional exercise, obese individuals do not. If consistent, then this would illustrate a very effective homeostatic control of calorific balance which should result in an appropriate body composition. In addition, there is the suggestion by some authorities that exercise can enable obese individuals to become more 'sensitive' to their calorific needs and hence reduce their calorific intake (Allen and Quigley, 1977).

Another area of controversy and misconception concerns the topic of 'spot reduction'. It has been put forward by certain individuals that specific exercises can promote the reduction of body fat at specific sites around the body. One such example is that of recommending sit-ups to reduce subcutaneous fat in the abdominal region. However, to date there is no conclusive proof to support such ideas and various investigations have concluded that spot reduction exercises are ineffective. The reason for this can be explained by the way in which the fat stores of the body are mobilized and then utilized by the exercising muscles. During exercise the fat stores of the body may be used as an energy source. They are mobilized from the fat cells by the secretion of various hormones. These hormones are secreted from specific endocrine glands situated around the body. The hormones then travel aound the body in the blood and hence can promote the utilization of any fat stores that the blood passes through. Thus, fat stores which are some distance from the exercising muscle groups may be mobilized in the same way as those close to the exercising muscles. Therefore, any exercise is likely to reduce the fat stores at numerous sites around the body, and not just those close to the exercising muscles. However, whereas specific exercises may not reduce the fat stores around specific muscles they may well be effective in improving the general muscle tone of the muscles concerned and hence an area of the body may appear 'less flabby' owing to an improved muscle tone, rather than being specifically attributable to a reduction in the amount of subcutaneous fat covering the exercised muscles.

Therefore, in summary, current research suggests that the fat-reducing effects of exercise have a general effect in reducing the fat stores of the body rather than specifically reducing the fat stores around the exercising muscles (Noland and Kearney, 1978; Schade et al., 1962). This is supported by the research of Katch (1984) in a study looking at the effects of sit-ups on fat reduction. In addition, to further dispel the misconceptions over spot reduction, Gwinap (1971) compared the dominant and non-dominant arms of high-level tennis players. The results showed that whilst the muscles of the dominant arm were significantly larger, as may be expected considering the additional work they did, there was no significant difference in the skinfold thickness of the dominant and non-dominant arms. Hence, they concluded that there was no difference in the amount of fat stored in the highly exercised arm compared to that in the less exercised arm.

A further factor to consider when discussing the topic of obesity is the difference between body composition and body weight. In terms of health, body composition – or, more specifically, the percentage of the body that is fat – is the key issue rather than body weight. However, because it is easier to measure body weight than body composition this tends to be the measurement that concerns most individuals. Thus complications can occur when individuals, who may be extremely muscular with a very low percentage body fat, are stated to be 'overweight' according to height/weight charts. Conversely, and somewhat more commonly, a person may be of the correct weight, but in reality, too much of that weight may be fat, rather than lean tissue. Additional complications may occur when an individual diets. Research would indicate that during some forms of excessive dieting much of the initial weight loss is due to a reduction in muscle glycogen and the water content of the body. This is not considered to be a healthy situation and indeed most authorities would recommend that for most people a gradual reduction in weight (fat) of 1 to 2 lb per week to be optimal. Therefore, whilst a reduction in weight may indicate a reduction in body fat levels it may not be a good indicator of the actual amount of fat lost. For this reason alternative means of estimating body composition may be employed. These include: the use of hydrostatic weighing; body densitometry; anthropometric measurements including skinfold thickness; radiography; and various forms of technological instrumentation which use conductance, impedence and/or absorbance. Thus, by using these methods a more precise and specific monitoring of fat levels can be achieved, thereby helping to ensure a healthy reduction in fat levels rather than an inappropriate loss of lean tissue.

As mentioned above, for those attempting to lose weight via diet only, while the initial loss in weight may be encouraging, it may not be producing the desired effect of significantly reducing their fat stores. It also has the undesirable effect of making them feel physically tired (owing to a lack of muscle glycogen) and it is also temporary, since the water and muscle glycogen stores will be replenished once normal eating habits are recommenced. Exercise, however, promotes a reduction in the fat stores through an increased calorific expenditure, prevents a reduction in metabolic rate (thereby aiding further fat loss) and conveys numerous other health benefits. However, some additional care should be taken with the excessively obese because of their physical condition: apart from the health-related problems such as an increased risk of CHD, their lack of physical fitness may mean that they are not fit enough to exercise at an intensity and duration that is sufficient to utilize a significant number of calories and hence reduce their fat stores. In such cases exercise may still be included because of its health-promoting benefits and as a means of initiating long-term lifestyle changes; alternatively, it may be left until some fat reduction has already occurred. The choice of exercise also has many additional implications for the obese since weight-bearing activities such as jogging could put an excessive strain on their joints. For this reason, non-weight-bearing activities such as swimming and/or cycling may be preferable.

On a further practical, administrative point, it has been demonstrated in various investigations that exercise adherence and compliance with recommended exercise programmes are much higher in supervised programmes than in unsupervised ones (MacKeen *et al.*, 1983). Therefore, to help ensure that an exercise programme is effective it should be carefully designed, monitored and supervised throughout, with the therapist being in regular contact with the participant.

EXERCISE AND STROKE

A 'stroke' occurs when the blood, and hence oxygen supply, to the brain becomes restricted. If the deprivation of oxygen to brain cells is prolonged the cells may die and brain functions will be interfered with, resulting in disability. A stroke is commonly caused by a blockage in an artery supplying blood to the brain. Typically the blockage occurs in an artery which is already partially constricted by atheroma, making it more susceptible to complete blockage by a blood clot. In the brain this is termed a cerebral thrombosis. Alternatively, a stroke may be caused by the bursting of an artery supplying the brain. This is called a cerebral haemorrhage and, as a consequence, the cells normally supplied by the artery become deprived of oxygen and may die. The major risk factors for a stroke are therefore atherosclerosis and high blood pressure.

A stroke may have a number of effects upon the victim, which may be temporary or permanent, with the degree of severity varying according to the area of brain damaged. The effects can include paralysis of one side of the body (hemiparesis), loss of memory and a reduction in the ability to communicate.

In general, the risk factors associated with a stroke are the same as those for CHD (high blood pressure, smoking, age and poor blood lipid profiles) and therefore behavioural factors such as physical activity which can reduce the risk of CHD are also likely to reduce the risk of stroke. Paffenbarger et al. (1984) and Salonen et al. (1982) presented evidence to this effect, suggesting that exercise could indeed reduce the risk of stroke, with the major benefits being related to its effects upon reducing blood pressure and improving blood cholesterol profiles.

EXERCISE AND DIABETES MELLITUS

Diabetes mellitus is a condition found in both adults and children. It is a complex disease with many side effects. However, in summary, the primary effects of the disease on individuals include a failure to control blood sugar levels and an inability to store glucose in the form of muscle glycogen or liver glycogen.

There are two basic types of diabetes mellitus. The first is caused by the beta cells of the pancreas failing to produce sufficient amounts of the hormone insulin. This form of diabetes most commonly appears during childhood and, hence, is sometimes referred to as juvenile or primary diabetes. The second is caused by the cells of the body becoming less sensitive to insulin and, hence, failing to respond effectively to the insulin that is produced by the body. This type of diabetes more commonly occurs later in life and is sometimes referred to as secondary or maturity onset diabetes.

In both forms of diabetes the disorder results in the sufferer being unable to store glucose in the form of glycogen in organs such as the liver and muscles. During the digestive and absorptive processes of a non-diabetic, carbohydrates such as starch, glycogen and various sugars are ultimately converted into the simple sugar, glucose. As a result of this, the glucose levels in the blood stream begin to rise and stimulate the secretion of the hormone insulin. Insulin then promotes the uptake of glucose into the liver and muscles and its conversion into glycogen. This uptake prevents the blood levels from becoming too high (hyperglycemia) and ensures that the body has a readily available supply of carbohydrate between meals. However, in the case of the diabetic, as a result of an inability to store glucose, eating a meal containing large amounts of sugar causes the level of glucose in the blood to rise rapidly. At very high levels of blood glucose the kidneys are unable to reabsorb all the glucose that passes through them and, consequently, the individual excretes glucose in the urine. A further consequence is that the individual has a very limited supply of glucose available between meals. The lack of stored glycogen means that the diabetic is unable to release glucose back into the blood as the blood glucose levels fall. This can result in a state of excessively low blood glucose (hypoglycemia), which causes certain metabolic disturbances and the incomplete breakdown of certain fats into ketones to provide energy. The production of ketones alters the acidic balance of the body, which in extreme cases can induce a diabetic coma that can be fatal.

People with diabetes mellitus may also suffer from additional side effects, including problems with their eyesight and an increased risk of CHD in both men and women. Diabetes mellitus may be treated by the careful control of an individual's diet and/or the injection of the hormone insulin.

Aerobic exercise can play an important role in preventing and/or controlling diabetes. Exercise can help by reducing an individual's weight, or more specifically their percentage of body fat. This may be significant since obese individuals appear to be more at risk of getting the disorder. In addition, exercise can also improve an individual's sensitivity to the hormone insulin, which can help in the control of the disorder and enable the insulin-dependent diabetic to substantially reduce the daily amount of insulin required. For some diabetics the severity of their disorder and complicating factors may preclude them from exercising. However, many should be encouraged to exercise because of its diverse benefits upon their general health as well as its specific implications for their diabetic condition.

Whilst exercise may be of benefit to diabetics, the nature of the disorder requires that certain specific precautions should be taken when they exercise:

1. The diabetic should ensure that their blood sugar level is normal prior to commencing an exercise session.
2. They should be in possession of a supply of sugar when they exercise; this is especially important during prolonged forms of exercise when their blood sugar levels are most likely to become depleted.
3. They should try to ensure that they do not exercise alone, in case they become hypoglycemic.
4. When exercising, the person accompanying a diabetic should be aware of the condition and know what to do in the event of collapse.

If a diabetic does feel hypoglycemic (or collapses) during exercise, sugar should be taken (or given) immediately in order to restore the blood glucose levels. In practice, most diabetics are fully aware of their condition and the symptoms they should look out for. Therefore, provided that diabetics adhere to these additional safety aspects, they should be able to exercise in the same manner as non-diabetics and gain all the desired health-related benefits as well as using it as a means to assist with the control of their disorder.

Recommended further reading for this section is given at the end of the book.

EXERCISE AND OSTEOPOROSIS

Another reported benefit of exercise is its effect upon bones. Bone, like other tissues of the body, is capable of adapting to the physical stresses that are placed upon it and, conversely, is liable to regress and become weak if unused. Significant losses in bone strength are observed in those who are bedridden for some time and even amongst astronauts in zero gravity.

The participation in exercise promotes favourable adaptations because of the stresses placed upon the bone when the muscles attached to it contract, and also the pressure placed upon the bone in weight-bearing forms of activity. The implications of exercise upon the strength of the skeleton begin in childhood, and it is generally considered that the strength of the skeleton reaches a peak between the late teens and early thirties. Strengthening the skeleton through exercise at this age may prevent it from becoming weak later in life. Exercise during adult life should help to maintain this strength or enhance it if the skeleton is already weak.

It has been demonstrated in various studies that regular exercise can strengthen bones and prevent the unwanted loss of calcium and other minerals, which can occur as part of the ageing process. This is particularly applicable to women who may experience a loss of calcium from the bones following the menopause, resulting in the condition of osteoporosis. Osteoporosis is a bone disease which affects men, women and children; however, it is most common in women. The condition of osteoporosis occurs when minerals such as calcium are gradually lost from the bone, making it weak and vulnerable to fracture. This may be caused by a number of factors including diet, ageing and hormonal disturbances. Osteoporosis is a major problem which is considered to be a contributing factor in over a million fractures a year, some of which can cause serious permanent disability. Exercise throughout life is important in reducing the risk of this condition.

In the context of osteoporosis the condition of amenorrhoea may cause some concern because of its implications for reduced oestrogen levels, and hence a risk of calcium loss from the bone. Ironically, one of the causes of amenorrhoea in athletic women may be the extreme levels of training they undertake, coupled with low levels of body fat and even psychological stress. Therefore, the therapist and medical practitioner should be aware of this possibility amongst this group of individuals. In some cases oestrogens may be prescribed to combat the potential effects upon bone density and, hence, the risk of osteoporosis in later life. Thus, whilst exercises may increase bone density and reduce the risk of osteoporosis in most individuals, in extreme cases the reverse may occur.

Further benefits of exercise on the musculoskeletal system include the strengthening of tendons, ligaments and their points of attachment to bones, all of which help to ensure an overall healthy physical condition. Recommended further reading for this section is given at the end of the book.

EXERCISE AND ASTHMA

The condition of an 'asthmatic attack' is characterized by a constriction of the airways of the lungs (bronchi) and the production of excess fluid by the membranes associated with these airways. The constriction of the airways and excess fluid or mucus causes breathing to be more difficult and a characteristic 'wheezing' may occur as the sufferer breathes.

Asthma varies considerably in its severity and may be induced by numerous factors, some of which are associated with an allergic response, an illness or emotions; alternatively, an asthmatic attack may be exercise induced. Chronic asthmatics may be restricted in the type of exercise in which they can participate, whilst others who are less severely affected can achieve a high level of physical performance, which is illustrated by the number of asthmatics who reach an élite level in sport. Therefore, asthmatics need not be precluded from exercise and the administration of broncho-dilator drugs can often be used to control the problem. Exercise-induced asthma appears to be most frequent when the exercise is performed in a cold dry environment. Conversely, it is relatively infrequent in environments where the air is warm and moist. Therefore, activities such as swimming are far less likely to induce an attack than, for example, jogging on a cold winter's morning.

Since the effects of an asthmatic attack may be prevented or minimized by appropriate medication, and if an attack does occur its effects are not considered to be harmful, most asthmatics can be encouraged to participate in appropriate forms of exercise which will provide all the previously discussed health benefits.

EXERCISE AND CORONARY REHABILITATION

Over the past two decades the inclusion of appropriately supervised exercises into coronary rehabilitation programmes has become widely accepted and previously advocated extended bedrest is now considered to be inadvisable for most individuals. With a number of exceptions, exercises are therefore recommended for most individuals who are rehabilitating after a myocardial infarction or coronary bypass surgery. This rehabilitation process will be supervised and guided by a team of individuals which may include a combination of cardiac specialists, physiotherapists, occupational therapists and nurses. The functions of such programmes are to restore patients' confidence in their capabilities, restore their physical capacity to its full potential and minimize the chances of further complications or another coronary event.

The prescribed exercise programme can sometimes result in individuals becoming fitter than they were before the coronary event or operation. Indeed, in a number of cases, some individuals have gone on to complete marathons after a heart attack and, whilst this extreme form of physical activity is not advocated by all authorities or recommended for all individuals, it does illustrate the potential capabilities of the heart attack victim if given the correct exercises.

Following a heart attack or surgery the initial stages of the rehabilitation process will be under the guidance of the cardiac specialist. In the case of a minor uncomplicated myocardial infarction this may include gentle walking within a week of the event, although slightly more vigorous forms of exercise are unlikely to be recommended until 3 to 6 weeks later. Any rehabilitation programme will also include advice on lifestyle habits such as diet, smoking, drinking, stress and relaxation, as well as exercise. Prior to the commencement of any exercise programme the patient is likely to undergo a graded exercise test, conducted by the specialist, during which the responses of the patient's heart to exercise will be monitored. The results of such tests will give the specialist information concerning exercise-induced arrythmias and the extent of angina. From this information the specialist will then be able to make recommendations concerning the type, duration and intensity of exercise which the patient should undertake. The specialist may also specify a specific heart rate training zone which should be attained during subsequent exercise sessions. This is therefore likely to be the stage at which the therapist becomes involved with the exercise programme.

An exercise programme for coronary rehabilitation should be conducted with the same basic principles as almost any other programme. Sessions should include warm-up and cool-down phases, and gradual progression should be evident within the programme. A cardiac rehabilitation programme is likely to emphasize the aerobic component of the exercises. In the early stages of a programme many authorities advise that the patient's cardiovascular responses should be monitored using ECG telemetry and that a defibrillation unit should be available. The basic components of the exercise programme should be based upon exercises which involve large rhythmic contractions and avoid isometric work or exercises which primarily involve small muscle groups. The activity should also be non-competitive and, in the early stages, an increase in the heart rate of 30 bpm is often recommended although this may be modified in accordance with any medication being taken. The exercises are therefore likely to include loosening exercises such as arm and leg swings and activities such as walking and cycling on an ergometer. The exercise sessions should progress with the objective of reaching a level at which the aerobic component of the session lasts for 20 minutes and the participant exercises at least three times a week. Where possible, as the programme progresses it should take on the format of a basic aerobically orientated programme as described in Chapter 7, although modifications may be advised by the specialist according to the specific circumstances of the individual.

Recommended further reading for this section is given at the end of the book.

EXERCISE AND SUDDEN DEATH

It is unfortunate that if a person collapses and dies during or after some form of physical activity it very often becomes highly publicized. Such reporting may give the impression that exercise is a major risk factor in causing sudden death and may deter many people from exercising. With such occurrences it is often forgotten that many people die in their sleep or from a heart attack whilst watching television. However, unlike the exercise case these deaths receive little or no publicity and there follows no media investigation into the 'dangers' of these more sedentary pastimes.

It is clear, however, that for some individuals suffering from certain cardiovascular disorders, extremely vigorous exercise such as very strenuous competitive sport may be neither advisable nor appropriate. For these individuals the effects of the exercise, combined with their medical condition, may make the participation in strenuous exercise 'risky'. However, for many of these sufferers it does not necessarily mean that they should do no exercise; just that it should be of a more appropriate intensity. If this is adhered to then it is likely to convey substantial benefits to the individual without being a major risk. Problems only usually occur when individuals attempt some strenuous activity for which they are not physically fit.

Indeed, as emphasized throughout this text, the vast majority of individuals are more at risk from underactivity than from overactivity. Prolonged underactivity will result in a reduced physical capacity and, perhaps, an increased risk of hypokinetic disease. If the individual then attempts an inappropriately strenuous activity then he or she may be at risk, and hence it is the combination of poor physical fitness, presence of disease and inappropriate levels of exercise that may cause problems, and not just the exercise itself. In fact the incidence of sudden death in élite athletes and regular exercises is very rare (Zeppilli and Venerando, 1981; Kanel, 1982). Recommended further reading for this section is given at the end of the book.

References

Allen, D.W. and Quigley, B.M. (1977) The role of physical activity in the control of obesity. *Med. J. Aust.* **2**, 434–8.

American Heart Association (1984) *Exercise and Your Heart*, American Heart Association, New York.

Andrew, M., Carter, C., O'Brodovich, H. and Heigenhauser, G. (1986) Increases in factor VIII complex and fibrinolytic activity are dependent upon exercise intensity. *J. Appl. Physiol.*, **60**, 1917–22.

Astrup, T. (1973) The effects of physical activity on blood coagulation and fibrinolysis, *Exercise Testing and Training in Coronary Heart Disease*, (eds J. Naughton and H.K. Hellerstein). Academic Press, New York, pp. 169–92.

Barnard, R.J. (1975) Long term effects of exercise on cardiac function. *Exer. and Sports Sci. Rev.*, **3**, 113–33.

Binkhorst, R.A., Kemper, H.C.G. and Saris, W.H.M. (eds) (1985) *Children and Exercise*, XI. Human Kinetics Publications.

Bjorntorp, P. (1974) Effects of age, sex and clinical conditions on adipose tissue cellularity in man. *Metabolism*, **23**, 1091.

Bjorntorp, P. (1978) Physical training in the treatment of obesity. *Int. J. Obesity*, **2**, 149–56.

Bjorntorp, P. (1983) Physiological and clinical aspects of exercise in obese patients. *Exer. Sports Sci. Rev.*, **11**, 159–80.

Blair, S.N., Goodyear, N.N., Gibbons, L.W. and Cooper, K.H. (1984) Physical fitness and incidence of hypertension in healthy normotensive men and women. *J. Amer. Med. Assoc.*, **252**, 487–90.

Bloor, C.M. and Leon, A.S. (1970) Interaction of age and exercise on the heart and its blood supply. *Lab. Invest.*, **22**, 16–4.

Blumenthal, J., Williams, R., Williams, R. and Wallace, A. (1980) Effects of exercise on Type A (coronary prone) behaviour pattern. *Psychosom. Medi.*, **42**, 289–96.

Blumenthal, S., Epps, R.P., Heavenrich, R., Lauer, R.M., Lieberman, E., Mirkin, B., Mitchell. S.C., Naito, V.B., O'Hare, D., Smith, W.M., Tarazi, R.C. and Upson, D. (1977) Report of the task force on blood pressure control in children. *Pediatrics* **59** (5), Part 2.

Blumgart, H.L., Schlesinger, M.J. and Davis, D. (1940) Studies on relation of clinical manifestations of angina pectoris, coronary thrombosis and myocardial infarction to pathogenic findings with particular reference to significance of collateral circulation. *Amer. Heart J.*, **19**, 1-91.

Boileau, R.A., Buskirk, E.R., Horstman, P.H., Mendez, J. and Nicholas, W.C. (1971) Body composition changes in obese and lean men during physical conditioning. *Med. Sci. Sports*, **3** (4), 183-9.

Bonnet, F., Gosselin, L., Chantraine, J. and Senterre, J. (1970) Adipose cell number and size in normal and obese children. *Rev. Eur. Etudes. Clin. Bio.*, **15**, 1101-4.

Borg, G. (1974) Psychological aspects of physical activities, in *Fitness, Health and Work Capacity* (ed. L.A. Larson). Macmillan, New York.

Boyer, J.L. and Kasch, F.W. (1970) Exercise therapy in hypertensive men. *J. American Med. Assoc.*, **211**, 1668-71.

British Cardiac Society (1987) Report of the British Cardiac Society working group on coronary disease prevention.

British Heart Foundation (1986) Reducing the risk of a heart attack. *Heart Research Series*, **14**, 5-7.

Brook, C.G.D. (1972) Evidence for a sensitive period in adipose cell replication in man. *Lancet*, **2**, 624.

Bruce, R.A. (1984) Exercise, functional aerobic capacity and aging: another viewpoint. *Med. Sci. Sports Exer.*, **16** (8).

Butler, J.R. (1987) *An Apple a Day*. Health Services Research Unit, Univ. of Kent at Canterbury.

Castelli, W.P., Garrison, R.J., Wilson, P.W.F., Abbott, R.D., Kalousdian, S. and Kanel, W.B. (1986) Incidence of coronary heart disease and lipoprotein cholesterol levels. The Framingham Study. *J. Amer. Med. Assoc.*, **256**, 2835-8.

Charney, H.C. (1976) Childhood antecedents of adult obesity. *N. Engl. J. Med*, **195**, 6.

Chirico, A.M. and Stunfard, A.J. (1976) Physical activity and human obesity. *N. Engl. J. Med.*, **263**, 935.

Choquette, G. and Ferguson, R.J. (1973) Blood pressure reduction in 'borderline' hypertensives following following physical training. *Can Med. Assoc. J.* **108**, 699-703.

Connor, J.F., LaCamera, F., Swanick, E.J., Oldham, M.J., Holzaepfel, D.W. and Lyczkowskyi, O. (1976) Effects of exercise on coronary collateralisation, angiographic studies of six patients in a supervised exercise programme. *Med. Sci. Sports*, **8** (3), 145-51.

Corbin, C.B. and Pletcher, P. (1968) Diet and physical activity patterns of obese and non-obese elementary school children. *Res. Quart.*, **39**, 922-8.

Coronary Prevention Group (UK) (1987) *Exercise – Heart – Health*. Conference Report.

Cowan, G.O. (1983) Influence of exercise on high density lipoprotein. *Amer. J. Cardiol.*, **52** (4), 138.

Currens, J.H. and White, P.D. (1961) Half a century of running: clinical, physiologic and autopsy findings in the case of Clarence DeMar (Mr Marathon). *N. Engl. J. Med.* **265**, 988-93.

Davis, G.L., Abildgaard, C.F., Bernauer, E.M. and Britton, M. (1976) Fibrinolytic and hemostatic changes during and after maximal exercise in males. *J. Appl Physiol.*, **40**, 287-92.

Donahoe, C.P., Lin, D.H., Kirschenbaum, D.S. and Keesey, R.E. (1984) Metabolic consequences of dieting and exercise in the treatment of obesity. *J. Consult. Clin Psychol.*, **52** 827-36.

Duncan, J.J., Farr, J.E., Upton, S.J., Hagon, R.D., Oglesby, M.E. and Blair, S.N. (1985) The effects of aerobic exercise on plasma catecholamines and blood pressure in patients with mild essential hypertension. *J. Amer. Med. Assoc.*, **254**, 2609–13.

Eckstein, R.W. (1957) Effects of exercise on coronary heart narrowing and coronary collateral circulation. *Circ. Res.* **5**, 230–5.

Enos, W.F., Holmes, R.H. and Beyer, J. (1953) Coronary disease amongst United States soldiers killed in action in Korea. *J. Amer. Med. Assoc.*, **152**, 1090–3.

Fentem, P. and Turnbull, N.B. (1987) Benefits of exercise for heart health: report on the scientific basis, in *Exercise – Heart – Health*. Coronary Prevention Group, pp. 110–25.

Ferguson, R.J., Petitclerc, R., Choquette, G., Chaniotis, L., Gauthier, P., Huot, R., Allard, C., Jankowski, L. and Campeau, L. (1974) Effect of physical training on treadmill capacity, collateral circulation and progression of coronary disease. *Amer. J. Cardiol.*, **34**, 764–9.

Folkins, C.M. and Amsterdam, E.A. (1977) Control and modification of stress emotions through chronic exercise. Chapter 20 in *Exercise, Cardiovascular Health and Disease* (eds E.A. Amsterdam, J.H. Wilmore and A.N. DeMaria). Medical Books, New York.

Friedman, M. (1969) *Pathogens of Coronary Artery Disease*. McGraw-Hill, New York.

Friedman, M., and Rosenman, R.H. (1959) Association of specific overt behaviour patterns with blood and cardiovascular findings. *J. Amer. Med. Assoc.*, **169**, 1286–96.

Friedman, M. and Rosenman, R.H., (1974) *Type A Behaviour and Your Heart*. Alfred A. Knopf, New York.

Fry, R.C. (1953) A comparative study of obese children selected on the basis of fat pads. *Amer. J. Clin. Nut.*, **1**, 453.

Gilliam, T.B. and Burke, M.B. (1978) Effects of exercise on serum lipids and lipoproteins in girls ages 8 to 10 years. *Artery*, **4**, 203.

Gilliam, T.B., Katch, V.L., Thorland, W. and Weltman, A. (1977) Prevalence of coronary heart disease risk factors in active children 7 to 12 years of age. *Med. Sci. Sports*, **9** (1), 21–5.

Gleeson, G. (1987) *The Growing Child in Competitive Sport*. Hodder and Stoughton.

Goldberg, L. and Elliot, D.L. (1985) The effect of physical activity on lipid and lipoprotein levels. *Med. Clin. N. Amer.*, **69** (1), 41–55.

Goldberg, A.P., Hagberg, J., Delemez, J.A., Carney, R.M., McKegitt, P.M., Ehsani, A.A. and Harter H.R. (1980) The metabolic and physiological effects of exercise training in hemodialysis patients. *Amer. J. Clin. Nut.*, **33**, 1620–8.

Gordon, D.J., Wiztum, J.L., Hunninhake, D.B., Gates, S. and Gluek, C.J. (1983) Habitual physical activity and high density lipoprotein cholesterol in men with primary hypercholesterolemia. *Circulation*, **67**, 512–20.

Grundy, S.M. (1986) Cholesterol and coronary heart disease. *J. Amer. Med. Assoc.*, **256**, 2849–58.

Gwinap, G. (1971) Thickness of subcutaneous fat and activity of underlying muscles. *Ann. Int. Med.*, **74**, 408.

Hartung, G.H. (1984) Diet and exercise and the regulation of plasma lipids and lipoproteins in patients at risk of coronary disease. *Sports Med.* **1**, 413–18.

Haskell, W.L. (1984a) The influence of exercise on the concentrations of triglyceride and cholesterol in human plasma. *Exer. Sports Sci. Rev.*, **12**, 205–44.

Haskell, W.L. (1984b) Exercise induced changes in plasma lipid and lipoprotein levels. *Prev. Med.* **13**, 23–36.

Hirsch, J. (1972) Can we modify the number of adipose cells? *Postgrad. Med.*, **51**, 83–6.

Hirsch, J. and Batchelor, B.R. (1976) Adipose cellularity in human obesity. *Clin. Endocrinol. Metab.*, **5**, 299.

Holloszy, J.O. (1983), Exercise, health and aging: a need for more information. *Med. Sci. Sports Exer.*, **15**, 1.

Hutchinson, R.G. (1985) *Coronary prevention: A clinical guide year book.* Medical Publications Inc., Chicago.

Huttunen, J.K., Lansimies, E., Voulilainen, E., Ehnholm, C., Hietanen, E., Penttila, I., Sitonen, O. and Rauramaa, R. (1979) Effect of moderate physical exercise on serum lipoproteins. A controlled clinical trial with special refrence to serum high density lipoproteins. *Circulation*, **60**, 1220–9.

Hyers, T.M., Martin, B.J., Pratt, D.S., Dreisin, R.B. and Franks, J.J. (1980) Enhanced thrombin and plasmin activity with exercise in man. *J. Appl. Physiol.*, **48** (5), 821–5.

Johnson, M.L., Burke, B.S. and Mayer, J. (1956) Relative importance of inactivity and overeating in the energy balance of obese high school girls. *Amer. J. Clin. Nut.*, **4**, 37.

Joye, K., DeMaria, A.N., Giddens, J., Kaku, R., Amsterdam, E., Mason, D.T. and Lee, G. (1978) Exercise induced decrease in platelet aggregation: comparison between normals and coronary patients showing similar physical activity related effects. *Amer. J. Cardiol.*, **41**, 432.

Kanel, W.B. (1982) Exercise and sudden death. *J. Amer. Med. Assoc.*, **248** (23), 3143.

Kannel, W.B. (1985) Physical activity and cardiovascular disease. *Amer. Heart J.*, **109** (4).

Kannel, W.B. and Dawber, T.R. (1972) Atherosclerosis as a pediatric problem. *J. Pediat.*, **80**, 544–54.

Karvonen, M.J., Klemola, H., Virkujarvi, J. and Kekkonen, A. (1974) Longevity of endurance skiers, *Med. Sci. Sports*, **6**, 49–51.

Kasch, F.W. (1976) Effects of exercise on the aging process. *Phys. Sportsmed.*, **4**, 64.

Kasch, F.W. and Wallace, J.P. (1976), Physiological variables during 10 years of endurance exercise. *Med. Sci. Sports*, **5**, 5–8.

Katch, F.I. (1969) Effects of physical training on body composition and diet of females *Res. Quart.*, **40**, 99.

Katch, F.I. (1984) Effects of sit up exercise training on adipose cell size and adipocytes *Res. Quart. Exer. Sport*, **55**, 242.,

Kiyonaga, A., Arakawa, K., Tanaka, H. and Shindo, M. (1984) Blood pressure and hormonal responses to aerobic exercise. *Hypertension*, **7**, 125–31.

Kukkonen, K., Pauramaa, R., Voutilainen, E. and Lansimies, E. (1982) Physical training of middle-aged men with borderline hypertension. *Ann Clin. Res.*, **14** (Suppl. 34), 139–45.

Ledwidge, B. (1980) Run for your mind: aerobic exercise as a means of alleviating anxiety and depression. *Can. J. Behav. Sci.*, **12**, 126–39.

Leon, A.S., Conrad, J., Hunninghake, D.B. and Serfass, R. (1979) Effects of a vigorous walking program on body composition and carbohydrate and lipid metabolism of obese young men. *Amer. J. Clin. Nut.*, **32**, 1776–87.

Linder, C.W. and DuRant, R.H. (1982) Exercise, serum lipids and cardiovascular disease risk factors in children. *Pediat. Clin. N. Amer.*, **29**, 1341–54.

Long, B.C. (1983) Aerobic conditioning and stress reduction: participation or conditioning? *Human Movement Sci.*, **2**, 171–86.

MacHeath, J. (1984) *Activity, Health and Fitness in Old Age.* St Martin's Press.

MacKeen, P.C., Franklin, B.A., Nicholas, W.C. and Buskirk, E.R. (1983) Body composition, physical work capacity and physical activity habits at 18-month follow-up of middle-aged women participating in an exercise intervention program. *Int. J. Obesity*, **7**, 61–71.

Martin, M.J., Hulley, S.B., Browner, W.S., Kuller, L.H. and Wentworth, D. (1986) Serum cholesterol, blood pressure and mortality implications from a cohort of 361,662 men. *Lancet*, 933–6.

Mayer, J. (1980) *Overweight: Causes, Cost and Control.* Prentice Hall, N.J.

Mayer, J. and Thomas, D.W. (1967) Regulation of food intake and obesity. *Science*, **156**, 328.

McNamara, J.J., Molot, M.A., Stremple, J.F. and Cutting, R.T. (1971) Coronary artery disease in combat casualties in Vietnam. *J. Amer. Med. Assoc.*, **216**, 1185–7.

Meade, T.W., Chakrabarti, R., Haines, A.P., North, W.R.S. and Stirling, Y. (1979) Characteristics affecting fibrinolytic activity and plasma fibrinogen concentration. *Brit. Med. J.*, **278** (i), 153–6.

Mole, P.A. , Stern, J.S., Schultz, C.L., Bernauer, E.M. and Holcomb, B.J. (1989) Exercise reverses depressed metabolic rate produced by severe caloric restriction. *Med. Sci. Sports Exer.*, **21** (1), 29–33.

Morris, J.N., Everitt, M.G. and Semmence, A.M. (1987) Exercise and heart disease, pp. 4–17, in *Exercise Benefits, Limits and Adaptations*, (eds D. Macleod, R. Maughan, M. Nimmo, T. Reilly and C. Williams) E & FN Spon.

Nizankowska-Blaz, T. and Abramowicz, T. (1983) Effects of intensive physical training on serum lipids and lipoproteins. *Acta. Pediat. Scand.*, **72**, 357–9.

Noakes, T.D., Opie, L.H. and Rose, A.G. (1984) Marathon running and immunity to coronary heart disease: Fact versus Fiction. *Clinics in Sport Med.*, **3** (2), 527–43.

Noland, M. and Kearney, J.T. (1978) Anthropometric and densitrometric responses of women to specific and general exercises. *Res. Quart.*, **49**, 322.

Pace, P.J., Webster, J. and Garrow, J.S. (1986) Exercise and obesity. *Sports Med.*, **3**, 89–113.

Paffenbarger, R.S., Hyde, R.T., Wing, A.L., Steinmetz, C.M. (1984) A natural history of athleticism and cardiovascular health. *J. Amer. Med. Assoc.*, **252**, 491–5.

Peckos, P.S. (1953) Caloric intake in relation to physique in children. *Science*, **117**, 631.

Qu Xia (1990) Morphological study of myocardial capillaries in endurance trained rats. *Brit. J. Sp. Med.*, **24** (2), 113–6.

Rikkers, R. (1986) *Seniors on the Move.* Human Kinetics Publications.

Roberts, W.C. (1984) An agent with lipid lowering, antihypertensive, positive, inotropic, negative chronotropic, vasodilating, diuretic, anorexigenic, weight

297

reducing, cathartic, hypoglycemic, tranquilising, hypnotic and antidepressive qualities. *Amer. J. Cardiol.*, **53** (1), 261.

Rognum, T.O., Rodahl, K. and Opstad, P.K. (1982) Regional differences in the lipolytic response of the subcutaneous fat depots to prolonged exercise and severe energy deficiency. *Eur. J. Appl. Physiol.*, **49**, 401.

Roman, O., Camuzzi, A.L., Villalon, E. and Klenner, C. (1984) Physical training program in arterial hypertension: a long term prospective follow-up. *Cardiology*, **67**, 230–43.

Rotkis, T.C., Cote, R., Coyle, E. and Wilmore, J.H. (1980) Relationship between high density lipoprotein cholesterol and weekly mileage.

Rutenfranz, J., Mocellin, R. and Klimt, F. (eds) (1987) *Children and Exercise*, XII. Human Kinetics Publications.

Salans, L.B., Cushman, S.W. and Weismann, R.E. (1973) Studies of human adipose tissue, adipose cell size and number in non-obese and obese patients. *J. Clin. Invest.*, **52**, 929.

Salonen, J.T., Puska, P. and Tuomileht, J. (1982) Physical activity and risk of myocardial infarction, cerebral stroke and death. *Amer. J. Epidemiol.*, **115** (4), 526.

Schade, M., Hellebrandt, F.A., Waterland, J.C. and Carns, M.C. (1962) Spot reducing in overweight college women. *Res. Quart.*, **33**, 461–71.

Schaible, T., Pehpargkul, S. and Scheuer, J. (1981) Cardiac responses to exercise in male and female rats. *J. Appl. Physiol., Res. Environ. Exer. Physiol.*, **50**, 112.

Schlesinger, M.J. (1938) An injection plus disection study of coronary artery occlusions and anastomoses. *Amer. Heart J.*, **15**, 528–68.

Seals, D.R. and Hagberg, J.M. (1984) The effect of exercise training on human hypertension: a review. *Med. Sci. Sports Exer.*, **16**, 107–15.

Segal, K.R. and Pi-Sunyer, F.X. (1989) Exercise and obesity. *Med. Clinics of N. Amer.*, **73** (1), 217–36.

Sims, E.A.H. (1974) Studies in human hyperphagia, in *Treatment and Management of Obesity* (eds G.A. Bray and J.E. Bethune) Harper & Row, New York.

Solomon, H. (1985) *The Exercise Myth*. Angus & Robertson.

Stevenson, J.A.F., Feleki, V., Rechnitzer, P. and Beaton, J.R. (1964) Effect of exercise on coronary tree size in the rat. *Circ. Res.*, **15**, 265–69.

Stirling, J. (1979) Characteristics affecting fibrinolytic activity and plasma fibrinogen concentrations. *Brit. Med. J.*, **278** (i), 153–6.

Strauzenberg, S.E. (1981) Sport in old age; advantages and risks. *J. Sports Med. Phys. Fit.* **21** (4), 309–19.

Tepperman, J. and Pearlman, D. (1961) Effects of exercise and anemia on coronary arteries of small animals as revealed by the corrosion-cast technique. *Circ. Res.*, **9**, 576–84.

Tharp, G.D. and Wagner, C.T. (1982) Chronic exercise and cardiac vascularisation. *Eur. J. Appl. Physiol.*, **48**, 97.

Thorland, W.G. and Gilliam, T.B. (1981) Comparison of serum lipids between habitually high and low active preadolescent males. *Med. Sci. Sports Exer.*, **13**, 316–21.

Thornton, E.W. (ed) (1984) *Exercise and Aging: An unproven relationship*. Liverpool Univ. Press.

Tipton, C.M. (1984) Exercise training and hypertension. *Exer. Sport. Sci. Rev.*, **12**, 245–306.

Udall, J.G. (1978) Interaction of maternal and neonatal obesity. *Pediatrics*, **62**, 17.

Valimaki, I., Hursti, M.L., Pihlaskoski, L. and Viikari, J. (1980) Exercise performance and serum lipids in relation to physical activity in school children. *Int. J. Sports Med.*, **1**, 132–8.

Vinten, J. and Galbo, H. (1983) Effect of physical training on transport and metabolism of glucose in adipocytes. *Amer. J. Physiol.*, **244** (2), E129.

Vogt, A. and Straub, P.W. (1979) Lack of fibrin formation in exercise induced activation of coagulation. *Amer. J. Physiol.*, **236** (4), H577–9.

Widhalm, K., Maxa, L. and Zyman, H. (1978) Effect of diet and exercise upon cholesterol and triglyceride control of plasma lipoproteins in overweight children. *Eur. J. Pediat.*, **127**, 121–6.

Wilmore, J.H. (1983) Body composition in sport and exercise: directions for future research. *Med. Sci. Sports Exer.*, **15** (1), 21–31.

Wilmore, J.H. and McNamara, J.J. (1974) The prevalence of coronary heart disease risk factors in boys 8 to 12 years. *J. Pediat.*, **84**, 527.

Woo, R., Garrow, J.S. and Pi-Sunyer, F.X. (1982a) Effects of exercise on spontaneous caloric intake in obesity. *Amer. J. Clin. Nut.*, **36**, 470–7.

Woo, R., Garrow, J.S. and Pi-Sunyer, F.X. (1982b) Voluntary food intake during prolonged exercise in obese women. *Amer. J. Clin. Nut.*, **36**, 478–84.

Woo, R. and Pi-Sunyer, F.X. (1985) Effects of increased physical activity on voluntary food intake in lean women. *Metab. Clin. Exp.*, **34**, 836–41.

Wood, P.D. and Haskell, W.L. (1979) The effect of exercise on plasma high density lipoproteins. *Lipids*, **14** (4), 417–27.

Wyatt, H.L. and Mitchell, J. (1978) Influences of physical conditioning and deconditioning on coronary vasculature of dogs. *J. Appl. Physiol.*, **45**, 619–35.

Zepilli, P., and Venerando, A. (1981) Sudden death and physical exertion. *J. Sports Med.*, **21**, 299.

Zoll, P.M., Wessler, S. and Schlesinger, M.J. (1951) Interarterial coronary anastomoses in the human heart with particular reference to anemia and relative anoxia. *Circulation*, **4**, 797–815.

Zuti, W.B. and Golding, L.A. (1976) Comparing diet and exercise as weight reducing tools. *Phys. Sports Med.*, **4**, 49–53.

FURTHER READING

Introductory aspects of exercise physiology

Brunnstrom's Clinical Kinesiology (1987) (4th edn). revised by L.D. Lehmkuhl and L.K. Smith. Davis Company, Philadelphia.

Hollis, M. (1989) *Practical Exercise Therapy* (3rd edn). Blackwell Scientific Publications, Oxford.

Nordin, M. and Frankel, V.H. (1989) *Basic Biomechanics of the Musculoskeletal System* (2nd edn). Lea & Febiger, Philadelphia.

Rasch, P.J. (ed.) (1989) *Kinesiology and Applied Anatomy* (7th edn). Lea & Febiger, Philadelphia.

Tortora, G.T. and Aganostakos, N.P. (1987) *Principles of Anatomy and Physiology* (5th edn). Harper and Row, New York.
Wirhead, R. (1984) *Athletic Ability and the Anatomy of Motion*. Wolfe Medical Publications, London.

Physiological aspects of nerves and muscles

Helal, B., King, J.B. and Grange, W.J. (1986) *Sports Injuries and their Treatment*. Chapman and Hall, London.
Hubbard, J.L. and Mechan, D.J. (1987) *Physiology for Health Care Students*. Churchill Livingstone, Edinburgh.
Moffat, D.B. and Mottram, R.F. (1987) *Anatomy and Physiology for Physiotherapists* (2nd edn). Blackwell Scientific Publications, Oxford.
Torg, J.S., Vegso, J.J. and Torg, E. (1987) *Rehabilitation of Athletic Injuries: an atlas of therapeutic exercise*. Wolfe Publishing Ltd, London.
Tortora, G.J. and Anagnostakos, N.P. (1987) *Principles of Anatomy and Physiology* (5th edn). Harper & Row, New York.
Tyldesley, B. and Grieve, J.I. (1989) *Muscles, Nerves and Movement: kinesiology in daily living*. Blackwell Scientific Publications, Oxford.
Schmidt, R.A. (1988) *Motor Control and Learning* (2nd edn). Human Kinetics Publications, Leeds.
Vander, A.J., Sherman, J.H. and Luciano, D.S. (1980) *Human Physiology* (3rd edn). McGraw-Hill, New York.

Nutrition, energy and exercise metabolism

Lamb, D. (1983) *Physiology of Exercise* (2nd edn). Macmillan, New York.
McCardle, W.D., Katch, F.I. and Katch, V .L. (1986) Exercise physiology: energy, nutrition and performance (2nd edn). Lea & Febiger, Philadelphia.
Sharkey, B.J. (1988) Physiology and physical activity, Harper & Row, New York.
Wootton, S. (1989) *Nutrition for Sport*. Simon & Schuster, London.

The principles of exercise and fitness training

American College of Sports Medicine (1988) *Resource Manual for Guidelines for Exercise Testing and Prescription*. Lea & Febiger, Philadelphia.
Fox, E.L., Bowers, R.W. and Foss, M.L. (1988) *The Physiological Basis of Physical Education and Athletics*. Saunders, Philadelphia.
MacDougal, J.D., Wenger, H.A. and Gree, H.J. (eds) (1982) *Physiological Testing of the Elite Athlete*. Canadian Association of Sport Sciences.
Skinner, J.S. (1987) *Exercise Testing and Exercise Prescription for Special Cases: theoretical basis and clinical application*. Lea & Febiger, Philadelphia.

Aerobic and activity-based exercises

Adams, R.C. and McCubbin, J.A. (1990) *Games, Sports and Exercises for the Physically Disabled* (4th edn). Lea & Febiger, Philadelphia.

American College of Sports Medicine (1978) The recommended quantity and quality of exercise for developing and maintaining fitness in healthy adults. *Med. Sci. Sports*, **10** (3), 7–10.

American College of Sports Medicine (1986) *Guidelines for Graded Exercise Testing and Prescription* (3rd edn). Lea & Febiger, Philadelphia.

American Heart Association (1975) The committee on exercise: *Exercise Testing and Training of Individuals with Heart Disease or at High Risk for its Development*. A handbook for physicians. American Heart Association, New York.

American Heart Association (1984) *Exercise and Your Heart*. American Heart Association, New York.

Badenhop, D.T., Cleary, P.A., Schaal, S.F., Fox, E.L. and Bartels, R.T. (1983) Physiological adjustments to higher or lower intensity exercise in elders. *Med. Sci. Sports Exer.*, **15** (6), 496–502.

Haskell, W.L., Montoye, H.J. and Orenstein, D. (1985) Physical activity and exercise to achieve health-related physical fitness components. *Public Health Reports* **100**, 202–11.

Kirkendall, D.T. (1984) Exercise prescription for the healthy adult. *Primary Care* **11** (1), 23–31.

MacDougall, J.D., Wenger, H.A. and Green, H.J. (eds) (1982) *Physiological Testing of the Elite Athlete*. Canadian Association of Sport Science.

Skinner, J.S. (ed.) (1987) *Exercise Testing and Exercise Prescription for Special Cases*. Lea & Febiger, Philadelphia.

The role of exercise in the promotion of good health

Aloia, J.F., Cohn, S.H., Ostuni, J.A., Cane, R. and Ellis, K. (1978) Prevention of involutional bone loss by exercise. *Ann. Int. Med.*, **89**, 356–8.

Amundsen, L. (ed.) (1981) *Cardiac Rehabilitation*. Churchill Livingstone.

Astrand, P.O. and Grimby, G. (eds) (1986) Physical activity in health and disease. *Acta Med. Scand. (Suppl)*, 711.

Bjorntorp, P. (1981) The effect of exercise on plasma insulin. *Int. J. Sports Med.*, **2**, 125–9.

Blackett, P.R. (1988) Child and adolescent athletes with diabetes. *Phys. Sports Med.*, **16** (3), 133–49.

Bouchard, C. (ed.) (1989) *Exercise, Fitness and Health: A concensus of current knowledge*. Human Kinetics Publications.

Campaigne, B.N., Landt, K.W., Mellies, M.J., James, F.W., Glueck, C.J. and Sperling, M.A. (1985) The effect of physical training on blood lipid profiles in adolescents with insulin dependent diabetes mellitus. *Phys. Sports Med.*, **13** (12), 83–9.

Cantu, R.C. (1982) *Diabetes and Exercise*. Mouvement Publications.

Carson, P. (1984) Activity after myocardial infarction. *Brit. Med. J.*, **288**, 6410–12.

Cohen, L.S., Mock, M.B. and Ringqvist, I. (1981) *Physical Conditioning and Cardiovascular Rehabilitation.* Wiley, New York.

DeBusk, R.F., Houston, N., Haskell, W., Fry, G. and Parker, M. (1979) Exercise training soon after myocardial infarction. *Amer. J. Cardiol.,* **44** (7), 1223–9.

Fardy, P.S., Yanowitz, F.G. and Wilson, P.K. (1988) *Cardiac Rehabilitation, Adult Fitness and Exercise Testing* (2nd edn). Lea & Febiger, Philadelphia

Fentem, P.H., Bassey, E.J. and Turnbull, N.B. (1988) *The New Case for Exercise.* The Sports Council and the Health Education Authority.

Fentem, P.H., Turnbull, N.B. and Bassey, E.J. (1990) *Benefits of Exercise: the Evidence.* Manchester Univ. Press.

Hartvig, J.T., Darre, E., Holmich, P. and Jahnsen, F. (1987) Insulin dependent diabetes mellitus and marathon running. *Brit. J. Sports Med.,* **21** (1), 51–2.

Haskell, W.L. (1978) Cardiovascular implications during exercise training of cardiac patients. *Circulation,* **57**, 920–4.

Holloszy J.O., Schultz, J., Kusmierkierkiewicz, J., Hagberg, J.M. and Ehsani, A.A. (1986) Effects of exercise on glucose tolerance and insulin resistance, in *Physical Activity in Health and Disease* (eds P.O. Astrand and G. Grimby). *Acta Med. Scand. (Suppl.),* **711**, 55–65.

James, D.E., Kraegen, E.W. and Chisholm, D.J. (1984) Effect of exercise training on whole body insulin sensitivity and responsiveness. *J. Appl. Physiol. (Resp. Env. Exer. Physiol.),* **56** (5), 1217.

Kavanagh, T. (1982) Evidence for the beneficial effect of exercise following myocardial infarction, in *Controversies in Cardiac Rehabilitation* (eds P. Mathes and M.J. Halhuber). Springer-Verlag, Berlin, pp. 43–52.

Kavanagh, T., Shephard, R.H. and Pandit, V. (1976) Marathon running after myocardial infarction. *J. Amer. Med. Assoc.,* **229**, 1602–5.

Maron, B.J., Roberts, W.C., McAlister, H.A., Rosing, D.R. and Epstein, S.E. (1980) Sudden death in young athletes. *Circulation,* **62**, 218–29.

Naughton, J. (1985) Role of physical activity as a secondary intervention for healed myocardial infarction. *Amer. J. Cardiol.,* **55**, 21D–26D.

Northcote, R.J., Flannigan, C. and Ballantyne, D. (1986) Sudden death and vigorous exercise. A study of 60 deaths associated with squash. *Brit. Heart J.,* **55**, 198–203.

Perper, J.A., Kuller, L.H. and Cooper, M. (1975) Arteriosclerosis of coronary arteries in sudden unexpected deaths. *Circulation* (Suppl. 3), **52**, 27–33.

Pollock, M.L., Wilmore, J.H. and Fox, E. (1984) Evaluation and prescription for prevention and rehabilitation. *Exercise in Health and Disease.* Saunders, Philadelphia.

Ruderman, N.B., Ganda, O.P. and Johanen, K. (1979) The effect of physical training on glucose tolerance and plasma lipids in maturity onset diabetes. *Diabetes,* **28** (Suppl. 1), 89–92.

Shephard, R.H. and Kavanagh, T. (1980) What exercise to prescribe for the post M.I. patient, in *Exercise, Science and Fitness* (ed. E.J. Burke). Mouvement Publications, New York, pp. 140–8.

Siscovick, D.S., Weiss, N.S., Fletcher, R.H. and Lasky, T. (1984) The incidence of primary cardiac arrest during vigorous exercise. *N. Engl. J. Med.,* **311**, 874–7.

Smith, E.L. and Babcock, S.W. (1973) Effects of physical activity on bone loss in the aged. *Med. Sci. Sports,* **5**, 68.

Smith, E.L. and Raab, D.M. (1986) Osteoporosis and physical activity, in *Physical Activity in Health and Disease* (eds P.O. Astrand and G. Grimby). *Acta Med. Scand.* (Suppl.) **711**, 149–56.

Soman, V.R., Koivisto, V.A., Diebert, O., Felig, P. and DeFronzo, R.A. (1979) Increased insulin sensitivity and insulin binding to monocytes after physical training. *N. Engl. J. Med.*, **301**, 1200–4.

Thompson, P.D. (1982) Cardiovascular hazards of physical activity. *Exer. Sports Sci. Rev.*, **10**, 208–35.

Thompson, P.D., Funk, E.J., Carleton, R.A. and Sturner, W.Q. (1982) Incidence of death during jogging in Rhode Island from 1975 through 1980. *J. Amer. Med. Assoc.*, **247**, 2535–8.

Van Camp, S.P. (1988) Exercise related sudden death. Risks and causes. *Phys. Sports Med.*, **16** (5),97–112.

Waller, B.F. and Roberts, W.C. (1980) Sudden death while running in conditioned runners aged 40 years or over. *Amer. J. Cardiol.*, **45**, 1292–1300.

Index